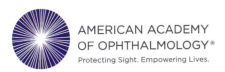

4 | Ophthalmic Pathology and Intraocular Tumors

Last major revision 2024–2025

2025–2026
BCSC
Basic and Clinical Science Course™

Published after collaborative review with the European Board of Ophthalmology subcommittee

The American Academy of Ophthalmology is accredited by the Accreditation Council for Continuing Medical Education (ACCME) to provide continuing medical education for physicians.

The American Academy of Ophthalmology designates this enduring material for a maximum of 10 *AMA PRA Category 1 Credits*™. Physicians should claim only the credit commensurate with the extent of their participation in the activity.

CME expiration date: June 1, 2027. *AMA PRA Category 1 Credits*™ may be claimed only once between June 1, 2024, and the expiration date.

To claim *AMA PRA Category 1 Credits*™ upon completion of this activity, learners must demonstrate appropriate knowledge and participation in the activity by taking the posttest for Section 4 and achieving a score of 80% or higher. For further details, please see the instructions for requesting CME credit at the back of the book.

The Academy provides this material for educational purposes only. It is not intended to represent the only or best method or procedure in every case, nor to replace a physician's own judgment or give specific advice for case management. Including all indications, contraindications, side effects, and alternative agents for each drug or treatment is beyond the scope of this material. All information and recommendations should be verified, prior to use, with current information included in the manufacturers' package inserts or other independent sources, and considered in light of the patient's condition and history. Reference to certain drugs, instruments, and other products in this course is made for illustrative purposes only and is not intended to constitute an endorsement of such. Some material may include information on applications that are not considered community standard, that reflect indications not included in approved FDA labeling, or that are approved for use only in restricted research settings. **The FDA has stated that it is the responsibility of the physician to determine the FDA status of each drug or device he or she wishes to use, and to use them with appropriate, informed patient consent in compliance with applicable law.** The Academy specifically disclaims any and all liability for injury or other damages of any kind, from negligence or otherwise, for any and all claims that may arise from the use of any recommendations or other information contained herein.

All trademarks, trade names, logos, brand names, and service marks of the American Academy of Ophthalmology (AAO), whether registered or unregistered, are the property of AAO and are protected by US and international trademark laws. These trademarks include, but are not limited to, AAO; AAOE; ACADEMY MOC ESSENTIALS; AMERICAN ACADEMY OF OPHTHALMIC EXECUTIVES; AMERICAN ACADEMY OF OPHTHALMIC PROFESSIONALS (AAOP); AMERICAN ACADEMY OF OPHTHALMOLOGY; ANIMAL EYES; ART AND VISION: SEEING IN 3-D; BASIC AND CLINICAL SCIENCE COURSE; BCSC; DIGITAL-EYES; DISCOVER YOUR EYE Q!; EYECARE AMERICA; EYENET; EYESMART; EYEWIKI; FOCAL POINTS; Focus Design; IRIS; IRIS REGISTRY; LEO; LEO LIFELONG EDUCATION FOR THE OPHTHALMOLOGIST; MUSEUM OF THE EYE; MUSEUM OF VISION; OJOSSANOS; OKAP; ONE; ONE NETWORK; ONE NETWORK THE OPHTHALMIC NEWS & EDUCATION NETWORK; OPHTHALMIC CODING COACH; OPHTHALMOLOGY; OPHTHALMOLOGY GLAUCOMA; OPHTHALMOLOGY RETINA; OPHTHALMOLOGY SCIENCE; OPHTHALMOLOGY WORLD NEWS; OPHTHPAC; PREFERRED PRACTICE PATTERN; PROTECTING SIGHT. EMPOWERING LIVES.; PROVISION; THE EYE M.D. ASSOCIATION; THE OPHTHALMIC NEWS AND EDUCATION NETWORK; TRUHLSEN-MARMOR MUSEUM OF THE EYE; UNDER PRESSURE; and WHERE ALL OF OPHTHALMOLOGY MEETS.

Ophthalmic researchers and others interested in using artificial intelligence (AI) technologies and Academy-owned materials, including material from the BCSC, should direct permission requests to permissions@aao.org. Without first seeking permission to use these copyrighted materials, individuals and organizations may infringe the Academy's rights, and such use is prohibited. The complete statement on the use of Academy materials and AI is available at aao.org/statement-on-artificial-intelligence.

Cover image: From BCSC Section 8, *External Disease and Cornea*. Slit-lamp photograph showing superotemporal displacement of the lens in Marfan syndrome. *(Courtesy of Arie L. Marcovich, MD, PhD.)*

Copyright © 2025 American Academy of Ophthalmology. All rights reserved. No part of this publication may be reproduced without written permission.

Printed in Slovenia.

Basic and Clinical Science Course

Christopher J. Rapuano, MD, Philadelphia, Pennsylvania
Senior Secretary for Education

J. Timothy Stout, MD, PhD, MBA, Houston, Texas
Secretary for Lifelong Learning and Assessment

Linda M. Tsai, MD, St Louis, Missouri
BCSC Course Chair

Section 4

Faculty for the Major Revision

Jesse L. Berry, MD
Co-Chair
Los Angeles, California

Nora V. Laver, MD
Boston, Massachusetts

Tatyana Milman, MD
Co-Chair
Philadelphia, Pennsylvania

Vivian Lee, MD
Philadelphia, Pennsylvania

Elaine M. Binkley, MD
Iowa City, Iowa

Amanda C. Maltry, MD
Minneapolis, Minnesota

Swathi Kaliki, MD
Hyderabad, India

The Academy acknowledges the *American Association of Ophthalmic Oncologists and Pathologists* for recommending faculty members to the BCSC Section 4 committee.

The Academy also acknowledges the following committees for review of this edition:

Committee on Aging: Claudia Maria Prospero Ponce, MD, El Paso, Texas

Vision Rehabilitation Committee: Marie A. Di Nome, MD, Scottsdale, Arizona

BCSC Resident/Fellow Reviewers: Sharon L. Jick, MD, *Chair,* St Louis, Missouri; Salma A. Dawoud, MD; Alexander H. De Castro-Abeger, MD; Maria Paula Fernandez, MD; Kalla A. Gervasio, MD; Hong-Gam T. Le, MD; Brittany Simmons, MD

Practicing Ophthalmologists Advisory Committee for Education: Bradley D. Fouraker, MD, *Primary Reviewer and Chair,* Tampa, Florida; George S. Ellis Jr, MD, New Orleans, Louisiana; Kevin E. Lai, MD, Carmel, Indiana; Philip R. Rizzuto, MD, Providence, Rhode Island; J. James Rowsey, MD, Largo, Florida; Gaurav K. Shah, MD, San Francisco, California; Scott X. Stevens, MD, Bend, Oregon; Troy M. Tanji, MD, Waipahu, Hawaii

The Academy also acknowledges the following committee for assistance in developing Study Questions and Answers for this BCSC Section:

Resident Self-Assessment Committee: Amanda D. Henderson, MD, *Chair,* Baltimore, Maryland; Jamie Rosenberg, MD, New York, New York

European Board of Ophthalmology: Anna P. Maino, MBBS, PGCert, *Liaison,* Manchester, England; Mandeep S. Sagoo, MB BChir, PhD, FRCS, FRCOphth, London, England

Recent Past Faculty

    Steffen Heegaard, MD
    Theresa Retue Kramer, MD
    Kirtee Raparia, MBBS
    Alison H. Skalet, MD, PhD
    Nasreen A. Syed, MD

The Academy also gratefully acknowledges the contributions of numerous past faculty and advisory committee members who have played an important role in the development of previous editions of the Basic and Clinical Science Course.

American Academy of Ophthalmology Staff

    Dale E. Fajardo, EdD, MBA, *Vice President, Education*
    Beth Wilson, *Director, Continuing Professional Development*
    Denise Evenson, *Director, Brand & Creative*
    Susan Malloy, *Acquisitions and Development Manager*
    Stephanie Tanaka, *Publications Manager*
    Jasmine Chen, *Manager, E-Learning*
    Sarah Page, *Online Education and Licensing Manager*

Rayna Ungersma, *Manager, Curriculum Development*
Lana Ip, *Senior Designer*
Amanda Fernandez, *Publications Editor*
Beth Collins, *Medical Editor*
Kenny Guay, *Program Manager, Publications*
Debra Marchi, *Online Education Specialist*

Financial Disclosures

Academy staff members who contributed to the development of this product state that within the 24 months prior to their contributions to this CME activity and for the duration of development, they have had no financial interest in or other relationship with any entity whose primary business is producing, marketing, selling, reselling, or distributing health care products used by or in patients.

The authors and reviewers state that within the 24 months prior to their contributions to this CME activity and for the duration of development, they have had the following financial relationships:*

Dr Berry: Castle Biosciences, Inc (C), BioTissue, Inc (C), Elsevier (P), Immunocore (C), Springer (P), UpToDate (P), US provisional patent PCT US19/26221 (P)

Dr Fouraker: AJL Ophthalmic, SA (C, L), Alcon Laboratories (C, L), OASIS Medical, Inc (C, L)

Dr Lai: Twenty/Twenty Therapeutics LLC (C)

Dr Lee: GlaxoSmithKline (C)

Dr Rowsey: HEO3 (C, P)

Dr Shah: Allergan (C, L, S), DORC International BV (S), Focus Vision Supplements (SO), Regeneron Pharmaceuticals, Inc (C, L, S)

All relevant financial relationships have been mitigated.

The other authors and reviewers state that within the 24 months prior to their contributions to this CME activity and for the duration of development, they have had no financial interest in or other relationship with any entity whose primary business is producing, marketing, selling, reselling, or distributing health care products used by or in patients.

*C = consultant fee, paid advisory boards, or fees for attending a meeting; L = lecture fees or honoraria, travel fees or reimbursements when speaking at the invitation of a commercial company; P = beneficiary of patents and/or royalties for intellectual property; S = grant support or other financial support from all sources, including research support from government agencies, foundations, device manufacturers, and/or pharmaceutical companies; SO = stock options in a public or private company

American Academy of Ophthalmology
655 Beach Street
Box 7424
San Francisco, CA 94120-7424

Contents

Introduction to the BCSC xv
Introduction to Section 4 xvii

Objectives 1

PART I Ophthalmic Pathology 3

1 Introduction to Part I 5
Highlights 5
Overview 5
Organizational Framework and Basic Pathologic Concepts 6
    Topography 6
    Disease Process 8
    Differential Diagnosis 18

2 Quick-Start Guide: Specimen Handling and Special Tests and Procedures in Pathology 19
Highlights 19
Glossary of Select Pathology Terminology 19
Introduction 21
Communication With the Pathologist 21
Handling and Transfer of Tissue 22
    Fixatives 22
    Tissue Submission 24
Gross (Macroscopic) Examination and Dissection 24
    Enucleation Specimens 24
    Eyelid and Conjunctival Biopsies 26
    Temporal Artery Biopsies 29
Tissue Processing and Staining 29
    Tissue Processing 29
    Slide Preparation and Tissue Staining 29
Special Techniques and Procedures 32
    Fine-Needle Aspiration Biopsy 32
    Frozen Section 34
Special Diagnostic Testing 36
    Immunohistochemistry 36
    Molecular Pathology 39
    Diagnostic Electron Microscopy 42

3 Wound Repair 43
Highlights 43
General Aspects of Wound Repair 43

Wound Repair in Specific Ocular Tissues 44
    Conjunctiva 45
    Cornea 45
    Sclera 47
    Lens 48
    Vitreous 48
    Retina 48
    Optic Nerve 49
    Uveal Tract 49
    Orbit and Ocular Adnexa 49
Types of Ocular Trauma and Their Sequelae 50

4 Conjunctiva 57
Highlights 57
Topography 57
Developmental Anomalies 59
    Choristomas 59
    Hamartomas 59
Inflammation 61
    Acute or Chronic Conjunctivitis 61
    Infectious Conjunctivitis 61
    Noninfectious Conjunctivitis 61
    Papillary Versus Follicular Conjunctivitis 63
    Granulomatous Conjunctivitis 64
    Pyogenic Granuloma 65
Degenerations 67
    Pinguecula and Pterygium 67
    Amyloid Deposits 68
    Epithelial Inclusion Cyst 69
    Conjunctivochalasis 70
Neoplasia 70
    Squamous Epithelial Lesions 70
    Melanocytic Lesions 75
    Lymphoid Lesions 86
    Glandular Neoplasms 89
    Other Neoplasms 89

5 Cornea 91
Highlights 91
Topography 91
Developmental Anomalies 93
    Dermoid 93
    Peters Anomaly 93
Inflammation 94
    Infectious Keratitis 94
    Noninfectious Keratitis 100
Degenerations, Depositions, and Ectasias 100
    Degenerations 100
    Depositions 105
    Ectatic Disorders 106

Dystrophies 108
   Epithelial and Subepithelial Dystrophies 109
   Epithelial–Stromal *TGFBI* Dystrophies. 109
   Stromal Dystrophies. 112
   Descemet Membrane and Endothelial
     Dystrophies 113
Neoplasia 118

6 Anterior Chamber and Trabecular Meshwork 119
Highlights 119
Topography 119
Developmental Anomalies 120
   Primary Congenital Glaucoma 120
   Anterior Segment Dysgenesis 121
Inflammation 122
Degenerations 122
   Iridocorneal Endothelial Syndrome 122
   Secondary Open-Angle Glaucoma. 124
Neoplasia 130

7 Sclera 131
Highlights 131
Topography 131
Developmental Anomalies 132
   Choristomas and Hamartomas 132
   Nanophthalmos. 132
   Microphthalmia 133
Inflammation 133
   Scleritis 133
Degenerations 136
   Age-Related Calcific Plaque 136
   Scleral Staphyloma 136
   Melanoma-Associated Spongiform Scleropathy 136
Neoplasia 137

8 Lens 139
Highlights 139
Topography 139
   Capsule 139
   Epithelium 141
   Cortex and Nucleus 141
   Zonular Fibers 141
Developmental Anomalies 142
   Congenital Aphakia 142
   Lenticonus and Lentiglobus 142
Inflammation 143
   Cutibacterium acnes Endophthalmitis 143
   Phacoantigenic Uveitis. 143
   Phacolytic Uveitis 144

  Degenerations 145
    Cataract and Other Lens Abnormalities 145
  Neoplasia and Associations With Systemic Disorders 149

9 Vitreous 151
Highlights 151
Topography 151
Developmental Anomalies 152
  Persistent Fetal Vasculature 152
  Bergmeister Papilla 153
  Mittendorf Dot 153
  Vitreous Cysts 153
Inflammation 153
Degenerations 155
  Synchysis, Syneresis, and Aging 155
  Posterior Vitreous Detachment 156
  Hemorrhage 159
  Asteroid Hyalosis 160
  Amyloidosis 160
Neoplasia 162
  Intraocular Lymphoma 162

10 Retina and Retinal Pigment Epithelium 167
Highlights 167
Topography 167
  Neurosensory Retina 168
  Retinal Pigment Epithelium 172
Developmental Anomalies 172
  Albinism 172
  Myelinated Nerve Fibers 172
  Vascular Anomalies 172
  Congenital Hypertrophy of the RPE 175
Inflammation 176
  Infectious Etiologies 176
  Noninfectious Etiologies 179
Degenerations 179
  Typical and Reticular Peripheral Cystoid Degeneration
    and Retinoschisis 179
  Lattice Degeneration 180
  Sequelae of Retinal Detachment 181
  Paving-Stone Degeneration 181
  Ischemia 182
  Abusive Head Trauma 192
  Age-Related Macular Degeneration 194
  Polypoidal Choroidal Vasculopathy 199
Dystrophies 200
  Macular Dystrophies 200
  Diffuse Photoreceptor Dystrophies 203

Neoplasia 204
　　　　Retinoblastoma 204
　　　　Retinocytoma 209
　　　　Medulloepithelioma 209
　　　　Nodular Hyperplasia of Ciliary Body Epithelium 211
　　　　Combined Hamartoma of the Retina and RPE 212
　　　　Adenomas and Adenocarcinomas of the Ciliary Body
　　　　　　Epithelium and RPE 213

11　Uveal Tract 215
　　Highlights 215
　　Topography 215
　　　　Iris 216
　　　　Ciliary Body 217
　　　　Choroid 218
　　Developmental Anomalies 218
　　　　Aniridia 218
　　　　Coloboma 219
　　Inflammation (Uveitis) 220
　　　　Infectious Uveitis 220
　　　　Noninfectious Uveitis 221
　　Degenerations 224
　　　　Neovascularization of the Iris (Rubeosis Iridis) 224
　　　　Hyalinization of the Ciliary Body 224
　　　　Choroidal Neovascularization 224
　　Neoplasia 225
　　　　Iris 225
　　　　Choroid and Ciliary Body 226
　　　　Metastatic Tumors 234
　　　　Other Uveal Tumors 236

12　Eyelids 239
　　Highlights 239
　　Topography 239
　　Developmental Anomalies 241
　　　　Distichiasis 241
　　　　Phakomatous Choristoma 241
　　　　Dermoid Cyst 241
　　Inflammation 242
　　　　Infectious Inflammatory Disorders 242
　　　　Noninfectious Inflammatory Disorders 244
　　Degenerations and Deposits 245
　　　　Xanthelasma 245
　　　　Amyloidosis 246
　　Cysts 247
　　　　Epidermoid Cysts 247
　　　　Ductal Cysts 247

Neoplasia 248
   Epidermal Neoplasms 248
   Dermal Neoplasms 254
   Neoplasms and Proliferations of the Dermal Appendages 255
   Merkel Cell Carcinoma 258
   Melanocytic Neoplasms 259

13 Orbit and Lacrimal Drainage System 265
Highlights 265
Topography 265
   Bony Orbit and Soft Tissues 265
Developmental Anomalies 266
   Cysts 266
Inflammation 267
   Noninfectious Inflammation 267
   Infectious Inflammation 271
Degenerations 273
   Amyloid 273
Neoplasia 273
   Lacrimal Gland Neoplasia 274
   Lymphoproliferative Lesions 277
   Soft-Tissue Tumors 280
   Vascular Tumors 280
   Tumors With Fibrous Differentiation 282
   Tumors With Muscle Differentiation 283
   Peripheral Nerve Sheath and Central Nervous System Tumors . . . 285
   Adipocytic Tumors 286
   Bony Lesions of the Orbit 286
   Lacrimal Sac Neoplasia 288
   Secondary Tumors 288

14 Optic Nerve 289
Highlights 289
Topography 289
Developmental Anomalies 291
   Colobomas 291
   Optic Nerve Pits 292
Inflammation 292
   Infections That Cause Optic Neuropathy 293
   Noninfectious Inflammations That Affect the Optic Nerve 295
Degenerations 298
   Optic Atrophy 298
   Optic Nerve Head Drusen 299
Neoplasia 301
   Melanocytoma 301
   Glioma 301
   Meningioma 303

PART II Intraocular Tumors: Clinical Aspects 305

15 Introduction to Part II 307

16 Melanocytic Tumors 309
Highlights 309
Introduction 309
Iris Nevus 310
Iris Melanoma 311
Ciliary Body and Choroidal Nevi 314
Melanoma of the Choroid and Ciliary Body 316
    Clinical Characteristics 318
    Diagnostic Evaluation 320
    Differential Diagnosis 324
    Classification 329
    Metastatic Evaluation 329
    Treatment 332
    Prognosis and Prognostic Factors 336
Melanocytoma of the Iris, Ciliary Body, and Choroid 338
Epithelial Tumors of the Uveal Tract and Retina 339
    Adenoma and Adenocarcinoma 339
    Simple Hamartoma 340
    Combined Hamartoma 340

17 Vascular Tumors 341
Highlights 341
Introduction 341
Choroidal Vascular Tumors 341
    Choroidal Hemangiomas 341
Retinal Vascular Tumors 345
    Prenatal Retinal Vascular Tumors: Nonleaking Lesions 345
    Postnatal Retinal Vascular Tumors: Leaking Lesions 347

18 Retinoblastoma 353
Highlights 353
Introduction 353
Diagnostic Evaluation 354
    Clinical Examination 354
    Ancillary Imaging 358
    Differential Diagnosis 360
Retinoblastoma Classification 365
    The International Intraocular Retinoblastoma Classification . . 365
    Other Retinoblastoma Classification Systems 365
Treatment 368
    Enucleation 369
    Chemotherapy 369
    Local Consolidation Therapy 371

Spontaneous Regression 374
Genetic Counseling 374
Associated Conditions 376
    Retinocytoma 376
    Primitive Neuroectodermal Tumor 376
Prognosis 377
    Ocular Prognosis 377
    Life Prognosis 378
    Second Nonocular Tumors 379

19 Ocular Involvement in Systemic Malignancies 381
Highlights 381
Secondary Tumors of the Eye 381
    Metastatic Carcinoma 381
    Direct Intraocular Extension 390
Lymphoid Tumors 390
    Primary Vitreoretinal Lymphoma 391
    Primary Uveal Lymphoma 393
    Secondary Involvement of Systemic Lymphoma 396
Ocular Manifestations of Leukemia 396

Additional Materials and Resources 399
Requesting Continuing Medical Education Credit 401
Study Questions 403
Answers 411
Index 419

Introduction to the BCSC

The Basic and Clinical Science Course (BCSC) is designed to meet the needs of residents and practitioners for a comprehensive yet concise curriculum of the field of ophthalmology. The BCSC has developed from its original brief outline format, which relied heavily on outside readings, to a more convenient and educationally useful self-contained text. The Academy updates and revises the course annually, with the goals of integrating the basic science and clinical practice of ophthalmology and of keeping ophthalmologists current with new developments in the various subspecialties.

The BCSC incorporates the effort and expertise of more than 100 ophthalmologists, organized into 13 Section faculties, working with Academy editorial staff. In addition, the course continues to benefit from many lasting contributions made by the faculties of previous editions. Members of the Academy Practicing Ophthalmologists Advisory Committee for Education, Committee on Aging, and Vision Rehabilitation Committee review every volume before major revisions, as does a group of select residents and fellows. Members of the European Board of Ophthalmology, organized into Section faculties, also review volumes before major revisions, focusing primarily on differences between American and European ophthalmology practice.

Organization of the Course

The Basic and Clinical Science Course comprises 13 volumes, incorporating fundamental ophthalmic knowledge, subspecialty areas, and special topics:

1. Update on General Medicine
2. Fundamentals and Principles of Ophthalmology
3. Clinical Optics and Vision Rehabilitation
4. Ophthalmic Pathology and Intraocular Tumors
5. Neuro-Ophthalmology
6. Pediatric Ophthalmology and Strabismus
7. Oculofacial Plastic and Orbital Surgery
8. External Disease and Cornea
9. Uveitis and Ocular Inflammation
10. Glaucoma
11. Lens and Cataract
12. Retina and Vitreous
13. Refractive Surgery

References

Readers who wish to explore specific topics in greater detail may consult the references cited within each chapter and listed in the Additional Materials and Resources section at the back of the book. These references are intended to be selective rather than exhaustive, chosen by the BCSC faculty as being important, current, and readily available to residents and practitioners.

Multimedia

This edition of Section 4, *Ophthalmic Pathology and Intraocular Tumors*, includes multimedia—videos and interactive content ("activities")—related to topics covered in the book. The multimedia content is available to readers of the print and electronic versions of Section 4 (aao.org/bcscvideo_section04 and aao.org/bcscactivity_section04). Mobile-device users can scan the QR codes below (a QR-code reader may need to be installed on the device) to access this content.

Videos

Activities

Self-Assessment and CME Credit

Each volume of the BCSC is designed as an independent study activity for ophthalmology residents and practitioners. The learning objectives for this volume are given on page 1. The text, illustrations, and references provide the information necessary to achieve the objectives; the study questions allow readers to test their understanding of the material and their mastery of the objectives. Physicians who wish to claim CME credit for this educational activity may do so by following the instructions given at the end of the book.*

Conclusion

The Basic and Clinical Science Course has expanded greatly over the years, with the addition of much new text, numerous illustrations, and video content. Recent editions have sought to place greater emphasis on clinical applicability while maintaining a solid foundation in basic science. As with any educational program, it reflects the experience of its authors. As its faculties change and medicine progresses, new viewpoints emerge on controversial subjects and techniques. Not all alternate approaches can be included in this series; as with any educational endeavor, the learner should seek additional sources, including Academy Preferred Practice Pattern Guidelines.

The BCSC faculty and staff continually strive to improve the educational usefulness of the course; you, the reader, can contribute to this ongoing process. If you have any suggestions or questions about the series, please do not hesitate to contact the faculty or the editors.

The authors, editors, and reviewers hope that your study of the BCSC will be of lasting value and that each Section will serve as a practical resource for quality patient care.

---

*There is no formal American Board of Ophthalmology (ABO) approval process for self-assessment activities. Any CME activity that qualifies for ABO Continuing Certification credit may also be counted as "self-assessment" as long as it provides a mechanism for individual learners to review their own performance, knowledge base, or skill set in a defined area of practice. For instance, grand rounds, medical conferences, or journal activities for CME credit that involve a form of individualized self-assessment may count as a self-assessment activity.

Introduction to Section 4

For the 2024–2025 major revision of Section 4, *Ophthalmic Pathology and Intraocular Tumors,* the committee made a number of important changes and added new features, the most significant of which are summarized below.

Quick-Start Guide

Chapters 2 and 3 were combined into a new Chapter 2, "Quick-Start Guide: Specimen Handling and Special Tests and Procedures in Pathology." This chapter's easy-to-follow format outlines approaches that pathology laboratories commonly use to process and analyze tissue specimens. The "Take Note" boxes in the Quick-Start Guide highlight information that should not be missed.

> **TAKE NOTE**
>
> *Conjunctival biopsies should be unrolled and placed flat on a dry piece of filter paper or similar material and allowed to adhere to the paper for several seconds. The paper with the tissue can then be gently submerged in a container of appropriate fixative or media.*

Feature Boxes

Feature boxes highlight important concepts throughout the book.

> **Key Antibodies at a Glance**
> - **Cytokeratins** (multiple subtypes): diagnosis of epithelial tumors (eg, adenoma, carcinoma)
> - **Desmin, myoglobin, or actin:** diagnosis of smooth muscle or skeletal muscle (eg, rhabdomyosarcoma, leiomyoma)
> - **S-100 protein:** diagnosis of tumors of neuroectodermal and neural crest origin (eg, schwannoma, neurofibroma, melanoma)
> - **Melan A and HMB-45:** diagnosis of melanocytic tumors (eg, nevus, melanoma)

Online *Pathology Atlas*

To supplement the figures in select chapters, annotated slides are available in the online *Pathology Atlas,* accessed at aao.org/education/resident-course/pathology-atlas. This URL is provided at the beginning of each relevant chapter. An icon (▣) also appears in the legend of each image in the book for which a related virtual slide image can be explored in the *Atlas.*

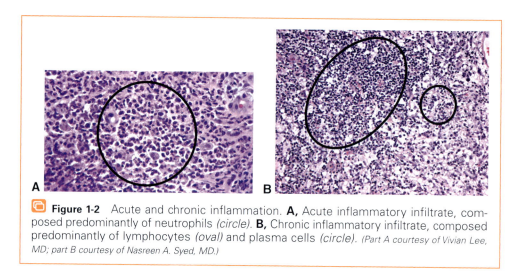

▣ **Figure 1-2** Acute and chronic inflammation. **A,** Acute inflammatory infiltrate, composed predominantly of neutrophils *(circle).* **B,** Chronic inflammatory infiltrate, composed predominantly of lymphocytes *(oval)* and plasma cells *(circle).* *(Part A courtesy of Vivian Lee, MD; part B courtesy of Nasreen A. Syed, MD.)*

In addition, the online *Pathology Atlas* includes case studies covering *tumors of the eyelids and orbit, intraocular tumors,* and *corneal dystrophies and infections.* These case studies complement and enhance the material presented in Section 4 and are easily accessed via the URL in the chapter opener.

Multimedia

Additional educational multimedia, including self-assessment activities and videos, were created to increase the reader's understanding of key concepts in ophthalmic pathology.

 ACTIVITY 1-2 Histology of the eye and orbit: identify tissues.
Developed by Tatyana Milman, MD.
Available at: aao.org/bcscactivity_section04

Clinical Pearls

"Clinical Pearls" throughout the book present information that has direct relevance to clinical practice.

Clinical Pearl OSSN is a clinical term, while CIN, SCC in situ (CIS), and SCC are histopathologic terms that are used to denote specific pathophysiologic findings.

Objectives

Upon completion of BCSC Section 4, *Ophthalmic Pathology and Intraocular Tumors,* the reader should be able to

- describe a structured approach to understanding major ocular conditions based on a hierarchical framework of topography, disease process, and differential diagnosis

- list the steps for handling ocular specimens for pathologic study, including preoperative surgeon-pathologist communication and obtaining, appropriately submitting, dissecting, processing, and staining tissues

- explain the basic principles of special procedures and diagnostic testing used in ophthalmic pathology, such as immunohistochemistry, flow cytometry, and molecular genetic techniques

- describe the types of specimens and appropriate submission methods, processing, and techniques appropriate to the clinical situation

- list the steps in wound healing in ocular tissues

- state the main histologic features of common ocular conditions

- describe the relationship between clinical and pathologic findings in various ocular conditions

- discuss current diagnostic, prognostic, and treatment information for the most common primary tumors of the eye and ocular adnexa

- identify those ophthalmic lesions that indicate systemic disease and are potentially life threatening

- describe the methodologies used for diagnosing intraocular tumors

- describe the genetic information that would be important to provide to families affected by retinoblastoma

- describe the key clinical, pathologic, and genetic prognostic factors for uveal melanoma and retinoblastoma
- describe current treatment modalities for ocular tumors in terms of patient prognosis and ocular function

PART I
Ophthalmic Pathology

CHAPTER 1

Introduction to Part I

 This chapter includes related activities. Go to aao.org/bcscactivity_section04 or scan the QR codes in the text to access this content.

 Indicates that supplemental figures are available in the Pathology Atlas *(aao.org/education /resident-course/pathology-atlas).*

Highlights

- Ophthalmic pathology is a subspecialty recognized by the American Academy of Ophthalmology, as well as other North American and international ophthalmology organizations.
- Pathologic entities are generally divided into the following major categories: developmental anomaly, inflammation, dystrophy and degeneration, and neoplasia.
- Developmental anomalies usually involve abnormalities in size, location, organization, or amount of tissue.
- Inflammation can be broadly classified as acute or chronic, focal or diffuse, granulomatous or nongranulomatous, and infectious or noninfectious.
- The degeneration of a blind, traumatized eye involves a range of tissue alterations, including atrophia bulbi without shrinkage, atrophia bulbi with shrinkage, and phthisis bulbi.

Overview

Ophthalmic pathology is recognized as a subspecialty by the American Academy of Ophthalmology, the American Board of Ophthalmology, the Association of University Professors of Ophthalmology, and the International Council of Ophthalmology. The study of ophthalmic pathology has contributed significantly to our understanding of the pathogenesis of diseases of the eye and ocular adnexa. In the United States, ophthalmologists and pathologists may receive subspecialty fellowship training in ophthalmic pathology after completion of an ACGME (Accreditation Council for Graduate Medical Education)–accredited residency in ophthalmology or pathology; some ophthalmic pathologists are board certified in both ophthalmology and pathology.

Clinical Pearl Ophthalmic pathology plays an important role in the diagnosis of various ophthalmic diseases, in cancer staging, and in guiding clinical management.

BCSC Section 4, *Ophthalmic Pathology and Intraocular Tumors*, provides a general overview of ophthalmic pathology and oncology: common practices and pathologic processes, as well as some less common, but important, entities, are discussed. For more comprehensive reviews of these entities, please refer to the references listed in the Additional Materials and Resources section at the end of this volume.

This chapter describes the organizational framework used in Chapters 4 through 14. Chapter 2, the Quick-Start Guide, discusses specimen handling and processing and emphasizes the importance of communication between the ophthalmologist and the pathologist for providing good patient care. Chapter 2 also covers special testing modalities such as immunohistochemical staining, flow cytometry, and frozen sections. Chapter 3 discusses the basic principles and specific aspects of wound repair. The remainder of Part I, Chapters 4 through 14, is dedicated to specific anatomical regions and pathology.

Clinical Pearl Communication between the ophthalmologist and pathologist is essential for optimal patient care. In especially complex cases, the ophthalmologist is encouraged to review pathology specimen slides with the pathologist.

Organizational Framework and Basic Pathologic Concepts

As stated previously, Chapters 4 through 14 in this volume focus on specific ocular structures and disease processes. In these chapters, the text is organized from general to specific, with the following topics as the framework for the discussion:

- topography
- disease process
- differential diagnosis

Thus, the text also provides an organizational paradigm for the study of ophthalmic pathology (Table 1-1).

Topography

When used in ophthalmic pathology, the term *topography* refers to the description of the anatomical location and structural features of a particular tissue. Topographic identification is the first step in analysis of a pathologic specimen. Identifying normal tissue in a specimen helps clinicians to define the abnormal areas and narrow the differential diagnosis.

Table 1-1 Organizational Paradigm for Ophthalmic Pathology

Topography
  Conjunctiva
  Cornea
  Anterior chamber/trabecular meshwork
  Sclera
  Lens
  Vitreous
  Retina
  Uveal tract
  Eyelids
  Orbit
  Optic nerve

Disease process
  Developmental anomaly
    Choristoma and hamartoma
  Inflammation
    Acute or chronic
    Focal or diffuse
    Granulomatous or nongranulomatous
    Infectious or noninfectious
  Dystrophy and degeneration
  Neoplasia
    Benign or malignant
    Epithelial, mesenchymal, hematopoietic, or melanocytic

Differential diagnosis
  Identification of index feature
  Formulation of a focused list of conditions resulting from the pathologic processes identified above

---

Understanding the disorders that affect the eye and periocular structures requires an understanding of normal ocular structures and functions (Activities 1-1, 1-2).

 ACTIVITY 1-1 Topography of the eye and orbit: identify structures.
Developed by Tatyana Milman, MD.
Available at: aao.org/bcscactivity_section04

 ACTIVITY 1-2 Histology of the eye and orbit: identify tissues.
Developed by Tatyana Milman, MD.
Available at: aao.org/bcscactivity_section04

Using the topographic features of the specimen, an examiner can orient and identify the tissue in question. For example, collagenous tissue lined by keratinized stratified squamous epithelium with dermal appendages is typical of eyelid skin, whereas organized layers, including nonkeratinized stratified squamous epithelium, Bowman layer, collagenous stroma, Descemet membrane, and endothelium, are typical of the cornea. Recognition of characteristic features, such as the presence or absence of an epithelium, can be particularly helpful. See BCSC Section 2, *Fundamentals and Principles of Ophthalmology,* for a review of ophthalmic anatomy.

Disease Process

In the evaluation of a pathologic specimen, the examiner should attempt to determine the general disease process after surveying the topography (Activity 1-3). The major disease processes discussed in Chapters 4 through 14 include

- developmental anomaly
- inflammation
- dystrophy and degeneration
- neoplasia

ACTIVITY 1-3 Identify the disease process.
Developed by Vivian Lee, MD.
Available at: aao.org/bcscactivity_section04

Developmental anomaly

Developmental anomalies are structural or functional anomalies that develop in utero or during early childhood, while the body is developing. They may be detected prenatally, at birth, or later in life. Developmental anomalies usually involve abnormalities in the size, location, organization, or amount of tissue, such as those seen in congenital hypertrophy of the retinal pigment epithelium or eyelid coloboma. Often, these anomalies are classified as choristomas or hamartomas. A *choristoma* consists of normal, mature tissue (1 or 2 embryonic germ layers) at an abnormal location. An *epibulbar dermoid* is classified as a choristoma because it consists of normal, mature skin structures at an atypical location, the limbus. In contrast, the term *hamartoma* describes hypertrophy and hyperplasia (abnormal amount) of mature tissue in a normal location. One example of a hamartoma is an *orbital cavernous venous malformation,* which is an encapsulated mass of mature venous channels in the orbit. A tumor made up of tissue derived from all 3 embryonic germ layers is called a *teratoma* (Fig 1-1).

Inflammation

Inflammation can be classified in several ways (see Table 1-1), for example:

- *onset:* acute or chronic
- *location:* focal or diffuse
- *predominant cell type:* granulomatous or nongranulomatous
- *etiology:* infectious or noninfectious

A bacterial corneal ulcer, for instance, is generally an acute, focal, nongranulomatous inflammatory process, whereas sympathetic ophthalmia is a chronic, diffuse, granulomatous inflammatory disease.

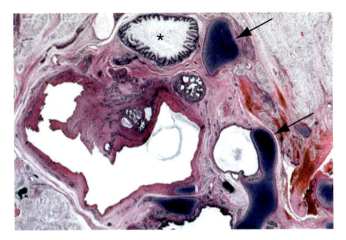

Figure 1-1 Orbital teratoma with tissue from the 3 germ layers. Note gastrointestinal mucosa *(asterisk)* and cartilage *(arrows)* in the tumor. *(Courtesy of Hans E. Grossniklaus, MD.)*

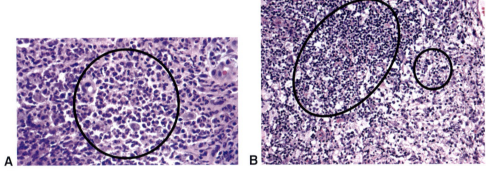

Figure 1-2 Acute and chronic inflammation. **A,** Acute inflammatory infiltrate, composed predominantly of neutrophils *(circle)*. **B,** Chronic inflammatory infiltrate, composed predominantly of lymphocytes *(oval)* and plasma cells *(circle)*. *(Part A courtesy of Vivian Lee, MD; part B courtesy of Nasreen A. Syed, MD.)*

In the early phases of the inflammatory process, polymorphonuclear leukocytes, which include neutrophils, eosinophils, and basophils, typically predominate (Fig 1-2). *Neutrophils* typify the acute inflammatory response and can be recognized by their multisegmented nuclei and intracytoplasmic granules (Fig 1-3). They are often associated with bacterial infections and may be found in blood vessel walls in some forms of vasculitis. *Eosinophils* are commonly associated with allergic reactions but may also be present in chronic inflammatory processes such as sympathetic ophthalmia. They have bilobed nuclei and prominent intracytoplasmic eosinophilic granules (Fig 1-4). *Basophils* and *mast cells* are also involved in allergic responses and contain basophilic intracytoplasmic granules (Fig 1-5). Mast cells are difficult to identify in tissue sections without the assistance of special stains.

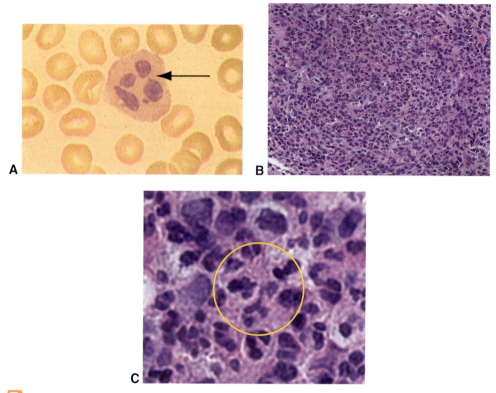

Figure 1-3 Polymorphonuclear leukocytes (PMNs). **A,** Blood smear shows a PMN with a multisegmented nucleus *(arrow).* **B,** Tissue section demonstrates PMNs (neutrophils) at low magnification. **C,** Tissue section (same as in part B) shows PMNs *(circle)* at high magnification. *(Part A courtesy of Hans E. Grossniklaus, MD; parts B and C courtesy of Vivian Lee, MD.)*

Inflammatory cells that are characteristic of a chronic inflammatory response include lymphocytes, plasma cells, and monocytes (see Fig 1-2B). *Lymphocytes* are small cells with round, hyperchromatic nuclei and scant cytoplasm (Fig 1-6). Lymphocytes mature either in the thymus *(T cells)* or in the bone marrow *(B cells).* It is not possible to distinguish between B and T lymphocytes with routine histologic stains in tissue sections; thus, specific immunohistochemical stains are required. T cells can be classified into several subtypes based on their surface markers, with each subtype having a different function. B cells can differentiate into *plasma cells* that produce immunoglobulins. Plasma cells are characterized by eccentric nuclei with a "cartwheel" or "clock-face" chromatin pattern and a perinuclear halo corresponding to the Golgi apparatus (Fig 1-7A, B). These cells may become completely distended with immunoglobulin and form *Russell bodies* (Fig 1-7C). See BCSC Section 9, *Uveitis and Ocular Inflammation,* for in-depth discussion of the mechanisms involved in inflammatory processes.

Monocytes can differentiate into histiocytes (also known as *macrophages*) when they migrate from the intravascular space into tissue (Fig 1-8). *Histiocytes* have eccentrically located, indented nuclei and abundant eosinophilic cytoplasm (see Fig 1-8C). Histiocytes

CHAPTER 1: Introduction to Part I • 11

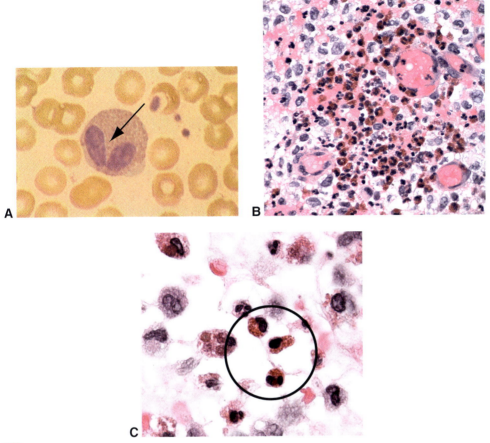

Figure 1-4 Eosinophils. **A,** Blood smear shows an eosinophil with bilobed nucleus *(arrow)* and granular cytoplasm. **B,** Tissue section demonstrates eosinophils at low magnification. **C,** Tissue section (same as in part B) shows eosinophils *(circle)* at high magnification. *(Part A courtesy of Hans E. Grossniklaus, MD; parts B and C courtesy of Nasreen A. Syed, MD.)*

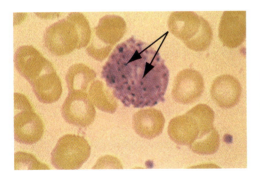

Figure 1-5 Blood smear demonstrates a basophil with intracytoplasmic basophilic granules *(arrows)*. *(Courtesy of Hans E. Grossniklaus, MD.)*

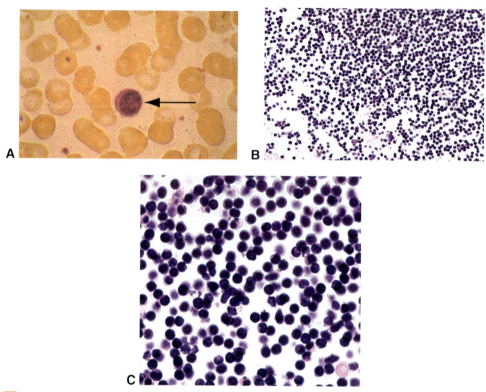

Figure 1-6 Lymphocytes. **A,** Blood smear shows a lymphocyte *(arrow)* with a small, hyperchromatic nucleus and scant cytoplasm. **B,** Tissue section demonstrates lymphocytes at low magnification. **C,** Higher magnification of lymphocytes shown in part B. Note again the small, round uniformly staining nuclei with minimal cytoplasm. *(Part A courtesy of Hans E. Grossniklaus, MD; parts B and C courtesy of Vivian Lee, MD.)*

activated by an antigen are referred to as *epithelioid histiocytes* because of their resemblance to epithelial cells. Epithelioid histiocytes are the hallmark of granulomatous inflammation and may aggregate into a spheroid formation known as a *granuloma*. Granulomas may consist completely of viable epithelioid histiocytes ("hard" tubercles; Fig 1-9A), or they may exhibit necrotic centers ("caseating" granulomas; Fig 1-9B). Epithelioid histiocytes may coalesce to form a *multinucleated giant cell,* of which there are several varieties:

- *Langhans cells,* characterized by a horseshoe arrangement of the nuclei (Fig 1-10A)
- *Touton giant cells,* characterized by an annulus of nuclei surrounded by a foamy, lipid-filled pale zone (Fig 1-10B)
- *foreign body giant cells,* characterized by haphazardly arranged nuclei (Fig 1-10C)

For more on cells that are part of the inflammatory response, see Activity 1-4.

 ACTIVITY 1-4 Identify the cell type.
Developed by Vivian Lee, MD.
Available at: aao.org/bcscactivity_section04

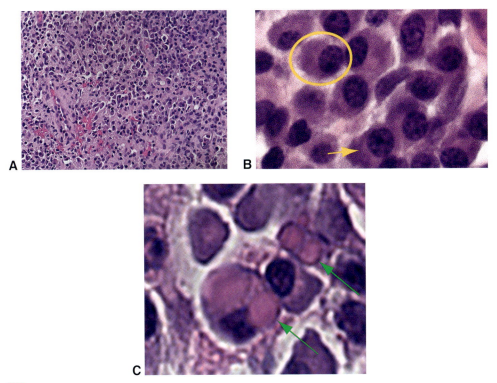

Figure 1-7 Plasma cells. **A,** Plasma cell–rich infiltrate in tissue. **B,** High magnification highlights eccentric nuclei and the clock-face arrangement of nuclear chromatin *(circle).* The lucent curvilinear area adjacent to the nucleus is the Golgi apparatus *(arrow).* Plasma cells are typically found in soft tissue and are rarely found in the blood. **C,** Plasma cell with intracellular accumulation of immunoglobulin (Russell bodies) *(arrows). (Parts A and C courtesy of Vivian Lee, MD; part B courtesy of Tatyana Milman, MD.)*

Dystrophy and degeneration

Dystrophies are bilateral, often symmetric, inherited conditions that appear to have little or no relationship to environmental or systemic factors. Dystrophies affecting the eye typically involve abnormal deposition of material in ocular tissues or characteristic patterns of degeneration. Dystrophies frequently affect the cornea and retina and are discussed in detail in Chapters 5 and 10 in this volume.

Degeneration refers to a wide variety of changes that may occur in tissue over time. It is usually characterized by accumulation of acellular material or loss of tissue mass rather than proliferation of cells. Extracellular deposits may result from cellular overproduction of normal material or metabolically abnormal material. These findings may occur in response to injury or inflammation or as part of a systemic process. Examples include calcification of the lens in congenital cataract (developmental anomaly) and corneal amyloid deposition in trachoma (inflammatory process). To streamline the discussion and avoid using multiple subcategories, such as aging, trauma, and vasculopathies, in this book, the concept of degeneration encompasses a wide range of tissue alterations.

14 • Ophthalmic Pathology and Intraocular Tumors

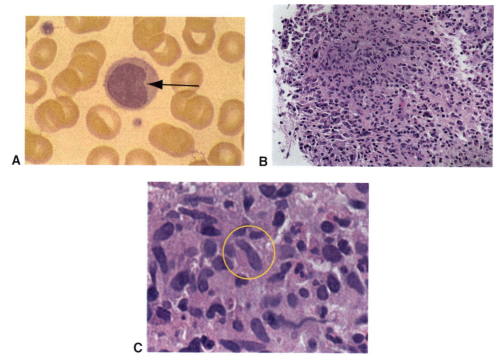

Figure 1-8 Monocytes. **A,** Blood smear demonstrates a monocyte with indented nucleus *(arrow).* **B,** Tissue section shows monocytes (histiocytes, macrophages) in soft tissue at low magnification. **C,** Tissue section (same as in part B) shows histiocytes *(circle)* in soft tissue at high magnification. *(Part A courtesy of Hans E. Grossniklaus, MD; parts B and C courtesy of Vivian Lee, MD.)*

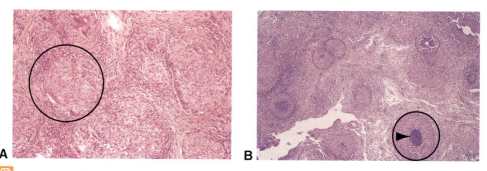

Figure 1-9 Granulomas. **A,** Numerous nonnecrotizing granulomas *(example circled),* or "hard" tubercles, formed by aggregates of epithelioid histiocytes surrounded by a cuff of lymphocytes. **B,** Caseating granuloma *(circle)* with necrotic center *(arrowhead). (Courtesy of Hans E. Grossniklaus, MD.)*

Degeneration of the eye The globe can undergo a unique range of tissue alterations secondary to trauma and chronic disease processes. *Phthisis bulbi* is defined as atrophy, shrinkage, and disorganization of the eye and intraocular contents. Not all eyes rendered sightless by trauma become phthisical. If the nutritional status of the eye and near-normal intraocular pressure (IOP) are maintained during the repair process, the globe

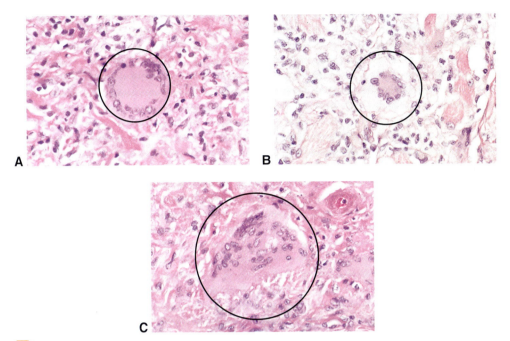

Figure 1-10 Types of multinucleated giant cells. **A,** Langhans cell *(circle)*. Note the peripheral arrangement of nuclei. **B,** Touton giant cell *(circle)*. Note the central eosinophilic cytoplasm and annulus of nuclei surrounded by a foamy, lipid-filled pale outer ring. **C,** Foreign body giant cell *(circle)*. Note the haphazardly arranged nuclei.

will remain clinically stable. However, blind eyes are at high risk for repeated trauma, with cumulative destructive effects. Slow, progressive functional decompensation may also prevail.

STAGES OF OCULAR DEGENERATION Many blind eyes pass through several stages of atrophy and disorganization before progressing to the end stage of phthisis bulbi:

- *Atrophia bulbi without shrinkage.* In this initial stage, the size and shape of the eye are maintained despite the atrophy of intraocular tissues. The following structures are most sensitive to loss of nutrition:
  - the lens, which becomes cataractous
  - the retina, which atrophies and becomes separated from the retinal pigment epithelium (RPE) by serous fluid accumulation
  - the aqueous outflow tract, where anterior and posterior synechiae develop
- *Atrophia bulbi with shrinkage.* In this stage, the eye becomes soft because of ciliary body dysfunction and progressive reduction of IOP. The globe becomes smaller and assumes a squared-off configuration as a result of the influence of the 4 rectus muscles. The anterior chamber collapses. Associated corneal endothelial cell damage initially results in corneal edema, followed by opacification with degenerative pannus, stromal scarring, and vascularization. Most of the remaining internal structures of the eye are atrophic but remain recognizable on histologic examination.

16 • Ophthalmic Pathology and Intraocular Tumors

- *Phthisis bulbi* (Fig 1-11). In this end stage, the size of the globe shrinks from a normal average diameter of 23–25 mm to an average diameter of 16–19 mm. Most of the ocular contents become disorganized. In areas of preserved uvea, the RPE proliferates, and nodular drusen may develop. In addition, extensive dystrophic calcification of the lens, retina, Bowman layer, and drusen usually occurs. Osseous metaplasia of the RPE with bone formation may be a prominent characteristic. Finally, the sclera becomes markedly thickened, particularly posteriorly.

Neoplasia

A *neoplasm* is a new growth of a specific tissue phenotype and may be either benign or malignant. General histologic signs of malignancy include nuclear hyperchromatism and pleomorphism; prominent nucleoli; necrosis; hemorrhage; and increased, sometimes atypical, mitoses. Some neoplastic proliferations are called *borderline* or *indeterminate* because they exhibit both malignant and nonmalignant characteristics. An example is a melanocytic nevus with atypical features that cannot be precisely classified as benign

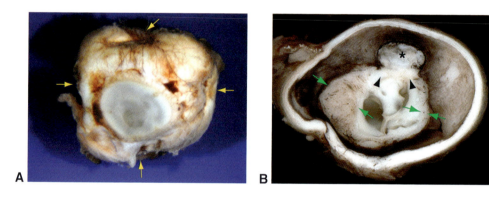

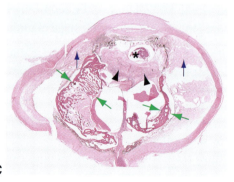

Figure 1-11 Phthisis bulbi. **A,** Gross photograph of a whole globe. Note the squared-off shape of the globe *(arrows)*, resulting from hypotony and the force of the 4 rectus muscles on the sclera. **B,** Gross photograph of a phthisical globe that has been opened. Note the irregular contour, cataractous lens with calcification *(asterisk)*, cyclitic membrane with adherent retina *(arrowheads)*, and bone formation *(between green arrows)*. **C,** Photomicrograph demonstrates the histopathologic correlation with the gross photograph shown in part B. In addition, organized ciliochoroidal effusions are apparent histologically *(blue arrows)*. *(Part A courtesy of Ralph C. Eagle Jr, MD; parts B and C courtesy of Robert H. Rosa Jr, MD.)*

or malignant. Many examples in this book are presented as definitively benign or malignant, but for some cases in clinical practice, the diagnosis is less certain or may evolve over time. Table 1-2 summarizes the origin and general classification of neoplasms and includes clinical examples of neoplasms found in various tissues. Figure 1-12 illustrates neoplastic growth patterns.

Table 1-2 Classification of Neoplasia

Tissue Origin	Terminology		Clinical Examples
	Benign	Malignant	
Epithelial	Papilloma Adenoma	Carcinoma Adenocarcinoma	Squamous papilloma, squamous cell carcinoma
Mesenchymal	Cell type + -oma	Cell type + *sarcoma*	Schwannoma, leiomyoma, rhabdomyosarcoma[a]
Hematopoietic	Hyperplasia Infiltrate	Leukemia Lymphoma	Lymphoid hyperplasia, extranodal marginal zone lymphoma of mucosa-associated lymphoid tissue (EMZL)
Melanocytic	Nevus Melanosis/melanocytosis	Melanoma	Primary acquired melanosis, melanoma

[a] *Note:* This nomenclature is not always consistent. For example, although the term *melanoma* contains the suffix *-oma*, this tumor is malignant.

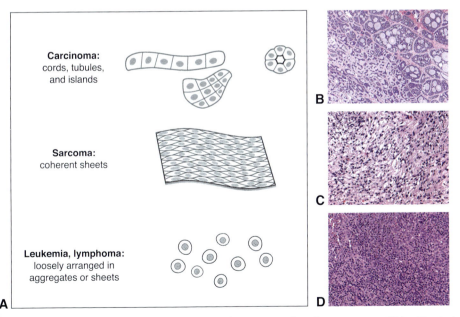

Figure 1-12 General classification and growth patterns of malignant tumors **(A)** with photomicrographs depicting adenoid cystic carcinoma of the lacrimal gland **(B)**, rhabdomyosarcoma **(C)**, and large B-cell lymphoma **(D)**. *(Illustrations by Christine Gralapp and Mark Miller; parts B and D courtesy of Vivian Lee, MD; part C courtesy of Nasreen A. Syed, MD.)*

Differential Diagnosis

Formulating a differential diagnosis begins after evaluation of the topography of the specimen and determination of the disease process. Recognizing an *index feature,* a morphological characteristic that helps define a disease process more specifically, can be extremely useful in establishing the correct diagnosis. For example, a tumor in the uveal tract composed of atypical cells containing cytoplasmic pigment is suggestive of uveal melanoma, whereas a small, round, blue cell tumor at the posterior pole of the eye of an infant or child is highly suggestive of retinoblastoma. The index feature should differentiate the specimen from others demonstrating the same general disease process. Returning to the example above, both uveal melanoma and retinoblastoma are malignant intraocular tumors, but the former is characterized by atypical, pigmented cells while the latter is characterized by small blue cells. Although very basic index features can be recognized without great difficulty, recognition of other index features requires familiarity and experience. For example, the differential diagnosis for a melanocytic proliferation of the conjunctiva includes nevus, primary acquired melanosis, and melanoma. Narrowing the differential diagnosis in this case requires recognition of the key histologic features of each of these entities.

If a key index feature is absent, forming a focused differential diagnosis based on the topography of the specimen and the disease process is necessary before a definitive or specific diagnosis can be established. Special stains or other ancillary pathology studies may provide information that narrows the differential. For instance, the differential diagnosis that can be constructed from the features of noncaseating granulomatous inflammation of the conjunctiva includes sarcoidosis, foreign body, and fungal and mycobacterial infections. Some of these entities can be excluded from the differential diagnosis with the use of special stains for acid-fast and fungal organisms.

Readers are encouraged to practice using the hierarchical framework presented in this chapter by reviewing each step in sequence when examining histologic images and pathologic specimens. Chapters 4 through 14 of this volume provide tissue-specific examples of the differential diagnoses for each of the major disease process categories. Refer to Table 1-1 for the expanded organizational paradigm.

CHAPTER 2

Quick-Start Guide: Specimen Handling and Special Tests and Procedures in Pathology

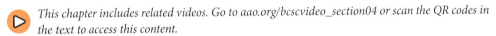 *This chapter includes related videos. Go to aao.org/bcscvideo_section04 or scan the QR codes in the text to access this content.*

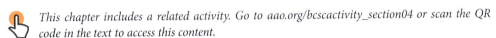 *This chapter includes a related activity. Go to aao.org/bcscactivity_section04 or scan the QR code in the text to access this content.*

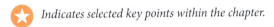 *Indicates selected key points within the chapter.*

Highlights

- Clear communication between the ophthalmologist and pathologist via the pathology request form and pathology report is essential for obtaining an appropriate specimen, ensuring proper handling, and facilitating an accurate diagnosis.
- In special circumstances, such as suspicion of malignancy or determination of a critical diagnosis, direct discussion with the pathologist during preoperative planning is vital.
- Although some histopathologic tests and procedures require fresh tissue, tissue fixation is typically required to arrest decomposition and preserve cellular morphology.
- Histochemical stains allow contrasting color staining of various cellular and extracellular elements and/or identification of specific material in tissue sections.
- Special procedures, such as immunohistochemistry and molecular genetic techniques, have led to improvements in the diagnosis of eye diseases.

Glossary of Select Pathology Terminology

Circulating tumor cells (CTCs) Cells shed from a primary tumor that may be detected in the blood of patients with early or advanced cancers using antibody-based assays or molecular methods. The presence of CTCs has been linked to unfavorable prognosis, and detection offers opportunities for individualized risk assessment.

Cytology fixatives Examples include ethanol, methanol, and Saccomanno fixatives, which are used to fix and preserve cells in smears and liquid-based cytology specimens (eg, corneal scrapes, aqueous and vitreous fluid, and fine-needle aspiration biopsies) (see Table 2-1). Direct smears are air-dried and stained without fixatives.

Direct immunofluorescence Similar to indirect immunohistochemistry, except that this method uses a single antibody directly conjugated to a fluorophore that binds to the selected antigen(s). Fluorophores emit a signal that can be visualized using a fluorescence microscope. This technique requires fresh tissue samples (see Table 2-1).

Flow cytometry A method used to analyze the physical and chemical properties of cells moving in single file in a fluid stream. This is the most used method for immunophenotyping hematopoietic proliferations and requires fresh tissue (see Table 2-1).

Formalin fixative The most used fixative, 10% neutral-buffered formalin, is a 40% formaldehyde solution that stabilizes proteins, lipids, and carbohydrates and crosslinks proteins to prevent the destruction of tissue by enzymes (autolysis) (see Table 2-1).

Glutaraldehyde fixative Fixative used for electron microscopy that quickly penetrates tissues, preserving proteins, glycogen, and structures such as microtubules and smooth endoplasmic reticulum (see Table 2-1).

Histochemical stains Tissue dyes, principally hematoxylin and eosin (H&E) and periodic acid–Schiff (PAS), used to stain tissue sections for microscopy (see Table 2-2).

In situ hybridization Localization of a specific DNA or RNA sequence in a tissue section using a labeled complementary DNA, RNA, or modified nucleic acid strand (or probe). This method can be used on paraffin-embedded formalin-fixed tissue.

Indirect immunohistochemistry A method that detects the presence of 1 or more selected antigen(s) in cells using a primary antibody that can bind specifically to the queried antigen(s). A secondary antibody is then applied to bind with the primary antibody, producing a colored compound (chromogen) that can be detected with a light microscope. This method typically utilizes paraffin-embedded formalin-fixed tissue sections or cytology specimens (see Table 2-1).

Microarray A molecular biology technique used to survey the expression of thousands of genes in a single assay, the output of which is called a gene expression profile (GEP).

Polymerase chain reaction (PCR) A molecular biology technique used to amplify a single strand of nucleic acid by several orders of magnitude, generating thousands to millions of copies of a particular DNA sequence.

Roswell Park Memorial Institute (RPMI) medium Cell culture medium that supports cell viability in biological samples (ie, "fresh tissue media"). RPMI is used when laboratory testing requires fresh, unfixed specimens (eg, flow cytometry to rule out lymphoma) (see Table 2-1).

Tissue processing An automated process involving the dehydration of tissues to allow infiltration with paraffin to make a tissue block, which can then be sectioned onto glass slides.

Introduction

This chapter covers the approaches that pathology laboratories commonly use to process and analyze tissue specimens, such as globes, intraocular contents, and ocular adnexal tissues. Glass slide preparations are typically used for histopathologic diagnosis and additional tests. In addition to diagnosis, tissues are evaluated for prognosis and therapeutic suitability. The main steps involved are

- communication with the pathologist
- appropriate handling and transfer of tissue, including submission of a requisition form containing relevant clinical information
- gross dissection to prepare the specimen for histologic sectioning
- tissue processing, slide preparation, and histochemical tissue staining
- consideration of special histological techniques and molecular clinical diagnostics

> **TAKE NOTE**
>
> *Prior to biopsy or surgery, it is critical to communicate with the attending pathologist to plan for appropriate specimen collection and tissue fixation.*

Communication With the Pathologist

Communication with the pathologist before, during, and after surgical procedures is an essential component of quality patient care. The ophthalmologist is responsible for providing relevant details regarding the clinical history when submitting the specimen to the laboratory. This history facilitates clinicopathologic correlation and enables the pathologist to provide the most accurate interpretation of the specimen.

Information is usually sufficiently conveyed by the pathology request form and pathology report. However, if there are any special circumstances, such as suspicion of malignancy or identification of a critical diagnosis, direct and personal communication between the ophthalmologist and the pathologist is essential. Discussion prior to surgery allows all involved physicians to consider the best way to collect a specimen and submit it to the laboratory. Checklist 2-1 is a preoperative checklist for handling routine specimens.

CHECKLIST 2-1

Ophthalmic Pathology Consultation Checklist for Routine Specimens

1. Fill out requisition form or electronic order, providing
   a. two patient identifiers
   b. sex and age of patient
   c. location of lesion (laterality and exact location)
   d. previous biopsies of the site and diagnosis

(Continued on next page)

(continued)
> e. pertinent clinical history
> f. clinical differential diagnosis
> g. ophthalmologist phone, pager, and/or fax number
2. Submit specimen in adequately sealed container with
   a. ample amount of 10% formalin (at least 10 times the volume of the biopsy specimen)
   b. label with 2 patient identifiers and location of biopsy site on the container itself, not the cap
3. If relevant, include diagram indicating the biopsy site and landmarks for orientation of resection margins (eg, complete resection of eyelid or conjunctival malignancies, ciliary body/iris tumors)

If a previous biopsy has been performed, the clinician should request a review of the prior slides, especially if there is a history of malignancy. The pathologist can compare the current and prior morphological features and diagnoses, and the subsequent treatment plan can be tailored based on the findings.

> **TAKE NOTE**
>
> If there is a significant discrepancy between the clinical diagnosis and the histologic diagnosis or between the initial and subsequent histologic diagnoses, the ophthalmologist should promptly contact the pathologist to resolve the discrepancy.

> **EXAMPLE 2-1**
>
> If the initial diagnosis was squamous cell carcinoma in situ but the repeat biopsy reveals a poorly differentiated, invasive squamous cell carcinoma, a more aggressive resection with lymph node biopsy may be more appropriate.

College of American Pathologists. Cancer protocol templates. Accessed June 10, 2023. www.cap.org/protocols-and-guidelines/cancer-reporting-tools/cancer-protocol-templates

Couce M, Dharamraj AM, Saad EAH, et al. Eye. PathologyOutlines.com. Accessed June 10, 2023. www.pathologyoutlines.com/eye.html

Handling and Transfer of Tissue

Fixatives

Table 2-1 lists many of the fixatives and transport media and their indications. Formalin is the most used fixative and diffuses quickly through tissues. In general, a specimen should be submerged in a volume of fixative that is at least 10 times the volume of the tissue. Tissue fixation time varies depending on the size and composition of the specimen. When a globe is sent for pathologic evaluation, for example, it should be suspended in formalin for at least 24–48 hours before processing. However, it is not necessary or desirable to open

Table 2-1 Fixatives Used in Ophthalmic Pathology

Fixative	Color	Examples of Use
10% neutral-buffered formalin (NBF)	Clear	Routine fixation of all tissues
Bouin solution	Yellow	Small biopsy specimens (eg, conjunctiva)
Absolute ethanol or methanol	Clear	Crystals (eg, corneal urate crystals)
Cytology fixatives (ethanol, methanol, or Saccomanno fixative)	Variety of colors	Liquid specimens or smears (eg, vitreous, aqueous humor, fine-needle aspirates, corneal smears)
Glutaraldehyde (2.5%)	Clear	Electron microscopy (eg, corneal microsporidia)
Michel or Zeus transport medium[a]	Clear	Immunofluorescence (eg, conjunctival biopsy for mucous membrane pemphigoid)
Roswell Park Memorial Institute (RPMI) tissue culture medium[a]	Pink, salmon	Tissue culture and fresh media (eg, orbital tumor for cytogenetics or flow cytometry) or transport medium for molecular studies

[a] Not a true fixative but prolongs tissue decomposition.

the eye, inject fixative, or create a scleral window to ensure adequate fixation despite the relatively large size and volume of the globe. Opening an eye before fixation may damage or distort sites of pathology, making histologic interpretation difficult or impossible.

While most pathology tests can be performed on fixed tissue, some situations require a fresh specimen. For example, biopsies to rule out lymphoproliferative disorders or conjunctival biopsies for suspected ocular cicatricial pemphigoid typically require ancillary diagnostic testing that can only be performed on fresh tissue. In these cases, tissue should be either submitted in a small volume of saline, wrapped in saline-soaked gauze, or submerged in tissue culture media (see Table 2-1). Because different institutions may use different protocols, preoperative consultation with the pathologist is critical to determine the appropriate approach.

> **TAKE NOTE**
>
> *Direct immunofluorescence studies for the evaluation of ocular cicatricial pemphigoid and other blistering disorders are usually performed in specialized pathology laboratories. Preoperative communication with the pathology laboratory is essential to ensure appropriate tissue submission and handling.*

Ocular cytology specimens, such as corneal or conjunctival scrapings, aqueous fluid samples, vitreous fluid samples, and fine-needle aspiration biopsies (see further discussion under Special Techniques and Procedures), may require specific fixatives or special tissue handling (Activity 2-1). For example, conjunctival and corneal scrapings are usually submitted as direct smears or may be alcohol-fixed like cytology specimens.

ACTIVITY 2-1 Quiz: Tissue fixative and special stains in ocular pathology.
Developed by Nora V. Laver, MD.
Available at: aao.org/bcscactivity_section04

Tissue Submission

Specimens are typically submitted to the pathology laboratory in a container with the appropriate fixative. The container should be labeled with 2 patient identifiers, specifically on the body of the container and not the cap, where it can be separated from the specimen. The container label should ideally provide the specimen laterality and location. A requisition form or order, again with 2 patient identifiers and an up-to-date and reliable contact method for the ophthalmologist (eg, phone, pager, and/or fax number), is submitted with the specimen. Pertinent clinical history, including history of a previous biopsy, and clinical differential diagnosis should also be provided on the form. If relevant, a diagram indicating the biopsy site and landmarks for orientation of resection margins (eg, complete resection of eyelid or conjunctival malignancies, ciliary body/iris tumors) should be included with the specimen when submitted to the pathology laboratory (see Checklist 2-1).

> **TAKE NOTE**
>
> Labeling both the specimen container and the paperwork with 2 patient identifiers is mandatory before submission to the pathology laboratory (see Checklist 2-1).

Gross (Macroscopic) Examination and Dissection

Enucleation Specimens

It is critical to confirm the laterality of a globe even if laterality is provided on the requisition form since discrepancies do occur. Globes may be oriented by identifying the long posterior ciliary arteries and nerves and the superior and inferior oblique muscles. The long posterior ciliary arteries and nerves, discernible as straight blue-gray lines on both sides of the optic nerve, establish the horizontal meridian (Fig 2-1). The laterality of the globe can be identified by isolating the superior and inferior oblique muscles. The superior oblique muscle inserts into the superotemporal post-equatorial sclera and is identified by its longest tendinous insertion. The inferior oblique muscle inserts temporally over the macula and has the shortest tendinous insertion, almost appearing as if the muscle belly is inserting directly into the sclera (see Fig 2-1). Although fixation may affect tissue architecture and therefore landmarks, the rectus muscles can be used to confirm laterality—the medial, inferior, lateral, and superior rectus muscles insert progressively farther from the limbus.

Once laterality is verified, the orientation of any pathology can be determined. The globe should be dissected in such a way as to display as many of the pathologic changes as possible on a single slide. Usually, globes are cut so that the pupil and optic nerve are present in the same section, called the *pupil–optic nerve (PO) section*. In routine cases, globes with no prior surgery or intraocular neoplasm are typically opened on the horizontal

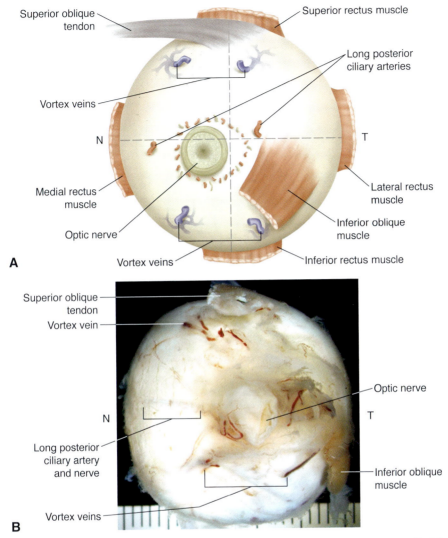

Figure 2-1 Posterior view of the right globe. N=nasal; T=temporal. **A,** Diagram. **B,** Macroscopic photograph. Note that the long posterior ciliary artery and nerve appear as a subtle blue-gray line as they pass through the sclera, marking the horizontal meridian of the globe. Also note that the rectus muscle insertions are not present. The rectus muscles are typically incised at their scleral insertion during enucleation so that they may be attached to the orbital implant. *(Part A modified by Cyndie C. H. Wooley from an illustration by Thomas A. Weingeist, MD, PhD; part B courtesy of Nasreen A. Syed, MD.)*

meridian, which includes the macula in the same section as the pupil and optic nerve (Fig 2-2). However, globes with a surgical or nonsurgical wound should be opened such that the wound is perpendicular to, and included in, the PO section. Before the dissection, the globe is *transilluminated* with a bright light. Intraocular lesions such as tumors usually block the light and cast a shadow, which can be outlined on the sclera with a marking pencil. This mark can then be used to guide the globe dissection so that the center of the section includes the maximum extent of the area of interest (Fig 2-3; Video 2-1).

26 • Ophthalmic Pathology and Intraocular Tumors

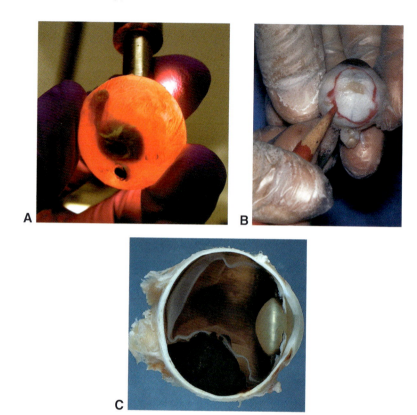

Figure 2-2 Preparation of an intraocular tumor enucleation specimen. **A,** Transillumination shows blockage of light due to an intraocular tumor. **B,** The shadow is traced with a marking pencil. **C,** The opened eye shows the intraocular tumor that was demonstrated by transillumination. *(Part A courtesy of Nasreen A. Syed, MD; part B courtesy of Hans E. Grossniklaus, MD.)*

 VIDEO 2-1 Gross dissection of the eye.
Courtesy of Ralph C. Eagle Jr, MD.
Available at: aao.org/bcscvideo_section04

Eyelid and Conjunctival Biopsies

When eyelid or conjunctival tissue is sent for pathologic evaluation, it may be important to evaluate the resection margins (ie, determine whether the lesion is present in the margins of resection).

> **TAKE NOTE**
>
> *Evaluation of the margins is highly dependent on specimen size and tissue handling. The smaller a tissue sample is, the more difficult it will be to accurately assess the surgical margins. Thus, an adequate tissue biopsy should include a relevant biopsy of lesional tissue and be of sufficient size for evaluation of the margins, taking into consideration the 10% tissue shrinkage that will occur from fixation.*

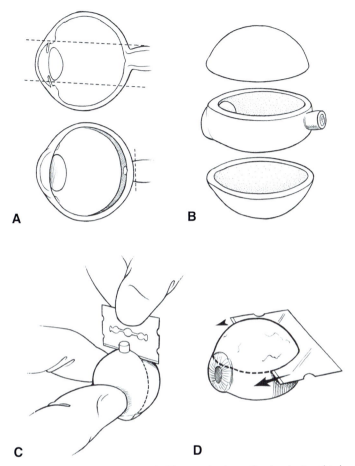

Figure 2-3 Gross dissection of a globe. **A,** The goal of sectioning is to obtain a pupil–optic nerve (PO) section that contains the maximum area of interest. **B,** Two caps, or calottes, are removed to obtain a PO section. **C,** Both cuts are generally performed from posterior (by the optic nerve head) to anterior. **D,** The second cut yields the PO section. *(Illustration by Christine Gralapp.)*

If the tissue rolls up or folds, it can be difficult to orient, and once fixed in formalin, it cannot be reshaped. The specimen should be spread out as far as possible and unfurled before fixation. This is particularly important for conjunctival biopsies because conjunctiva tends to roll and curl up.

> **TAKE NOTE**
>
> Conjunctival biopsies should be unrolled and placed flat on a dry piece of filter paper or similar material and allowed to adhere to the paper for several seconds. The paper with the tissue can then be gently submerged in a container of appropriate fixative or media.

To properly orient a specimen without innate landmarks, the tissue needs to be marked to discriminate the surgical margins before it is submitted to the pathology lab.

Sutures (long and short or of different colors) positioned 90° apart are commonly used to mark the margins (Fig 2-4A–C). The clinician should note that small sutures placed under surgical magnification may be difficult to see with the naked eye in the pathology laboratory; therefore, the length of the sutures should be visualized and cut without the assistance of magnifiers. In cases where the pathology laboratory is on-site, fresh tissue spread on filter paper and oriented with a diagram can be submitted (Fig 2-4D). For tissues that will be fixed, permanent marker and surgical marking ink are not recommended as they may dissolve in fixative. A diagram indicating the meaning of the marks should accompany the specimen. Once in the surgical pathology lab, the specimen edges are inked, and the specimen is submitted for tissue processing.

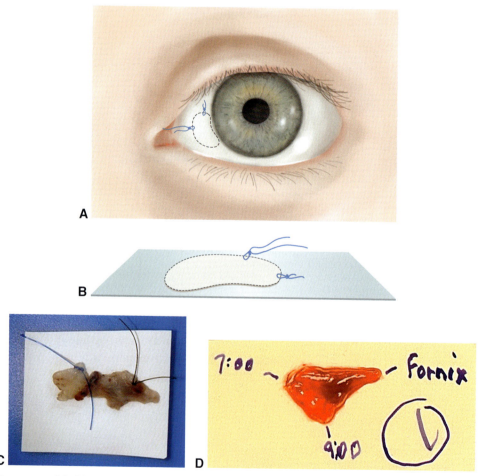

Figure 2-4 Marking the orientation of excised tissue for analysis of surgical margins. **A,** Sutures, 1 long and 1 short, are placed 90° apart. **B,** The tissue is carefully placed on a piece of filter paper and allowed to adhere for several seconds before it is placed in a container of formalin. **C,** Example of conjunctival biopsy submitted with 2 differently colored sutures for orientation. **D,** Example of a fresh conjunctival biopsy submitted with the orientation marked on filter paper. *(Parts A–B illustrations by Cyndie C. H. Wooley; part C courtesy of Vivian Lee, MD; part D courtesy of Sara Lally, MD, and Carol Shields, MD.)*

Temporal Artery Biopsies

The gold standard for histologic diagnosis of giant cell arteritis (GCA) is a superficial temporal artery biopsy. It is critical to obtain a specimen of adequate length, approximately 2 cm, because the areas of involvement can be patchy (ie, skip lesions). During grossing, the artery is transversely sectioned every millimeter, and each section is submitted for evaluation. Careful histologic examination requires stepped sections (levels) through the tissue, where a minimum of 4 levels are typically evaluated.

Tissue Processing and Staining

Tissue Processing

Tissue processing involves dehydrating the specimen to allow paraffin to infiltrate the tissue. The tissue is then made into a paraffin block, which mechanically stabilizes the tissue for sectioning (Fig 2-5A). The organic solvents used in tissue processing—for example, ethanol and xylene—dissolve lipids and some synthetic materials, such as intraocular lenses made of acrylic or silicone, but do not dissolve sutures made of silk or nylon.

> **TAKE NOTE**
>
> Routine specimen processing usually takes a day. Techniques for rapidly processing surgical pathology material are generally reserved for small biopsy specimens that require urgent handling. Rapid processing might result in inferior tissue preparations and therefore should not be routinely requested. Surgeons should communicate directly with their pathologists about the availability and shortcomings of such techniques.

Slide Preparation and Tissue Staining

Tissue sections in paraffin are usually 4–6 μm thick. Cut sections are colorless except for areas of innate pigmentation. Various tissue dyes—principally hematoxylin and eosin (H&E; Fig 2-5B, Fig 2-6A) and periodic acid–Schiff (PAS; Fig 2-6B)—are used to stain the tissue for visualization under the microscope. The stains provide contrast and color, enabling pathologists to identify cellular elements, such as nuclei and cytoplasm. The stains

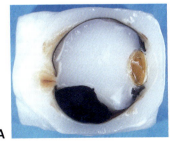
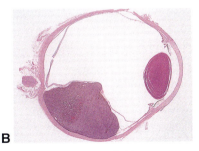

Figure 2-5 Processing an intraocular tumor enucleation specimen. **A,** The paraffin-embedded eye shows the intraocular tumor. **B,** The hematoxylin and eosin (H&E)–stained section shows that the maximum dimension of the tumor is in the center of the section, which also includes the pupil and optic nerve.

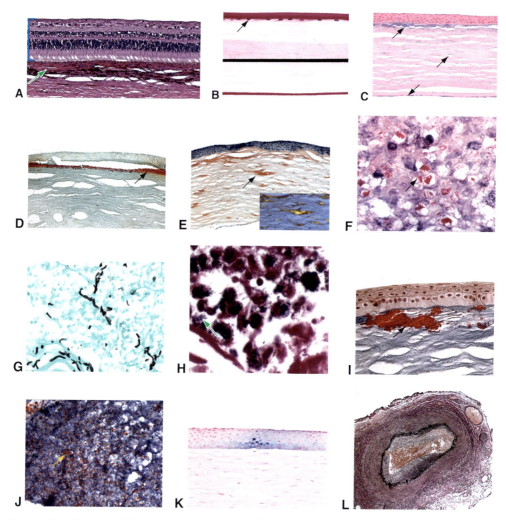

Figure 2-6 Common histochemical stains. **A,** H&E stain of the normal retina and retinal pigment epithelium *(blue bracket)*, choroid *(arrow)*, and sclera. **B,** PAS stain highlights the anterior (top) and posterior (bottom) lens capsule. The lens epithelial cells are located directly under the anterior lens *(arrow)*. **C,** Alcian blue–positive mucopolysaccharide material *(arrows)* in macular dystrophy. **D,** Alizarin red stain highlights calcium deposits in Bowman layer *(arrow)* in band keratopathy. The epithelium and stroma stain a bluish-green color as a counterstain. **E,** Congo red–positive stromal deposits *(arrow)* in lattice corneal dystrophy. *Inset:* Deposits demonstrate apple-green birefringence under polarized light. **F,** Fite-Faraco stain highlights *Mycobacterium leprae* in red *(arrow)*. **G,** GMS stain shows filamentous fungi elements in black. **H,** Gram-positive coccoid bacteria stain blue *(arrow)*. **I,** Masson trichrome–stained red positive corneal deposits *(arrow)* in granular dystrophy. **J,** Oil red O stain performed on a frozen section of a tumor. The tumor cells stain blue, and the intracellular lipid vacuoles stain red *(arrow)*. **K,** Prussian blue iron stain of corneal epithelial cells in a Fleischer ring in keratoconus. **L,** Verhoeff–van Gieson (elastin) stain of a normal temporal artery biopsy highlights the internal lamina elastica in black. *(Parts A–B, D–J, and L courtesy of Nora V. Laver, MD; parts C and K courtesy of Tatyana Milman, MD.)*

also highlight various cellular and extracellular structures depending on their chemical composition (Video 2-2; Table 2-2). After staining, a small amount of resin is placed over the section, and the slide is cover slipped to protect and preserve the tissue.

 VIDEO 2-2 Ocular tissue processing and staining.
Courtesy of Ralph C. Eagle Jr, MD.
Available at: aao.org/bcscvideo section04

Special histochemical stains

Pathologists employ special histochemical stains to identify organisms and substances that are not detected with routine stains. Special stains are typically performed when indicated by findings on routine stains or when a particular diagnosis is suspected clinically. These stains are performed on permanent sections cut from processed tissues, except for oil red O, which requires a frozen tissue section. See Activity 2-1.

Table 2-2 Histochemical Stains Commonly Used in Ophthalmic Pathology

Stain	Material Stained: Color	Examples of Use
Hematoxylin and eosin (H&E)	Nucleus: blue Cytoplasm: pink	General tissue stain (see Fig 2-5B and Fig 2-6A)
Periodic acid–Schiff (PAS)	Glycogen and proteoglycans: magenta	Basement membranes: Descemet membrane (see Fig 5-14B), lens capsule (see Fig 2-6B), Bruch membrane Mucin: goblet cells (see Fig 4-1C) Glycogen: lacy vacuolization (see Fig 10-25A)
Alcian blue	Acid mucopolysaccharide: blue	Corneal macular dystrophy (see Fig 2-6C), cavernous optic atrophy (see Fig 14-10B)
Alizarin red	Calcium: red	Band keratopathy (see Fig 2-6D)
Colloidal iron	Acid mucopolysaccharide: blue	Corneal macular dystrophy (see Fig 5-24C,D)
Congo red	Amyloid: red orange, apple green with polarized light (dichroism)	Lattice corneal dystrophy (see Fig 2-6E and Fig 5-21C,D)
Fite-Faraco	Some acid-fast organisms: red	*Mycobacterium leprae* (see Fig 2-6F)
Ziehl-Neelsen, Kinyoun	Acid-fast organisms: red	*Mycobacterium tuberculosis* and most other mycobacteria
Giemsa, Wright-Giemsa	Some bacteria and parasites: blue	Conjunctival *Chlamydia* (eg, trachoma; see Fig 4-3), *Acanthamoeba* keratitis
Gomori or Grocott methenamine silver (GMS)	Fungal elements: black	Fungal *Fusarium* (see Fig 2-6G and Fig 5-5B)
Gram stain for tissue (Brown and Brenn [B&B], Brown and Hopps [B&H])	Gram-positive bacteria: blue Gram-negative bacteria: red	Bacterial infection (see Fig 2-6H and Fig 5-3C)

(Continued)

Table 2-2 *(continued)*

Stain	Material Stained: Color	Examples of Use
KOH with calcofluor white	Fungal elements	Fungal infections (stain usually performed in microbiology laboratory)
Masson trichrome	Collagen: blue Muscle: red Granular dystrophy deposits: red	Granular corneal dystrophy (see Fig 2-6I and Fig 5-22C)
Oil red O	Lipid: red	Sebaceous carcinoma of eyelid (see Fig 2-6J)
Perls Prussian blue	Iron: blue	Fleischer ring (see Fig 2-6K), corneal blood staining (see Fig 5-16C)
Thioflavin T (ThT)	Amyloid: fluorescent yellow-white	Lattice corneal dystrophy
Verhoeff–van Gieson (elastin)	Elastic fibers: black	Temporal artery elastic layer (see Fig 2-6L and Fig 14-6C)
von Kossa	Calcium phosphate salts: black	Band keratopathy (see Fig 5-10C)

Special Techniques and Procedures

Fine-Needle Aspiration Biopsy

Diagnostic intraocular fine-needle aspiration biopsy (FNAB) is a biopsy technique in which a needle is used to acquire a small tissue sample (Checklist 2-2). FNAB is useful for diagnosing or prognosticating intraocular tumors. The procedure is performed under direct visualization through a dilated pupil, transvitreally or transsclerally (see Chapter 16, Videos 16-1 and 16-2, respectively). Iris tumors may be accessible for FNAB via sampling through the anterior chamber.

> **CHECKLIST 2-2**
>
> **Ophthalmic Pathology Consultation Fine-Needle Aspiration Biopsy and Cytology Checklist**
>
> Initiate communication with pathologist prior to the procedure to discuss goals and logistics:
>
> 1. Check adequacy of tissue, particularly intraocular tumors, for this approach (ie, Is there enough tissue to sample?).
> 2. Select appropriate fixative.
> 3. Determine whether fresh tissue is needed for molecular testing or flow cytometry.
> 4. Select the appropriate cytology form or electronic order to be filled out.

Special cytology fixatives, typically alcohol-based, are used for FNAB specimens (see Table 2-1). Cells obtained through FNAB can be processed using various cytopathologic techniques, such as a cytospin preparation, in which cells are centrifuged onto a glass slide. When enough cells are obtained, they can be centrifuged and processed into a paraffin block (cell block) (Fig 2-7). A cell block allows the pathologist to perform special stains, immunohistochemistry, in situ hybridization, microarray, and gene expression profiling if needed and as cellular material permits. In cases of suspected uveal melanoma, biopsy specimens can undergo genetic analysis to identify prognostic chromosomal abnormalities and gene expression profiling patterns. Intraocular FNAB has also facilitated the diagnosis of primary vitreoretinal lymphoma (PVRL). In cases of suspected PVRL, the FNAB specimen can undergo flow cytometric, immunocytologic, cytokine, or molecular biology analyses, depending on the sample volume. See also Chapters 16 and 19.

When properly performed, FNAB does not pose a major risk for tumor seeding. However, retinoblastoma is a notable exception where FNAB has been shown to increase the risk of local and distant tumor spread.

Some orbital surgeons use FNAB to diagnose orbital lesions, especially optic nerve tumors and presumed metastases. However, FNAB is not ideal for adequately sampling the representative areas of an orbital mass because it is difficult for the surgeon to make several passes through an intraorbital tumor without risking complications. Specific indications for performing intraocular or intraorbital FNAB are beyond the scope of this discussion, but some of these indications are discussed in Chapters 16 and 19 of this volume.

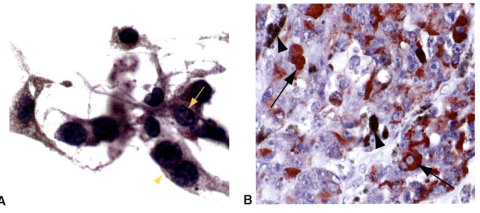

Figure 2-7 Fine-needle aspiration biopsy (FNAB) of a choroidal tumor. **A,** Cytology preparation displaying pigmented spindle cells with prominent nucleoli *(arrow)* and large binucleated epithelioid cells *(arrowhead)* consistent with a diagnosis of malignant melanoma. **B,** Sections from a cell block. Aspirated cells stained with HMB-45 immunohistochemical stain using a red chromogen are positive, confirming the diagnosis of melanoma. Note the difference between the red chromogen color product *(arrows)* and the brown melanin *(arrowheads)*. *(Part A courtesy of Nora V. Laver, MD; part B courtesy of Patricia Chévez-Barrios, MD.)*

> **TAKE NOTE**
>
> Ophthalmic FNAB should be performed with the assistance of an ophthalmic pathologist or cytopathologist experienced with these types of cases because of the small amount of tissue/cells often obtained.

Bellerive C, Biscotti CV, Singh N, Singh AD. Fine-needle aspiration biopsy for suspected uveal metastases. *Can J Ophthalmol.* 2019;54(6):694–698.

Frozen Section

A *frozen section* is tissue that is snap-frozen and immediately sectioned in a cryostat. It is indicated when the results of the study will affect intraoperative management of the patient (Checklist 2-3). *Permanent sections,* which are made from tissue processed into paraffin prior to sectioning, are always preferred in ophthalmic pathology because of the superior morphological preservation achieved with this technique. In addition, frozen sectioning may damage small specimens.

> **CHECKLIST 2-3**
>
> **Ophthalmic Pathology Consultation Frozen Section Checklist**
>
> 1. Unfixed, fresh tissue is required.
> 2. If possible, initiate communication with pathologist before requesting frozen sections.
> 3. Fill out requisition form or electronic order, specifying the reason for the service, such as
>   a. exact and adequate sampling of tissue
>   b. assessment of margins
>   c. diagnosis
>   d. determination for other molecular testing (eg, retinoblastoma, rhabdomyosarcoma, metastatic neuroblastoma)
> 4. Include map/diagram of margins and orientation.
> 5. Indicate tissue landmarks (eg, sutures) to orient specimen according to the diagram (for analysis of margins).

The most frequent indication for a frozen section is to determine whether the resection margins are free of tumor, especially in eyelid carcinomas. When tissue is submitted for margin evaluation, appropriate orientation of the specimen, correlated with documentation (through drawings of the excision site, labeled margins, or margins of the excised tissue that are tagged with sutures or other markers), is crucial (Fig 2-8). Two techniques can be used for assessing the margins in eyelid carcinomas (eg, basal cell carcinoma,

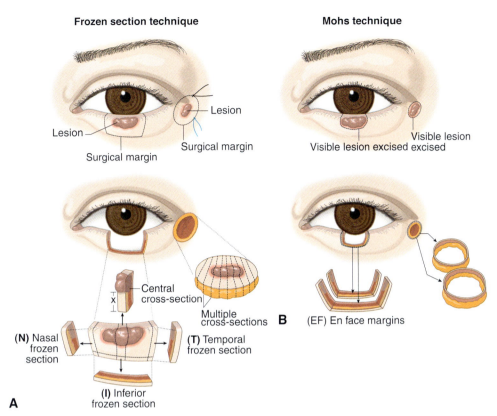

Figure 2-8 Frozen section and Mohs micrographic surgery techniques. **A,** To prepare a frozen section, the surgeon excises the lesion, typically a malignancy, with surgical margins denoted for the pathologist. For an eyelid margin lesion, the surgeon often performs a pentagonal wedge eyelid resection. Note that when the anatomy of the eyelid margin is easily recognizable, appropriate tissue identification as in this example, *left lower eyelid*, is sufficient for orientation by the pathologist. The pathologist samples the nasal, temporal, and inferior margins to assess for the presence of tumor. A central cross section may be performed to demonstrate the distance of the tumor from the inferior surgical margin. An elliptical excision of a skin tumor requires orientation with sutures (1 long, 1 short or different colors) placed 90° apart. An elliptical excision can be evaluated by frozen section using the bread-loaf technique, in which multiple cross sections are prepared. **B,** In Mohs micrographic surgery performed on an eyelid margin tumor, the surgeon excises the visible lesion. Then, additional thin shavings of tissue are prepared by frozen section from the bed of the residual defect, allowing the surgeon to evaluate en face margins. In another variation of Mohs surgery, the surgeon performs an elliptical excision of the visible tumor and obtains frozen en face sections from the undersurface and the edges of the excised lesion. The tumor locations are marked on a map for a subsequent second-stage excision. *(Illustration developed by Tatyana Milman, MD, and rendered by Mark Miller.)*

squamous cell carcinoma): (1) routine frozen sections (as discussed previously) and (2) Mohs micrographic surgery (see Fig 2-8), which preserves normal tissue while obtaining clear margins. Tissue conservation during the excision of eyelid lesions, especially those located in the canthal areas, is required to maintain adequate cosmetic and functional results.

Another indication for obtaining frozen sections is to determine whether adequate diagnostic tissue has been obtained by the surgeon. In some centers, frozen sectioning of representative tissue is performed to assess whether the tissue is appropriate for *flow cytometry* studies (Checklist 2-4; also see Fig A-1 in the online appendix on molecular pathology at aao.org/bcscappendix_section04). As frozen sections are a time-intensive and costly process, they should be used with discretion.

> **CHECKLIST 2-4**
>
> **Ophthalmic Pathology Consultation Flow Cytometry Checklist**
>
> 1. Unfixed, fresh, unfrozen tissue is required.
> 2. Initiate communication with pathologist before the biopsy to discuss the necessity of the test and logistics.
>   a. Select appropriate fresh tissue transport (no media vs nutrient media, such as RPMI).
>   b. Determine size of sample needed.
>   c. Consider geographic proximity to the laboratory for transportation of tissue.

See the section on eyelid disorders in BCSC Section 7, *Oculofacial Plastic and Orbital Surgery*, for more information.

> **EXAMPLE 2-2**
>
> A conjunctival biopsy of a salmon patch lesion suspicious for lymphoma is best submitted fresh so the tissue can be divided for flow cytometry and routine paraffin embedding. Communication is especially important for specimens like these, which are very small and require careful handling. In some cases, careful selection of the surgical facility is also necessary to ensure proper specimen handling.

Special Diagnostic Testing

Immunohistochemistry

A given cell type can express specific antigens, a property that pathologists use to identify cell type or cell of origin, typically in tumors. Immunohistochemistry (IHC) is a common method used to detect specific antigens. In most cases, the process involves a primary antibody that binds to a specific antigen expressed in or on the cell surface and a secondary antibody linked to a chromogen (a compound that produces a particular color as a result of a chemical reaction) that binds to the primary antibody (Fig 2-9).

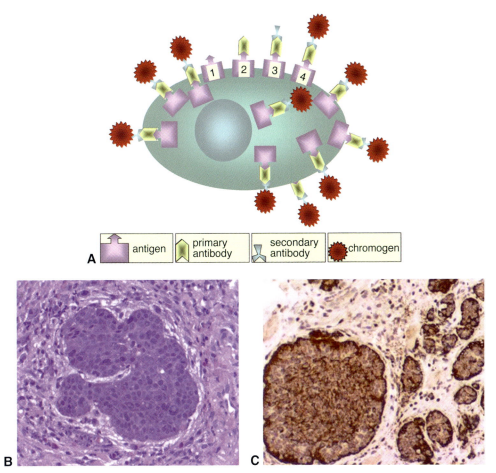

Figure 2-9 Immunohistochemistry. **A,** Schematic representation of the general immunohistochemistry method. (1) The cell expresses its specific antigen; (2) the cellular antigen is recognized by the specific primary antibody; (3) a secondary antibody targeting the primary antibody is added and attaches to the primary antibody; and (4) the secondary antibody reacts with the enzymatic complex, thereby activating the chromogen. The final product allows visualization of the cell containing the antigen based on identification of the color product of the activated chromogen in the tissue section. **B–C,** A metastatic carcinoid to the orbit seen with H&E staining **(B)** shows bland epithelial characteristics. In **C,** an antibody directed against chromogranin highlights the neuroendocrine nature of the cells. *(Courtesy of Patricia Chévez-Barrios, MD.)*

The most common chromogen color products are brown (see Fig 2-9C) or red (see Fig 2-7B). A red chromogen is especially advantageous when dealing with pigmented ocular tissues and melanomas because it contrasts with the brown melanin pigment in the uveal tissue or tumor.

A specific antigen can be identified using this method, and depending on the antigen profile, the specific cell type can be ascertained. Many antibodies are routinely used for diagnosis, treatment, and prognosis. However, antibodies can vary in their specificity and sensitivity, affecting interpretation. Therefore, it is critical to compare results with appropriate standardized controls. New antibodies are continually being manufactured to improve specificity and sensitivity. In addition, automated equipment and antigen retrieval techniques can be modified to increase sensitivity and decrease turnaround time.

The Key Antibodies at a Glance box lists some common antibodies used in IHC stains; a more comprehensive list can be found in Table 2-3.

Table 2-3 Common Immunohistochemical Stains in Ophthalmic Pathology

Associated Condition	Antibodies
Primary tumors	
Carcinomas	Various cytokeratins (CK7, CK20, pancytokeratin, CK5/6), EMA, other markers of squamous lineage (p40, p63)
Melanoma and melanocytic lesions	Melan A, HMB-45, S-100, SOX-10, MITF
Lymphoma and reactive lymphoid hyperplasia	CD3, CD20, kappa and lambda light chains, CD43, CD5, CD10, BCL-2, BCL-6, CD21, CD23, cyclin D1, Ki-67
• B lymphocytes	CD19, CD20, PAX-5
• T lymphocytes	CD3, CD4, CD8
Schwannoma	S-100, GFAP
Rhabdomyosarcoma	MSA, desmin, myogenin, myoglobin, Myo-D1
Neuroblastoma	Neuron-specific enolase, CD56, Leu-7, ALK-1, synaptophysin, chromogranin, GFAP
Retinoblastoma	Synaptophysin, neuron-specific enolase
Meningioma	EMA, somatostatin receptor 2a, PR
Optic nerve glioma	GFAP, S-100, SOX-10, p16, OLIG2
Metastatic tumors	
Carcinoma (nonspecific)	CK AE1/AE3, CK7, CK20, CAM5.2, CK5/6, EMA, p63
Lung carcinoma	TTF-1, napsin A
Breast carcinoma	ER, PR, GATA-binding protein 3, GCDFP-15, mammaglobin
Prostate carcinoma	PSA, AMACR, NKX3.1
Gastrointestinal tract carcinomas	CDX2
Neuroendocrine tumors	Chromogranin, synaptophysin
Infection	
Retinitis	Herpes simplex virus, herpes zoster virus, cytomegalovirus, *Toxoplasma*

ALK-1 = anaplastic lymphoma kinase 1; AMACR = alpha-methylacyl-coenzyme-A racemase; BCL = B-cell lymphoma; CAM5.2 = anti-cytokeratins 7 and 8; CD = cluster of differentiation/designation; CDX2 = homeobox protein CDX2; CK = cytokeratin; EMA = epithelial membrane antigen; ER = estrogen receptor; GCDFP-15 = gross cystic disease protein 15; GFAP = glial fibrillary acidic protein; HMB-45 = human melanoma black 45; Ki-67 = cellular proliferation marker; Leu-7 = anti-CD57 antibody; MITF = microphthalmia transcription factor; MSA = muscle-specific antigen; Myo-D1 = myogenic differentiation gene 1; OLIG2 = oligodendrocyte transcription factor; p63 = tumor protein 63; PR = progesterone receptor; PSA = prostate-specific antigen; TTF-1 = thyroid transcription factor.

Key Antibodies at a Glance

- **Cytokeratins** (multiple subtypes): diagnosis of epithelial tumors (eg, adenoma, carcinoma)
- **Desmin, myoglobin, or actin:** diagnosis of smooth muscle or skeletal muscle (eg, rhabdomyosarcoma, leiomyoma)
- **S-100 protein:** diagnosis of tumors of neuroectodermal and neural crest origin (eg, schwannoma, neurofibroma, melanoma)
- **Melan A and HMB-45:** diagnosis of melanocytic tumors (eg, nevus, melanoma)
- **Chromogranin and synaptophysin:** diagnosis of neuroendocrine tumors (eg, metastatic carcinoid [see Fig 2-9B, C] and small cell carcinoma)
- **Leukocyte common antigen:** diagnosis of hematopoietic-origin tumors (eg, leukemia, lymphoma)
- **CD** (cluster of differentiation/designation): antigen for subtyping white blood cells, particularly lymphocytes
- **BAP1:** diagnosis and prognosis of neoplasia (eg, prognosis of uveal melanoma)

Molecular Pathology

Molecular biology techniques are used increasingly in diagnostic ophthalmic pathology and extensively in experimental pathology (see Table A-1 in the online appendix at aao.org/bcscappendix_Section04). These techniques require special tissue handling (see Checklist 2-5 later in this chapter). More recently, the use of molecular pathology techniques has expanded to include disease prognostication and treatment selection. For example, molecular pathology tests such as comparative genomic hybridization (CGH), polymerase chain reaction (PCR), or array CGH have been used to identify tumor-promoting or tumor-inhibiting genes (eg, the retinoblastoma gene), and tests such as PCR or in situ hybridization (ISH) have been used to identify viral DNA or RNA strands, such as those seen in herpesviruses and Epstein-Barr virus. Molecular pathology techniques have made it possible not only to recognize the presence or absence of a strand of nucleic acid but also to localize precise DNA sequences within specific cells (eg, via fluorescence in situ hybridization [FISH] or ISH). In addition, 2 major techniques, PCR (and its variations) and microarray (and its subtypes), have markedly advanced our knowledge of developmental biology and tumorigenesis. These techniques are described in more detail in the following sections.

Polymerase chain reaction

A common molecular biology technique is the PCR method, which amplifies a single strand of nucleic acid by several orders of magnitude, generating thousands to millions of copies of a particular DNA sequence (see Fig A-2 in the online appendix at aao.org/bcscappendix_section04 for discussion of PCR reaction). This method relies on thermal cycles of repeated heating and cooling of the DNA sample for thermal denaturation and enzymatic replication. The components required for selective and repeated amplification are *primers,* which are short DNA fragments that contain sequences complementary to the target region (cDNA), DNA polymerase, and nucleotides. The selectivity of PCR is determined by the specificity of these primers. Successful DNA extraction from various tissues and fluids with PCR techniques is dependent on the condition of the specimen.

PCR techniques have advanced considerably in recent years, and there are now many variations, including reverse transcription PCR, touchdown PCR, real-time PCR, nested PCR, strand displacement amplification, rolling circle amplification, ligase chain reaction, helicase-dependent DNA amplification, and multiplex PCR, among others. The clinical relevance of detecting a PCR product depends on numerous variables, including the primers selected, laboratory controls, and demographic considerations. Thus, for clinicians making a clinicopathologic diagnosis, PCR is best used as an adjunct to routine pathologic diagnostic techniques. See also Part III, Genetics, in BCSC Section 2, *Fundamentals and Principles of Ophthalmology.*

Clinical use of PCR

Routine clinical use of PCR was traditionally limited to the diagnosis of leukemias, lymphomas, soft-tissue neoplasms, and tumors with nondiagnostic histopathology results. PCR procedures are now increasingly used in the detection of infectious agents (eg, the herpesvirus family), tumor prognostication (eg, uveal melanoma), and the detection of genetic alterations that are amenable to targeted therapies (eg, cutaneous melanoma and hematologic malignancies).

> **EXAMPLE 2-3**
>
> Real-time PCR/DNA probe hybridization can be used to rule out infectious agents. A diagnostic vitrectomy, where an undiluted sample (0.5–1 cc) of vitreous is obtained, can be submitted for molecular diagnosis, for instance, to rule out herpes simplex virus types I and II, varicella-zoster virus, cytomegalovirus, toxoplasmosis, and *Mycobacterium tuberculosis* complex.

> **EXAMPLE 2-4**
>
> A diagnostic vitrectomy performed in a patient with chronic vitritis can be submitted for molecular diagnosis to rule out primary vitreoretinal lymphoma. An undiluted or diluted vitreous sample (0.5–1 cc) can be tested for an immunoglobulin heavy-chain rearrangement for B-cell lymphoma by PCR and for *MYD-88* L265P somatic gene mutation by DNA allele-specific PCR.

Microarray

Scientists and clinicians use microarrays to survey the expression of thousands of genes in a single assay, the output of which is called a *gene expression profile.* Microarray technology has been used to advance our understanding of fundamental aspects of human growth and development, explore the molecular mechanisms underlying normal and dysfunctional biological processes, and elucidate the genetic causes of many human diseases. Although DNA microarrays were initially developed to quantify the expression of a limited number of genes of clinical relevance, the technology has since been applied to tumor diagnosis and drug resistance in malignancies. A variety of microarrays are currently available, including DNA microarrays (the most common type), microRNA microarrays (eg, MMChips), protein microarrays, and tissue microarrays (see Fig A-3 in the online appendix at aao.org/bcscappendix_section04). However, the fundamental process underlying all DNA microarray platforms is the hybridization of oligonucleotides or DNA fragments (called *probes*) that represent specific gene-coding regions with fluorescently or chemiluminescently labeled purified cDNA or cRNA (called *target*). The raw data are obtained by laser scanning, entered into a database, and analyzed with statistical methods. Validating the results of microarray experiments is a critical step in the analysis of gene expression. Quantitative (real-time) PCR is the preferred method for validating gene expression profiling.

Clinical use of microarray

The selection of commercially available microarray kits continues to grow. The ongoing refinement and wider commercial availability of molecular genetic techniques will likely lead to broader integration of these modalities into clinical practice and the pathologic evaluation of biopsy specimens. Some current commercial microarray and PCR platforms can be used to stratify biopsy-sized tumor samples based on the metastatic potential of the tumor. However, the cost of these testing modalities is often significantly higher than that of more traditional diagnostic modalities and should be discussed with patients before tests are ordered.

> **EXAMPLE 2-5**
>
> Gene expression profiling can be performed on uveal melanoma material collected via fine-needle aspiration biopsy to stage the 5-year metastatic risk into 3 prognostic groups: 1A, 1B, and 2. See also Chapters 11 and 16 in this volume.

Circulating tumor cells

Tumor cells can become detached from the primary tumor and extravasate into the bloodstream. Emerging technologies for the detection of circulating tumor cells (CTCs) have contributed to a deeper understanding of the biology of these cells and their clinical significance. CTC detection is usually dependent on molecular markers, which can vary between different types of cancer. Nevertheless, the epithelial cell adhesion molecule is one of the most widely used molecular markers for CTC detection. Only a small proportion of CTCs survive and initiate metastases, suggesting that interaction and modulation between CTCs and the hostile blood microenvironment are essential for CTC metastasis. Extensive single-cell sequencing of CTCs has been applied to reveal the genome and transcriptome of CTCs—information that can be used for monitoring response to cancer treatment and evaluating prognosis.

Bustamante P, Tsering T, Coblentz J, et al. Circulating tumor DNA tracking through driver mutations as a liquid biopsy-based biomarker for uveal melanoma. *J Exp Clin Cancer Res.* 2021;40:196.

Lin D, Shen L, Luo M, et al. Circulating tumor cells: biology and clinical significance. *Signal Transduct Target Ther.* 2021;6(1):404.

Diagnostic Electron Microscopy

Historically, diagnostic electron microscopy (DEM) was used to identify the cell of origin of a tumor of questionable differentiation rather than distinguish between benign and malignant processes. In selected cases, DEM is now used to complement immunopathologic studies when IHC is not sufficient for accurate diagnosis. However, DEM is less widely available and more expensive than IHC. The surgeon should consult with the pathologist before surgery to determine whether DEM is necessary and available and ensure that the tissue is fixed appropriately (Checklist 2-5).

CHECKLIST 2-5

Ophthalmic Pathology Consultation Molecular Techniques and Electron Microscopy Checklist

Initiate communication with pathologist before the biopsy to deliberate on

1. differential diagnosis
2. fixative or transport medium (fresh vs alcohol vs glutaraldehyde vs other)
3. logistics of the biopsy, including
    a. availability of specialized personnel on decided date and time
    b. optimizing transportation based on geographic proximity to laboratory

EXAMPLE 2-6

An extraocular muscle biopsy to rule out progressive external ophthalmoplegia can be submitted fresh and triaged for conventional histological staining, special histochemical staining on frozen tissue (Gomori trichrome, oil red O, PAS, myosin heavy-chain antibody stains for fast and slow muscle fibers, Cox-10/SDH, and SBSD mitochondria stain), and DEM to study the number, size, and location of intracellular mitochondria.

CHAPTER 3

Wound Repair

Highlights

- Wound healing is an integral part of a tissue's ability to maintain function and homeostasis.
- Wound healing is a highly interdependent 4-stage process, consisting of hemostasis, inflammation, tissue proliferation, and tissue remodeling.
- Each stage depends on specific cell populations, which may be absent in certain tissues. If 1 or more stages are compromised, subsequent stages and outcome could be affected.
- Wound healing can produce undesirable consequences that can lead to decreased vision. Conversely, unique aspects of wound healing in specific ocular tissues can be utilized for therapeutic purposes.

General Aspects of Wound Repair

Wound healing is a common physiologic process in which the anatomical and functional integrity of an organ or tissue is restored as quickly as possible. It involves a complicated sequence of events that may take many months, and it typically results in a scar (Fig 3-1). Wound healing can be divided into 4 general phases:

1. *Hemostasis phase:* occurs within seconds to minutes to prevent blood loss. In this phase, the blood vessels constrict, the clotting pathway activates, and the tissue swells, acting like a tourniquet.
2. *Inflammatory phase:* may last from minutes to hours. Neutrophils and fluid enter the extravascular space. Histiocytes (also called *macrophages*) remove debris from the damaged tissues, and new vessels form. Fibroblasts begin to produce collagen, the main structural protein in connective tissues. Collagen plays multiple roles in wound healing, including interacting with platelets to initiate the inflammatory phase and functioning as a scaffold or guide for fibroblast migration.
3. *Proliferative phase* (eg, *regeneration*): the replacement of lost cells; occurs only in tissues composed of cells capable of undergoing mitosis throughout life (eg, epithelial cells, fibroblasts).
4. *Remodeling phase (reparative phase):* the process of restructuring of tissues to recapitulate normal tissue; it typically results in a fibrous scar. In this final phase, *contraction* causes the reparative tissues to shrink so that the scar is smaller than the

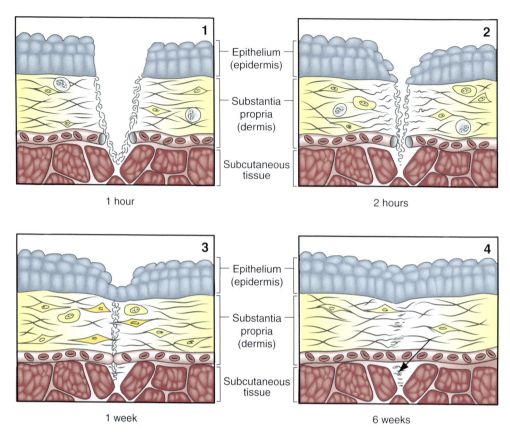

Figure 3-1 Sequence of general wound healing with an epithelial surface. **1,** The wound is created. Blood clots in the vessels; neutrophils migrate to the wound; the wounded edges begin to disintegrate. **2,** The wound edges are reapposed with the various tissue planes in good alignment. The epithelium is lost over the wound but starts to migrate. The stromal/dermal fibroblasts enlarge and become activated. Fibronectin is deposited at the wound edges. The blood vessels begin to produce buds. **3,** The epithelium seals the surface. Fibroblasts and blood vessels enter the wound and lay down new collagen. Much of the debris is removed by histiocytes. **4,** As the scar matures, the fibroblasts subside. Newly formed blood vessels canalize. New collagen strengthens the wound, which contracts. Note that the striated muscle cells in the subcutaneous tissue do not regenerate and are replaced by a scar *(arrow)*. *(Illustration by Cyndie C. H. Wooley.)*

surrounding uninjured tissues. This process may affect adjacent tissues and structures. Both repair and contraction of wounds are highly dependent on fibroblasts.

Wound Repair in Specific Ocular Tissues

Wound healing has variable mechanisms and consequences in different ocular tissues. See the relevant chapters within this volume as well as the other BCSC volumes for more information about the processes summarized in the following sections or about specific ocular tissues.

Clinical Pearl Following injury, surface ectoderm–derived epithelium (eg, conjunctival and corneal epithelium) generally regenerates without scarring. In contrast, traumatized neuroectoderm-derived tissues (eg, retina) do not regenerate. Neural crest–derived tissues (such as corneal stroma) have limited, if any, regenerative capacity.

Conjunctiva

The conjunctiva's response to injury embodies the typical wound response. The conjunctiva is lined by a constantly self-renewing nonkeratinized stratified squamous epithelium with goblet cells. The underlying stroma, called the *substantia propria,* is composed of blood vessels, lymphatic channels, fibroblasts, and collagen fibers that are randomly distributed in a relatively loose configuration. In response to a wound, activated platelets form hemostatic plugs within the vessels, and the epithelium migrates to cover the wound. At the edge of the wound, neutrophils migrate to the surface (see Fig 3-1), and stromal fibroblasts begin to proliferate and deposit fibronectin. Fibroblasts and blood vessels enter the wound and lay down new collagen. In the final phase of remodeling, new blood vessels canalize and collagen contracts, leading to a scar.

Cornea

The wound healing response of the cornea is distinct due to its unique attributes. A *corneal epithelial defect,* or *abrasion,* refers to a wound limited to the corneal epithelium, although Bowman layer and superficial stroma may be involved. The corneal epithelium is capable of rapid regeneration; on average, reepithelialization occurs at a rate of 2 mm per day. Within an hour of injury, the parabasilar epithelial cells begin to migrate across the denuded area until they touch other migrating cells, at which point contact inhibition stops migration. Simultaneously, the surrounding basal cells undergo mitosis to replenish the cell population. Although a large corneal abrasion is usually covered by migrating epithelial cells within 24–48 hours, complete healing, which includes restoration of the full thickness of epithelium (5–8 layers) and re-formation of the anchoring fibrils, takes 3–6 weeks. If a thin layer of the anterior corneal stroma is lost with the abrasion, epithelial cells will fill the shallow crater, forming a *facet* (Fig 3-2A). In contrast, Bowman layer is not replaced when it is incised or destroyed.

A *corneal ulcer* refers to a wound associated with loss of the corneal epithelium and stroma. Because the corneal stroma is avascular, corneal stromal healing occurs via the process of fibrosis rather than fibrovascular proliferation seen in other tissues (Fig 3-2B). Following a central corneal wound, growth factors from the epithelium stimulate and sustain healing. Neutrophils arrive at the site via the tears (Fig 3-3), and the edges of the wound swell. The 2 corneal matrix glycosaminoglycans, keratan sulfate and chondroitin sulfate, disintegrate at the edge of the wound. Stromal keratocytes (fibroblast-like cells) are activated and eventually migrate across the wound, laying down collagen and fibronectin. Because spacing of the keratocytes is not regular, collagen fibers are not laid down

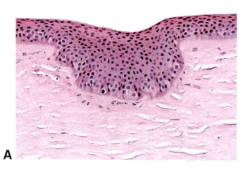 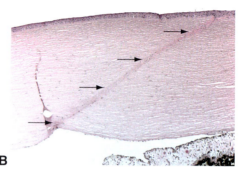

Figure 3-2 Corneal wound healing. **A,** Photomicrograph shows an epithelial facet. **B,** A full-thickness corneal wound *(arrows)* from cataract surgery. Note the mild hypercellularity of the wound due to fibrosis. There are no blood vessels in or around the wound. *(Part A courtesy of Ralph C. Eagle Jr, MD; part B courtesy of Nasreen A. Syed, MD.)*

parallel to the stromal lamellae, as they are in healthy tissue. Therefore, irregularity in the stroma will be visible microscopically and clinically as an opacity. If the wound edges are not well apposed, the proliferating keratocytes will not completely fill the gap, resulting in focal stromal thinning. In these cases, little of the lost stroma is replaced by fibrous tissue, while the surface of a healed ulceration is covered by epithelium. If the epithelium does not cover the wound within a few days of injury, healing of the subjacent stroma will be limited, and the resulting wound will be weak.

In full-thickness corneal wounds, the endothelium is critical for good wound healing. Endothelial cells typically respond to defects by migrating across the posterior cornea. Studies have shown that although most endothelial cells are postmitotic, few cells are replaced through mitosis, which may be enhanced with Rho kinase (ROCK) inhibitors. The endothelial cells eventually cover the wounded area with a new thin layer of Descemet membrane. If the wound is not covered by Descemet membrane, stromal keratocytes may continue to proliferate onto the posterior surface of the membrane as a fibrous ingrowth, or the posterior wound may remain open permanently. In the late months of healing, the initial fibrillar collagen is replaced by stronger, thicker collagen fibers.

In some cases, for example as in a laser-assisted in situ keratomileusis (LASIK) flap, stromal wounding results in predictable alterations in the corneal curvature as a result of stromal remodeling. Additionally, a fibrotic scar does not form and corneal clarity is maintained, which is advantageous for refractive procedures.

> Kopecny LR, Lee BWH, Coroneo MT. A systematic review on the effects of ROCK inhibitors on proliferation and/or differentiation in human somatic stem cells: A hypothesis that ROCK inhibitors support corneal endothelial healing via acting on the limbal stem cell niche. *Ocul Surf.* 2023;27:16–29.

CHAPTER 3: Wound Repair • 47

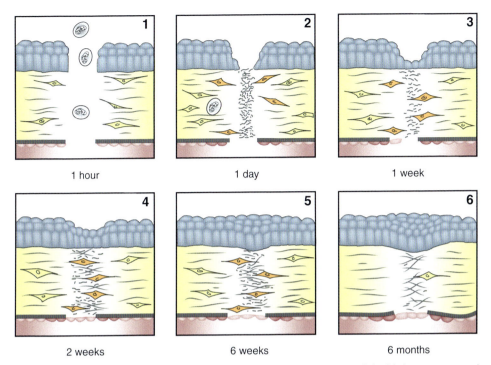

Figure 3-3 Clear corneal wound. **1,** Tears carry neutrophils *(white cells)* with lysozymes to the wound within an hour. **2,** Immediately after closure of the incision, the wound edge shows early disintegration and edema. The glycosaminoglycans at the edge are degraded. The nearby keratocytes are activated. **3,** At 1 week, migrating epithelial and endothelial cells partially seal the wound; keratocytes begin to migrate and supply collagen and fibronectin. **4,** Fibrocyte activity and collagen and matrix deposition continue. The endothelium, sealing the inner wound, lays down a new layer of Descemet membrane. **5,** Epithelial regeneration is complete. Keratocytes fill the wound with type I collagen and repair slows. **6,** The final wound contracts. The collagen fibers are not parallel with the surrounding lamellae, resulting in a wound that appears microscopically as scarring and clinically as an opacity. The number of keratocytes decreases. *(Illustration by Cyndie C. H. Wooley.)*

Sclera

In contrast to the cornea's collagen fibers, the collagen fibers in the sclera vary in thickness and are randomly distributed rather than laid down in orderly lamellae. Because the sclera is relatively avascular and hypocellular, the episclera, when stimulated by injury, migrates into the scleral wound, supplying vessels, fibroblasts, and activated histiocytes. The final wound contracts, creating a puckered appearance. If the adjacent uveal tract (also called *uvea*) is damaged, uveal fibrovascular tissue may enter the scleral wound, resulting in a scar with dense adhesion between the uvea and the sclera. Indolent episcleral fibrosis produces a dense coat around an extrascleral foreign body such as an encircling scleral buckling element or a glaucoma tube shunt. In certain clinical situations, such as glaucoma filtering surgeries, modifying the healing process through the use of topical antimetabolites such as 5-fluorouracil or mitomycin C may be desirable to prevent scar tissue from forming between the conjunctiva and the sclera at the surgical site (see BCSC Section 10, *Glaucoma*, Chapter 13).

Clinical Pearl   Because the wound healing processes in the cornea and sclera are relatively avascular, the tensile strength of wounds in these parts of the eye is less than that of the native, undisturbed tissue. Surgical wounds of the cornea remain susceptible to dehiscence indefinitely, for example, dehiscence of the scars from an old penetrating keratoplasty after blunt trauma.

Lens

Small tears in the anterior lens capsule are sealed by nearby lenticular epithelial cells, which are capable of multiple responses to injury. Under anoxic or hypoxic conditions, such as posterior synechiae or markedly elevated intraocular pressure, a metaplastic response may occur, producing fibrous plaques intermixed with basement membrane (also known as anterior subcapsular cataract).

Vitreous

The vitreous has few cells and no blood vessels. However, the collagen fibrils of the vitreous can provide a scaffold for glial, retinal pigment epithelium (RPE)–derived, and fibrovascular tissue from the retina and uveal tract to grow and extend into the vitreous and proliferate as membranes. These membranes usually have a contractile component, which can lead to traction on the retina and ciliary body.

Retina

The retina is made of terminally differentiated cells that typically do not regenerate when injured. Because the retina is part of the central nervous system, glial cells (eg, Müller cells, astrocytes), rather than fibroblasts, proliferate in response to retinal injury. Therefore, retinal wound healing induces gliosis, not fibrosis. The internal limiting membrane (ILM) and Bruch membrane provide the architectural anchors for glial scarring. Adhesions between the ILM and Bruch membrane may incorporate a rare residual glial cell, and variable numbers of retinal and RPE cells may be present between the membranes. If the wound contains damaged Bruch membrane, choroidal fibroblasts and vessels may participate in the formation of the final scar. The end result is a metaplastic fibrous or fibrovascular plaque in the sub–neurosensory retina and sub-RPE regions. The RPE usually undergoes hyperplasia in such scars, causing the dense pigmented clumps seen clinically on fundus examination.

Surgical techniques to close holes or tears in the neurosensory retina are successful when the retina and RPE are injured (eg, as a result of cryotherapy, photocoagulation), forming an adhesive, atrophic scar between the neurosensory retina and Bruch membrane (see Chapter 10, Fig 10-24).

Optic Nerve

Injury to the optic nerve may result in irreversible axonal degeneration and vision loss. There is ongoing research to modulate the innate immune response to injury, as well as axonal regeneration and remyelination, but effective therapies for optic nerve injury are not currently available.

Uveal Tract

In most circumstances, wounds of the uveal tract do not stimulate a healing response in either the stroma or epithelium. For example, the iris stroma does not produce granulation tissue to close a defect, even though it is richly endowed with blood vessels and fibroblasts. In some circumstances, the pigmented epithelium may be stimulated to migrate, but that migration is typically limited to the subjacent surface of the lens capsule, where subsequent adhesion of epithelial cells occurs (posterior synechia). When fibrovascular tissue forms, it usually does so on the anterior surface of the iris as a neovascular membrane that may cover iridectomy or pupillary openings. This fibrovascular tissue may arise from the iris, the anterior chamber angle, or the peripheral cornea. The stroma and melanocytes of the ciliary body and choroid do not regenerate after injury. Histiocytes remove debris, and a thin fibrous scar, which appears white and atrophic clinically, develops.

Clinical Pearl   Lack of wound healing in the iris is exploited when iridotomies, both surgical and laser, are performed.

Orbit and Ocular Adnexa

Like the conjunctiva, the wound response of the eyelid skin embodies a typical wound response. Its rich blood supply supports rapid healing. On approximately the third day after injury, myofibroblasts derived from vascular pericytes migrate around the wound and actively contract, decreasing the size of the wound. Because the eyelid and orbit are compartmentalized by intertwining fascial membranes that enclose muscular, tendinous, fatty, lacrimal, and ocular tissues, these tissues can become distorted by scarring. Exuberant contraction distorts muscle action, producing dysfunctional scars. The striated muscles of the orbicularis oculi and extraocular muscles are made of terminally differentiated cells that do not regenerate after injury, but the viable cells may hypertrophy.

Extraocular muscles

The extraocular muscles are composed of 2 different types of muscle fibers: slow, tonic type and fast, twitch type. The ratio of nerve fibers to muscle fibers is very high, which

50 • Ophthalmic Pathology and Intraocular Tumors

allows for precise, coordinated eye movements. Each extraocular muscle attaches to the sclera at a specific anatomical location via a tendinous insertion. As a response to injury or inflammation, strabismus may occur because of atrophy of the muscle belly itself or from scarring of the tendon to the sclera, which results in muscle restriction.

Types of Ocular Trauma and Their Sequelae

Ocular trauma can lead to a variety of sequelae, depending on the tissue affected and the nature of the trauma.

Rupture of Descemet membrane may occur after nonpenetrating injuries. For example, rupture can occur in association with keratoconus (Fig 3-4A) or during forceps delivery (Fig 3-4B).

Anterior chamber angle structures, especially the trabecular beams, are vulnerable when the anterior segment is distorted during trauma. *Traumatic recession of the anterior chamber angle* occurs when there is a tear in the anterior ciliary body between the longitudinal fibers and the circular fibers of the ciliary muscle with posterior displacement of the iris root (Fig 3-5). Concurrent damage to the trabecular meshwork with subsequent fibrosis may lead to glaucoma.

Iridodialysis is a tear in the iris root, the thinnest portion of the diaphragm where it inserts into the supportive tissue of the ciliary body (Fig 3-6). Only a small amount of supporting tissue surrounds the iris sphincter. If the sphincter muscle is torn, contraction of the remaining muscle will create a notch at the pupillary border.

Cyclodialysis results from disinsertion of the longitudinal ciliary muscle fibers from the scleral spur (Fig 3-7). This condition can lead to hypotony because the aqueous humor of the anterior chamber now has free access to the suprachoroidal space, resulting in increased outflow. In addition, because the blood supply to the ciliary body is reduced, production of aqueous humor is decreased.

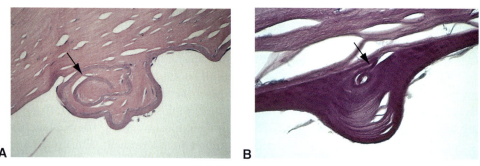

Figure 3-4 Rupture of Descemet membrane. **A,** A break in Descemet membrane in keratoconus shows anterior curling of Descemet membrane toward the corneal stroma *(arrow)* (hematoxylin and eosin [H&E] stain). **B,** A break in Descemet membrane due to forceps injury shows anterior curling of the original membrane *(arrow)* and production of a secondary thickened membrane (periodic acid–Schiff [PAS] stain). *(Courtesy of Hans E. Grossniklaus, MD.)*

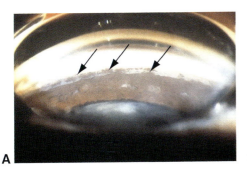 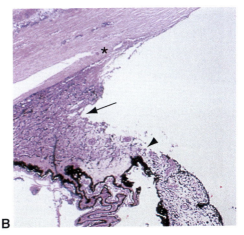

Figure 3-5 Anterior chamber angle recession. **A,** Gonioscopy image shows angle recession; the scleral spur is increasingly visible with localized depression in trabecular meshwork. Torn iris processes *(arrows)* are also visible. **B,** Photomicrograph of angle recession shows a tear in the ciliary body in the plane between the external longitudinal muscle fibers and the internal circular and oblique fibers *(arrow);* the iris root is displaced posteriorly *(arrowhead)*. Note the scleral spur *(asterisk)*. *(Part A courtesy of Steven T. Simmons, MD.)*

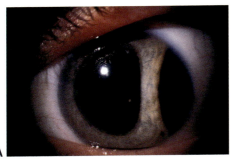 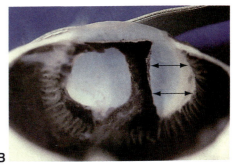

Figure 3-6 Iridodialysis. **A,** Clinical photograph of an eye shows iridodialysis, a disinsertion of the iris root from the ciliary body. **B,** Gross photograph shows a posterior view of iridodialysis *(arrows)*. *(Part A courtesy of Hans E. Grossniklaus, MD.)*

The uveal tract is attached to the sclera at 3 points:

1. the scleral spur
2. the internal ostia of the vortex veins
3. the peripapillary region

This anatomical arrangement is the basis of the evisceration technique and explains the vulnerability of the eye to expulsive choroidal hemorrhage. The borders of a dome-shaped suprachoroidal hemorrhage are delimited by the position of the vortex veins and the scleral spur (Fig 3-8).

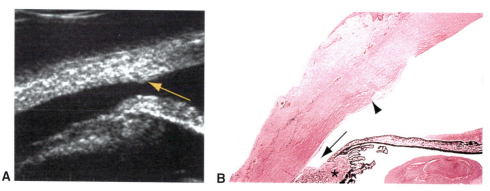

Figure 3-7 Cyclodialysis. **A,** Ultrasound biomicroscopy demonstrates disinsertion of the ciliary body from the scleral spur *(arrow)*. **B,** Photomicrograph from a different patient illustrates detachment of the ciliary body *(asterisk)* from the scleral spur *(arrowhead)*, creating a cleft *(arrow)*. *(Part A courtesy of David Rootman, MD; part B courtesy of Hans E. Grossniklaus, MD.)*

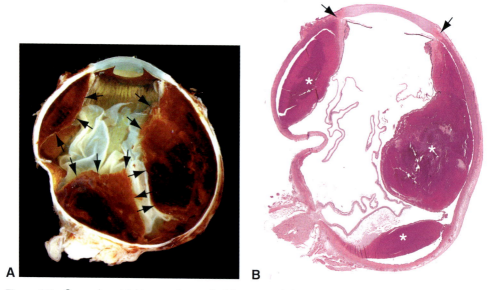

Figure 3-8 Suprachoroidal hemorrhage. **A,** Macroscopic image demonstrates multiple areas of suprachoroidal hemorrhage *(arrows)*. **B,** Microscopic image of the same eye with multiple areas of suprachoroidal hemorrhage *(asterisks)*. The anterior edge of the hemorrhages is delineated by the insertion of the choroid at the scleral spur *(arrows)*. *(Courtesy of Nasreen A. Syed, MD.)*

A *Vossius ring* appears when iris pigment epithelial cells are compressed against the anterior surface of the lens, depositing a ring of melanin pigment concentric with the pupil.

A *cataract* may form immediately if the lens capsule is disrupted. The capsule is thinnest at the posterior pole, the point farthest from the lens epithelial cells. The lens epithelium may be stimulated by trauma to form an anterior fibrous plaque just inside the capsule. The lens zonular fibers are points of relative weakness. If they rupture, lens displacement occurs, either partial (subluxation) or complete (luxation). Focal areas of zonular rupture may allow formed vitreous to enter the anterior chamber.

Commotio retinae (Berlin edema) often complicates blunt trauma to the eye. Although it is most prominent in the macula, commotio retinae can affect any portion of the retina. The retinal opacification seen clinically results from disruption in the architecture of the photoreceptor outer segments and the RPE, which can be seen with optical coherence tomography (OCT) or on histologic examination.

Retinal dialysis is most likely to develop in the inferotemporal or superonasal quadrant. The retina is anchored anteriorly to the nonpigmented epithelium of the ciliary pars plana. This union is reinforced by the attachment of the vitreous base, which straddles the ora serrata. Deformation of the eye can result in a circumferential retinal tear at the point of attachment of the ora serrata or immediately posterior to the point of attachment of the vitreous base (Fig 3-9). The interface between necrotic and normal neurosensory retina is also vulnerable to retinal tears. Retinal tears can incite proliferative vitreoretinopathy, characterized by the growth of RPE-derived and glial-derived membranes within the retina.

After a penetrating injury, intraocular *fibrous* or *fibrovascular proliferation* may occur. This proliferation may lead to vitreous, subretinal, and/or choroidal hemorrhage; tractional retinal detachment; proliferative vitreoretinopathy (PVR) including anterior PVR (Fig 3-10); hypotony; and phthisis bulbi (discussed in Chapter 1). Formation of proliferative intraocular membranes may affect the timing of vitreoretinal surgery. Sequelae of intraocular hemorrhage include hemosiderosis bulbi secondary to iron deposition from breakdown of red blood cells, and cholesterolosis, also as a result of red blood cell breakdown.

Rupture of Bruch membrane or a *choroidal rupture* may occur after direct or indirect injury to the globe. Choroidal neovascularization, granulation tissue proliferation,

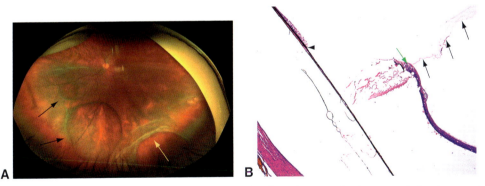

Figure 3-9 Retinal dialysis. **A,** Wide-field color fundus photograph shows an inferotemporal retinal dialysis *(yellow arrow)* and large nasal and inferior macrocysts *(black arrows)*. **B,** Photomicrograph of a different patient illustrates separation of the retina from its normal attachment to the posterior edge of the nonpigmented epithelium of the pars plana *(arrowhead)* at the ora serrata *(green arrow)*. The vitreous base is still attached to the ora serrata *(black arrows)*. *(Part A courtesy of Avni P. Finn, MD; part B courtesy of Tatyana Milman, MD.)*

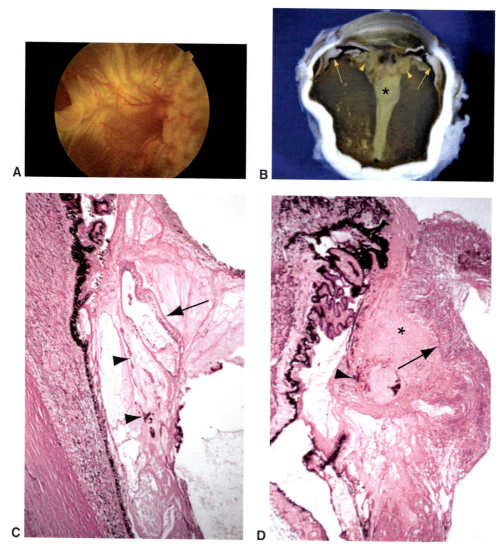

Figure 3-10 Anterior proliferative vitreoretinopathy (PVR). **A,** Fundus photograph demonstrates contractile membranes enveloping the retina and vitreous, resulting in a tractional funnel retinal detachment. **B,** Gross photograph shows membrane formation at the vitreous base *(arrowheads)* and funnel retinal detachment *(asterisk)*. Note thickening of the ciliary body *(arrows)*. **C,** Photomicrograph reveals incorporation of peripheral retinal *(arrow)* and ciliary body tissue *(arrowheads)* into the vitreous base. **D,** Photomicrograph shows condensed vitreous base *(asterisk)*, adherent retina *(arrow)*, and retinal pigment epithelium (RPE) hyperplasia *(arrowhead)*. *(Part A courtesy of Paul Griggs, MD; part B courtesy of Tatyana Milman, MD; parts C and D courtesy of Hans E. Grossniklaus, MD.)*

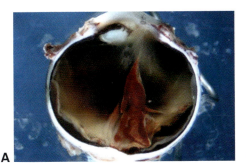 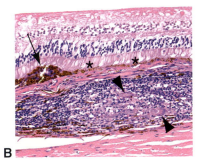

Figure 3-11 Focal posttraumatic choroidal granulomatous inflammation. **A,** Enucleated eye with perforating limbal injury extending to the posterior choroid from a projectile injury. **B,** Photomicrograph shows chronic inflammation with multinucleated giant cells *(arrowheads)* in the choroid, focal RPE hyperplasia *(arrow)*, and attenuation of photoreceptor outer segments *(asterisks)*. *(Part A courtesy of Hans E. Grossniklaus, MD; part B courtesy of Vivian Lee, MD.)*

and scar formation may occur in areas where the choroid has ruptured or where there are disruptions in Bruch membrane. A subset of direct choroidal ruptures, usually those occurring after a projectile injury, may result in *focal posttraumatic choroidal granulomatous inflammation* (Fig 3-11). This inflammation may be related to foreign material introduced into the choroid. A chorioretinal rupture and necrosis is known as *chorioretinitis sclopetaria*.

CHAPTER 4

Conjunctiva

 This chapter includes a related activity. Go to aao.org/bcscactivity_section04 or scan the QR code in the text to access this content.

 Indicates that supplemental figures are available in the Pathology Atlas *(aao.org/education /resident-course/pathology-atlas).*

Highlights

- The conjunctiva is a mucous membrane that lines the posterior surface of the eyelids and the anterior surface of the globe; it is composed of a nonkeratinized, stratified squamous epithelium overlying the substantia propria.
- Choristomas of the conjunctiva may be associated with developmental syndromes. For example, epibulbar dermoids and dermolipoma may be associated with oculoauriculovertebral dysgenesis (Goldenhar syndrome), and complex choristoma with linear nevus sebaceous syndrome.
- Inflammation of the conjunctiva, or conjunctivitis, is common and may be caused by infectious or noninfectious etiologies.
- Chronic environmental exposures can induce elastotic degeneration of the conjunctiva, which can lead to development of pinguecula and pterygium.
- Suspicion for a malignant conjunctival tumor often requires a biopsy to confirm diagnosis and determine the clinical course and treatment options. Conjunctival biopsies often require special handling, which necessitates communication and planning with the pathologist.

Topography

The conjunctiva is a contiguous mucous membrane that covers the posterior surface of the eyelids and the anterior surface of the globe up to the limbus. Conjunctiva can be divided into 3 anatomical regions:

- *palpebral:* lines the tarsi of the eyelids
- *bulbar:* covers the surface of the eyeball
- *forniceal:* comprises the junction between the bulbar and palpebral conjunctivae

The conjunctiva consists of nonkeratinized stratified squamous epithelium with goblet cells, a delicate basement membrane that rests on the underlying stroma (substantia propria) and scattered indistinct melanocytes (Fig 4-1A–C). Named after their cuplike shape, *goblet cells* are specialized cells that secrete mucin, which is incorporated into the tear film. The *substantia propria* is composed of loosely arranged collagen fibers, blood vessels, lymphatic channels, nerves, occasional accessory lacrimal glands, and resident inflammatory cells that include lymphocytes, plasma cells, histiocytes, and mast cells. In some areas of the substantia propria, lymphocytes are organized into lymphoid follicles, referred to as *conjunctiva-associated lymphoid tissue (CALT)*, a subtype of mucosa-associated lymphoid tissue (MALT).

The conjunctiva also contains 2 specialized anatomical areas: the *caruncle* and the *plica semilunaris*. The *caruncle* is the most medial aspect of the bulbar conjunctiva and, histologically, is a transitional zone between skin and conjunctiva. Its surface consists of nonkeratinized squamous epithelium with numerous goblet cells (similar to the conjunctiva), while its stroma contains hair follicles, sebaceous glands, and sweat glands like skin (Fig 4-1D). The *plica semilunaris* is a fold of bulbar conjunctiva just temporal to the caruncle and is a vestige of the nictitating membrane found in other species (Fig 4-1E). Its epithelium contains abundant goblet cells, and its stroma is richly vascular and often contains smooth muscle fibers.

A fascial sheath composed of collagen, referred to as *Tenon capsule (fascia bulbi)*, separates the conjunctiva and the sclera. This capsule surrounds the globe and the anterior portions of the extraocular muscles, partitioning them from the orbital fat. Anteriorly, Tenon capsule is connected to the sclera by fine bands of connective tissue posterior to the corneoscleral junction. Posteriorly, the capsule fuses with the optic nerve sheath. Between the capsule and the outer surface of the sclera is a potential space referred to as *episcleral*

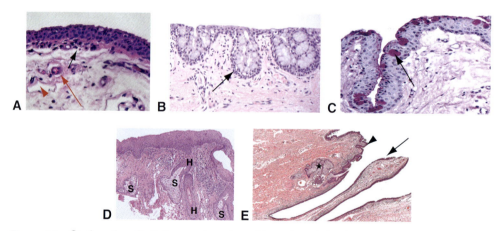

Figure 4-1 Conjunctiva. **A,** Bulbar conjunctiva with nonkeratinized stratified squamous epithelium. Note blood vessel *(red arrow)*, lymphatic vessel *(arrowhead)*, and resident lymphocytes *(black arrow)* in the substantia propria. **B,** Forniceal conjunctiva containing pseudoglands of Henle (infoldings of conjunctival epithelium with abundant goblet cells *[arrow]*). **C,** Periodic acid–Schiff (PAS) stain highlights the mucin in goblet cells *(arrow)*. **D,** Photomicrograph of caruncle with sebaceous glands (S) and hair follicles (H). **E,** Photomicrograph of plica semilunaris *(arrow)* and caruncle *(arrowhead)*. Note the pilosebaceous unit *(asterisk)* beneath the nonkeratinized epithelium of the caruncle. *(Parts A and B courtesy of Vivian Lee, MD; part C courtesy of Patricia Chévez-Barrios, MD; part D courtesy of George J. Harocopos, MD; part E courtesy of Tatyana Milman, MD.)*

(Tenon) space. See BCSC Section 2, *Fundamentals and Principles of Ophthalmology*, and Section 8, *External Disease and Cornea*, for further discussion of these structures.

Developmental Anomalies

Choristomas

A *choristoma* is a benign developmental proliferation of histologically mature tissue in an abnormal location; in other words, it is normal tissue in an abnormal place. On the ocular surface, choristomatous lesions range from simple to complex forms.

Simple choristomas include epibulbar dermoids and dermolipomas. *Epibulbar dermoids* are firm, dome-shaped, noncystic (solid) white-yellow nodules that are typically found at or straddling the limbus, most commonly in the inferotemporal quadrant (Fig 4-2A, B). Dermoids may occur in isolation or, particularly when bilateral, as a manifestation of a developmental syndrome such as oculoauriculovertebral dysgenesis (ie, Goldenhar syndrome) or linear nevus sebaceous syndrome (ie, a neurocutaneous syndrome). The former is characterized by upper eyelid coloboma, preauricular skin tags, and vertebral anomalies in addition to epibulbar dermoid.

Dermolipomas contain a substantial amount of mature adipose tissue, which makes them softer and yellower than dermoids. Similar to dermoids, dermolipomas may be associated with linear nevus sebaceous syndrome or oculoauriculovertebral dysgenesis. However, unlike dermoids, dermolipomas occur more commonly in the superotemporal quadrant, toward the fornix. They may also extend posteriorly into the orbit.

The common histologic feature of both epibulbar dermoids and dermolipomas is dense, obliquely arranged bundles of collagen in the substantia propria that is reminiscent of skin dermis. Dermal adnexal structures are often present, and the surface epithelium may or may not be keratinized (Fig 4-2C, D). In dermolipomas, adipose tissue is present deep to the dense collagenous tissue.

Complex choristomas are often clinically indistinguishable from simple choristomas. They may also be associated with linear nevus sebaceous syndrome and the histologic features of complex choristomas overlap with those of epibulbar dermoids and dermolipomas. However, complex choristomas also contain other types of tissue, such as lacrimal gland, cartilage, bone (osseous choristoma), and neural tissue (Fig 4-2E). In addition, they may involve deeper layers of the cornea and sclera.

See BCSC Section 6, *Pediatric Ophthalmology and Strabismus,* and Section 8, *External Disease and Cornea,* for additional discussion.

Hamartomas

Like choristomas, *hamartomas* are benign proliferations, but in contrast, they represent abnormal overgrowths of mature tissue normally present at a given location. In the conjunctiva, the most common type of hamartoma is the infantile (capillary) hemangioma, although this lesion most often involves the eyelid (see Chapter 12 for further discussion of infantile hemangioma).

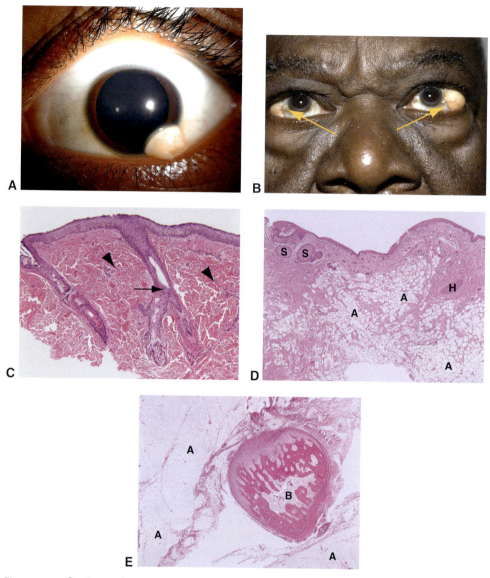

Figure 4-2 Ocular surface choristomas. **A,** Clinical photograph of a solid limbal dermoid. **B,** Clinical photograph of a dermolipoma. Note the yellowness of the dermolipoma due to its higher fat content *(arrows)*. **C,** Histology of the dermoid shows keratinized epithelium, dense bundles of collagen in the stroma *(arrowheads)* and hair follicles with associated sebaceous glands *(arrow)*. **D,** Unlike a dermoid, a dermolipoma contains a significant amount of mature adipose tissue (A). This dermolipoma also contains dermal adnexal structures, including sebaceous glands (S) and hair follicles (H). **E,** A complex choristoma combines features of multiple types of choristomas, in this case osseous, with the presence of bone (B), and dermolipoma, with the presence of adipose tissue (A). *(Part A courtesy of Morton E. Smith, MD; part B courtesy of Stephen E. Orlin, MD; parts C–E courtesy of George J. Harocopos, MD.)*

Inflammation

Because the conjunctiva is an exposed surface, it can be affected by a variety of organisms, allergens, and toxic agents, which can initiate an inflammatory response referred to as *conjunctivitis*. Depending on the onset, duration, etiology, constituents of the inflammatory infiltrate, or macroscopic and microscopic appearance of the conjunctiva, the response may be categorized as

- acute or chronic
- infectious or noninfectious
- papillary, follicular, or granulomatous

Acute or Chronic Conjunctivitis

Most cases of conjunctivitis do not require histopathologic examination; instead, they can be diagnosed clinically based on the presentation and chronicity of the symptoms. See BCSC Section 8, *External Disease and Cornea*, for additional discussion of acute and chronic conjunctivitis.

Infectious Conjunctivitis

A wide variety of pathogens can infect the conjunctiva, including viruses, bacteria, atypical bacteria (eg, chlamydiae), fungi, and parasites. Bacterial infections are more common in children (eg, *Haemophilus influenzae*, *Streptococcus pneumoniae*), whereas adenovirus and other viruses tend to be more common in adults. Recently, cases of conjunctivitis associated with SARS-CoV-2 have been reported; this may be the initial presenting symptom of systemic infection. SARS-CoV-2–related conjunctivitis can be unilateral or bilateral and is typically accompanied by fever. Infectious conjunctivitis may be diagnosed based on clinical history and examination findings (typically sufficient for viral disease), or it may require laboratory studies such as biopsy with special stains (eg, Gram, Giemsa), culture, polymerase chain reaction (PCR), or serology, depending on the suspected organism. In cases of diagnostic uncertainty or nonresponsiveness to initial treatment, cytologic evaluation of the ocular surface epithelium (Fig 4-3) or tissue biopsy may help establish a definitive diagnosis.

> Cheema M, Aghazadeh H, Nazarali S, et al. Keratoconjunctivitis as the initial medical presentation of the novel coronavirus disease 2019 (COVID-19). *Can J Ophthalmol.* 2020;55(4):e125–e129. doi:10.1016/j.jcjo.2020.03.003

Noninfectious Conjunctivitis

Noninfectious conjunctivitis has many potential etiologies, including toxic exposure, allergy/atopy, and autoimmune disease. The inflammation associated with these conditions is often histologically nonspecific, although the presence of eosinophils in the tissue suggests an allergic/atopic etiology.

Mucous membrane pemphigoid (MMP), also known as *ocular cicatricial pemphigoid* (OCP), is a form of autoimmune cicatrizing conjunctivitis. Typically, it involves the conjunctiva (Fig 4-4A) and other mucous membranes. In approximately 25% of affected

Figure 4-3 *Chlamydia trachomatis.* Conjunctival scraping for cytologic examination for infectious conjunctivitis, Giemsa stain. The cytoplasmic inclusion body *(asterisk),* composed of chlamydial organisms, can be seen capping the epithelial cell nucleus (N). A distinct space separates the inclusion body from the nuclear chromatin. Because this finding is often difficult to identify in conjunctival samples, other methods such as polymerase chain reaction are usually used to identify chlamydial infection.

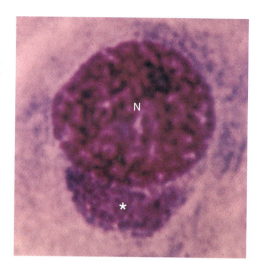

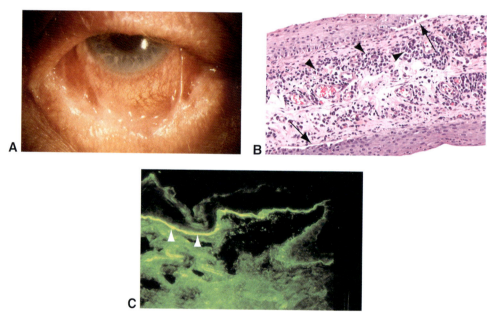

Figure 4-4 Mucous membrane pemphigoid (MMP)/ocular cicatricial pemphigoid (OCP). **A,** Clinical photograph. Note the conjunctival injection, symblepharon formation, shortening of the inferior fornix, and conjunctival/eyelid cicatrization. **B,** Histology shows epithelial bullae *(arrows)* and a dense chronic inflammatory cell infiltrate in the stroma *(arrowheads).* **C,** Direct immunofluorescent staining of unfixed tissue demonstrates immunoglobulin deposition along the epithelial basement membrane *(arrowheads)* in MMP. *(Part A courtesy of Andrew J. W. Huang, MD; part B courtesy of George J. Harocopos, MD.)*

patients, the skin is also involved. When this diagnosis is suspected clinically, a conjunctival biopsy is performed to establish the diagnosis. Biopsies for OCP typically require special handling: half of the specimen is submitted in formalin for routine histologic examination, while the other half is submitted fresh for direct immunofluorescence analysis. For fresh preparation, the tissue can be either placed in special media, such as Michel or Zeus, or wrapped in saline-soaked gauze (see Chapter 2). As mentioned, the histologic findings are generally nonspecific, but they typically show a subepithelial, band-like, mixed inflammatory cell infiltrate rich in plasma cells. The overlying epithelium may demonstrate squamous metaplasia with keratinization and loss of goblet cells. Bullae are occasionally present (Fig 4-4B). Direct immunofluorescence is the gold standard for the diagnosis of MMP; it demonstrates linear deposition of immunoglobulins (IgG, IgM, and/or IgA) and/or complement 3 (C3) along the epithelial basement membrane (Fig 4-4C). However, it is important to note that the sensitivity of immunofluorescence may be as low as 50% (particularly in long-standing cases with severe cicatrization). Thus, a negative result does not rule out MMP.

> Anesi SD, Eggenschwiler L, Ferrara M, Artornsombudh P, Walsh M, Foster CS. Reliability of conjunctival biopsy for diagnosis of ocular mucous membrane pemphigoid: redetermination of the standard for diagnosis and outcomes of previously biopsy-negative patients. *Ocul Immunol Inflamm.* 2021;29(6):1106–1113.
> Queisi MM, Zein M, Lamba N, Mees H, Foster CS. Update on ocular cicatricial pemphigoid and emerging treatments. *Surv Ophthalmol.* 2016;61(3):314–317.

Papillary Versus Follicular Conjunctivitis

Most cases of conjunctivitis can be divided into one of 2 types, papillary or follicular, depending on the macroscopic (Fig 4-5) and microscopic (Fig 4-6) appearances of the conjunctiva. Neither type is pathognomonic. In cases of *papillary conjunctivitis,* a cobblestone arrangement of small nodules with central vascular cores is visible clinically. Histologically, the papillae appear as closely packed, flat-topped epithelial projections, with inflammatory cells in the stroma surrounding a central vascular channel (see Fig 4-6A, B). *Follicular conjunctivitis* is characterized clinically by small, pink, dome-shaped nodules without a prominent central vessel (follicles). Histologically, a follicle appears as a dense oval aggregate of lymphocytes in the superficial stroma (see Fig 4-6C, D). The lymphocytes are occasionally arranged into reactive follicles with germinal centers composed of large proliferating B cells, surrounded by a mantle of smaller, more differentiated B cells.

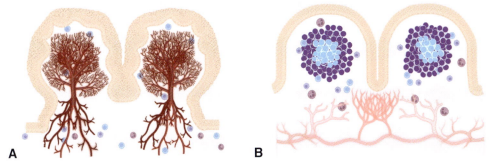

Figure 4-5 Schematic representations of papillary and follicular conjunctivitis. **A,** In papillary conjunctivitis, fine projections of blood vessels underlie the conjunctival epithelium. The stroma contains eosinophils, lymphocytes, and plasma cells. **B,** In follicular conjunctivitis, lymphoid follicles are present in the superficial stroma. They are distinguished by their paler germinal center surrounded by a darker corona. *(Courtesy of Vivian Lee, MD [images created with Biorender].)*

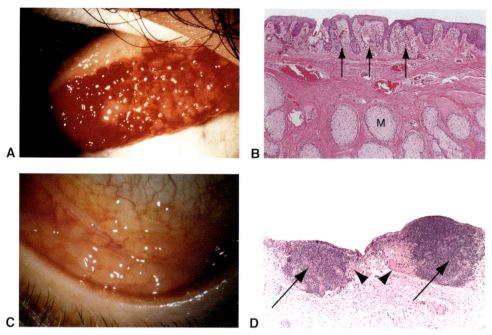

Figure 4-6 Papillary and follicular conjunctivitis. **A,** Clinical photograph of papillary conjunctivitis. Papillae efface the normal palpebral conjunctival surface and form a confluent cobblestone pattern. **B,** Photomicrograph of papillary conjunctivitis shows the characteristic closely packed, flat-topped papillae with central fibrovascular cores *(arrows)* in the palpebral conjunctiva. Note the meibomian glands (M) in the tarsus. **C,** Clinical photograph of follicular conjunctivitis, showing pale pink follicles. **D,** Photomicrograph of follicular conjunctivitis shows aggregates of lymphocytes *(arrows)* with blood vessels at the base *(arrowheads)*. *(Part A courtesy of Harry H. Brown, MD; part B courtesy of George J. Harocopos, MD; part C courtesy of Anthony J. Lubniewski, MD; part D courtesy of Vivian Lee, MD.)*

Granulomatous Conjunctivitis

Granulomatous conjunctivitis is less common than papillary and follicular conjunctivitis and has both infectious and noninfectious causes. Clinically, the nodular elevations of granulomatous conjunctivitis may be difficult to distinguish from follicles, but the clinical history and systemic symptoms may indicate the diagnosis.

Granulomatous conjunctivitis that occurs in association with ipsilateral regional lymphadenopathy is known as *Parinaud oculoglandular syndrome.* Many organisms, often atypical ones such as *Bartonella henselae,* can cause this syndrome. The diagnosis can be made by using cultures, serologic testing, PCR techniques, or a combination of these methods. In some cases, special stains such as Gram, acid-fast, or silver stain may be useful for identifying organisms in biopsied tissue. In cases of infectious granulomatous conjunctivitis, the granulomas typically display central necrosis (ie, necrotizing or caseating granulomas).

Sarcoidosis is thought to be a noninfectious cause of granulomatous conjunctivitis. Sarcoidosis, a systemic disease that may involve all ocular tissues, including the conjunctiva,

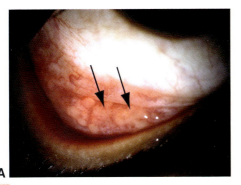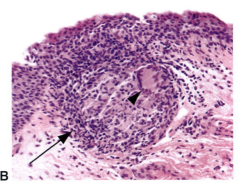

Figure 4-7 Sarcoidosis. **A,** Clinical photograph shows granulomas *(arrows)* of the conjunctiva in a patient with sarcoidosis. **B,** Histology shows a noncaseating granuloma with pale-staining histiocytes, including a multinucleated Langhans-type giant cell *(arrowhead)*. Note the small cuff of lymphocytes and plasma cells *(arrow)*. *(Courtesy of George J. Harocopos, MD.)*

manifests as small tan nodules without overt inflammatory signs, primarily in the lower forniceal conjunctiva (Fig 4-7A). Conjunctival biopsy may be a simple, minimally invasive way of providing diagnostic corroboration of this systemic disease. Histologically, nonnecrotizing granulomatous nodules, which are round to oval aggregates of epithelioid histiocytes with or without multinucleated giant cells, are present within the conjunctival stroma, typically with a narrow cuff of lymphocytes and plasma cells (Fig 4-7B). Central necrosis is not characteristic and, if present, suggests an infectious etiology. To ensure that granulomas are not missed, step-sectioning of the paraffin block is done, similar to a temporal artery biopsy. However, histologic findings are not pathognomonic for sarcoidosis and must be correlated with clinical findings after infectious causes of granulomatous inflammation have been excluded by special stains and/or cultures.

Because the ocular surface is continually exposed to dust, hair, or other foreign material, foreign bodies are another cause of granulomatous conjunctivitis. Some foreign bodies may be transient and/or inert; others may become embedded and incite a foreign-body reaction, visible histologically as epithelioid histiocytes and multinucleated giant cells surrounding the foreign body. Viewing the tissue section under polarized light may help reveal the presence of foreign material (Fig 4-8).

> Bui KM, Garcia-Gonzalez JM, Patel SS, Lin AY, Edward DP, Goldstein DA. Directed conjunctival biopsy and impact of histologic sectioning methodology on the diagnosis of ocular sarcoidosis. *J Ophthalmic Inflamm Infect.* 2014;4(1):8.

Pyogenic Granuloma

The term "pyogenic granuloma" is a misnomer because the lesion is neither pus-producing nor granulomatous. Rather, a pyogenic granuloma is an overgrowth of granulation tissue composed of acute and chronic inflammatory cells, as well as radially arranged, proliferating capillaries within loose connective tissue (Fig 4-9). Pyogenic granuloma typically occurs in association with a chalazion (on the palpebral conjunctiva) or a punctum or at

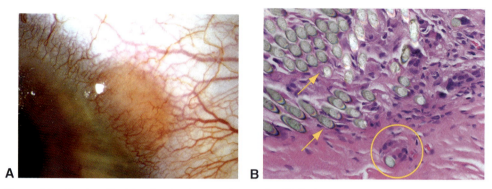

Figure 4-8 Conjunctival foreign-body granuloma. **A,** Clinical appearance on the bulbar conjunctiva. **B,** Histologic analysis of the specimen under polarized light shows multiple refractile foreign fibers *(arrows)* with a foreign body–type giant cell engulfing 1 fiber *(circle)*. *(Part A courtesy of Anthony J. Lubniewski, MD; part B courtesy of Tatyana Milman, MD.)*

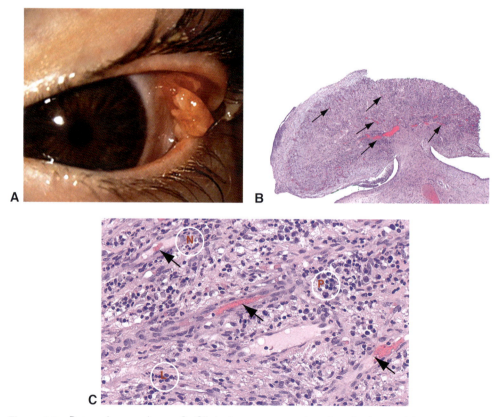

Figure 4-9 Pyogenic granuloma. **A,** Clinical appearance at a site of prior strabismus surgery. **B,** Low-magnification photomicrograph illustrates a pedunculated mass composed of granulation tissue with radiating, "spoke-wheel" vascular pattern *(arrows)*. **C,** High-magnification photomicrograph shows a mixture of acute and chronic inflammatory cells of pink fibrin and collagen and radiating small caliber vascular channels *(arrows)*. Note the neutrophils (N), lymphocytes (L), and plasma cells (P). *(Part A courtesy of Gregg T. Lueder, MD; parts B and C courtesy of Tatyana Milman, MD.)*

a site of prior accidental or surgical trauma. Clinically, pyogenic granuloma presents as a fleshy, red, pedunculated, nodular elevation on the conjunctival surface. The formulation of granulation tissue is part of the reparative process that is necessary for wound healing after inflammation or injury.

See BCSC Section 6, *Pediatric Ophthalmology and Strabismus,* and Section 8, *External Disease and Cornea,* for additional discussion of conjunctivitis.

Degenerations

See BCSC Section 8, *External Disease and Cornea,* for discussion of the clinical aspects of many of the topics covered in the following sections.

Pinguecula and Pterygium

A *pinguecula* (plural, *pingueculae*) is a small, yellow-tan bulbar conjunctival nodule, typically located at the nasal and/or temporal limbus, often bilaterally (Fig 4-10A). Pinguecula is commonly associated with actinic damage from chronic exposure to sunlight or other environmental factors, such as dust and wind, and its incidence increases with age. On histologic examination, the stroma contains basophilic fragmented and vermiform elastotic material, which consists of abnormal elastin fibers, fibrillin, proteoglycans, and degenerated collagen. Elastotic material is likely synthesized de novo by stromal cells in response to ultraviolet (UV) light damage and to a lesser extent may form from degradation of preexisting stromal collagen and elastin fibers, a process known as *actinic* or *solar elastosis*. Unlike normal elastin fibers, tissue that has undergone actinic elastosis stains positively with elastic stains, such as Verhoeff–van Gieson, even after it has been treated with elastase for digestion of normal elastin (Fig 4-10B).

A *pterygium* (plural, *pterygia*) is similar to a pinguecula in etiology and location but differs from the latter in that it invades the superficial cornea as a fibrovascular, wing-shaped growth (Fig 4-10C). Histologic examination typically demonstrates elastotic degeneration, as in a pinguecula, as well as fibrosis, variable degrees of chronic inflammation, and prominent blood vessels that correlate with the vascularity visible clinically (Fig 4-10D). A *recurrent pterygium* may lack the histologic feature of elastotic degeneration and is more accurately classified as pannus (discussed in Chapter 5) or a fibrovascular connective tissue response.

In both pingueculae and pterygia, the overlying epithelium may exhibit mild squamous metaplasia, loss of goblet cells, and surface keratinization resulting from ocular surface irregularity. Some studies have demonstrated abnormal expression of Ki-67, a proliferation marker; dysregulation of tumor suppressor genes such as *p53* and *p63,* and other genes associated with DNA repair; cell proliferation, migration, and angiogenesis; loss of heterozygosity; and microsatellite instability. These findings indicate the potential for malignant transformation of the conjunctival epithelium, similar to actinic damage to the skin, although this occurs in the conjunctiva only in rare cases. When conjunctival squamous neoplasia arises, it often overlies an area of preexisting elastotic degeneration. Therefore, it is important to examine pinguecula and pterygium

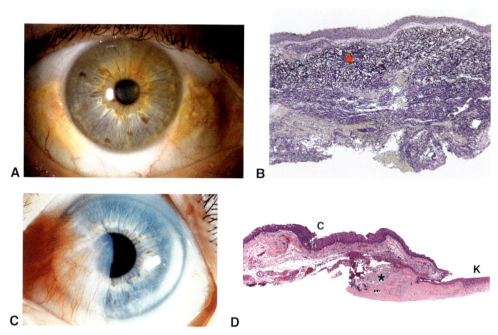

Figure 4-10 Pinguecula and pterygium. **A,** Clinical appearance of a pinguecula at the nasal and temporal limbus. In advanced cases of elastosis, lesions can appear quite yellow, as seen here. **B,** Histologically, both pinguecula and pterygium exhibit actinic elastosis, which presents as acellular, thick, curly fibers *(asterisk)* in the stroma that stain black with Verhoeff–van Gieson stain for elastin. **C,** Clinical appearance of a pterygium. **D,** Unlike a pinguecula, a pterygium crosses the limbus, as seen in this image where the conjunctival (C) and corneal (K) portions of the pterygium are evident. Note the lighter gray stroma demonstrating actinic elastosis *(asterisk)* in the hematoxylin and eosin (H&E)–stained preparation. *(Parts A and C courtesy of George J. Harocopos, MD; part B courtesy of Hans E. Grossniklaus, MD; part D courtesy of Tatyana Milman, MD.)*

specimens histologically when they are excised (see the section "Ocular surface squamous neoplasia" in this chapter).

> He S, Wu Z. Biomarkers in the occurrence and development of pterygium. *Ophthalmic Res.* 2022;65(5):481–492.

Amyloid Deposits

Amyloid deposition in the conjunctiva is most commonly a localized idiopathic process that occurs in healthy young and middle-aged adults. The deposits are typically composed of monoclonal immunoglobulin (AL amyloid) secreted by local clonal plasma cells. Conjunctival amyloidosis may also be induced by long-standing inflammation, as in cases of trachoma (ie, secondary localized amyloidosis, AA amyloid). In rare cases, conjunctival amyloidosis may occur in patients with primary conjunctival lymphoma or plasmacytoma or secondary to systemic lymphoma or plasma cell myeloma.

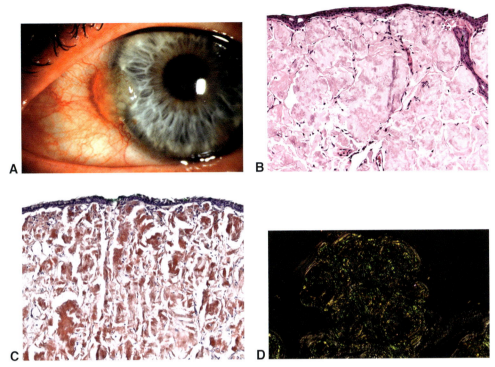

Figure 4-11 Conjunctival amyloidosis. **A,** Clinical appearance at the limbus and adjacent bulbar conjunctiva. **B,** Histologic examination reveals diffuse, amorphous, extracellular eosinophilic material throughout the stroma. **C,** Congo red stain under standard light stains the amyloid red orange. **D,** Under polarized light, Congo red–stained amyloid exhibits apple-green birefringence. *(Part A courtesy of George J. Harocopos, MD; parts B–D courtesy of Tatyana Milman, MD.)*

Clinically, conjunctival amyloidosis typically presents as a salmon-colored nodular elevation that may be associated with hemorrhage (Fig 4-11A). On histologic examination, amyloid appears as a glassy pink, extracellular stromal deposit, sometimes in a perivascular distribution. With Congo red stain, under standard light, these deposits appear red orange, and under polarized light, they exhibit birefringence with dichroism, changing from red orange to apple green depending on the plane of light (Fig 4-11B–D). Other useful stains for identifying conjunctival amyloidosis include crystal violet and the fluorescent stain thioflavin T.

Characteristic fibrils are visible under electron microscopy. Techniques used in amyloid subtyping include immunohistochemical methods, sequencing, and mass spectrometry–based proteomic analysis. Mass spectrometry is particularly sensitive. See Chapter 12 for more information on amyloid subtypes.

Epithelial Inclusion Cyst

A conjunctival epithelial inclusion cyst may form at a site of prior accidental or surgical trauma (eg, after strabismus surgery, retinal surgery, or enucleation). Clinically, the lesion

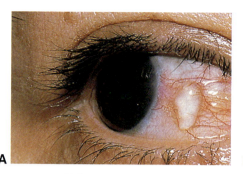 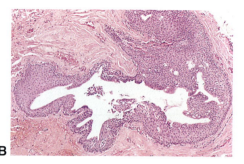

Figure 4-12 Epithelial inclusion cyst. **A,** Clinical photograph. **B,** Histologically, the cyst is lined by nonkeratinized stratified squamous epithelium with goblet cells, characteristic of the conjunctiva.

presents as a clear, translucent cystic elevation on the ocular surface, occasionally in association with prominent vascularity. Histologic examination shows a cystic space in the stroma lined by nonkeratinized stratified squamous epithelium with or without goblet cells (Fig 4-12). The lumen may be empty or may contain proteinaceous material and cellular debris.

Conjunctivochalasis

Conjunctivochalasis is a chronic condition characterized by loose, redundant, nonedematous bulbar conjunctival folds that may overhang the lower eyelid margin. This condition is often associated with aging. Some histologic studies have revealed stromal inflammation and/or dilated lymphatic vessels in cases of conjunctivochalasis.

Neoplasia

Conjunctival specimens, particularly those involving potential malignancies, often require special tissue handling. Clear communication with the pathologist prior to the procedure is essential for optimizing the quality of the specimen and its evaluation, yielding the best diagnostic and prognostic information for the patient. Techniques such as immunohistochemistry (IHC), flow cytometry, and in situ hybridization, as well as molecular studies, may be required not only for diagnoses and prognostication, but may also be necessary for determining the appropriate targeted therapy for the patient. See Chapter 2 for more information.

Squamous Epithelial Lesions

Squamous papilloma
Epithelial tumors are the most common ocular surface neoplasms. Of these, the most common benign variant is *squamous papilloma*. Clinically, squamous papillomas may be divided into pedunculated and sessile subtypes.

Pedunculated squamous papilloma is an exophytic, pink-red, strawberry-like mass composed of translucent epithelial fronds with hairpin-like central vascular loops, frequently localized to the caruncle (Fig 4-13A), plica semilunaris, or forniceal conjunctiva. It occurs most commonly in children and young adults, sometimes presenting with multiple lesions. Pedunculated papillomas have been associated with human papillomavirus (HPV) infection, subtypes 6 and 11. Histologic examination demonstrates fingerlike projections of hyperplastic squamous epithelium with a central fibrovascular core (Fig 4-13B). Goblet cells may be present as in normal conjunctival epithelium. However, when the overlying tear film is disrupted, resulting in exposure, the number of goblet cells may be reduced and the surface keratinized. Neutrophils may be found within the epithelium, and a chronic inflammatory infiltrate is frequently present in the stroma. Pedunculated papillomas typically exhibit benign behavior and rarely undergo malignant transformation.

A *sessile squamous papilloma* generally arises on the bulbar conjunctiva, especially at the limbus, and occurs more commonly in adults. This type of papilloma has also been associated with HPV infection, subtypes 16 and 18, which are the same subtypes associated with squamous malignancies. Clinical features worrisome for malignant transformation include leukoplakia (ie, white patches indicative of keratinization), inflammation, atypical vascularity, and corneal involvement. Histologically, a sessile papilloma exhibits a broad base and lacks the prominent fingerlike projections seen in a pedunculated papilloma. The epithelium is hyperplastic with intervening fibrovascular cores but is otherwise normal. The presence of nuclear hyperchromatism and pleomorphism, altered maturation (dysplasia), dyskeratosis, and frequent mitotic figures suggests a diagnosis of ocular surface squamous neoplasia.

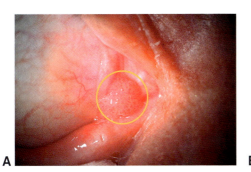
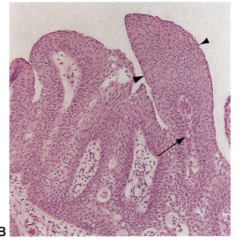

Figure 4-13 Squamous papilloma. **A,** Clinical photograph shows squamous papilloma located at the caruncle *(circle).* **B,** The epithelium is hyperplastic *(arrowheads)* with fingerlike projections surrounding fibrovascular cores *(arrow). (Part A courtesy of George J. Harocopos, MD.)*

Ocular surface squamous neoplasia

Ocular surface squamous neoplasia (OSSN) is the clinical term that encompasses the wide histopathologic spectrum of dysplastic changes of the ocular surface epithelium, including *conjunctival and corneal intraepithelial neoplasia (CIN), squamous cell carcinoma in situ (SCCIS),* and *squamous cell carcinoma (SCC),* which, by definition, has invaded through the epithelial basement membrane. In addition, *spindle cell carcinoma,* a rare variant of conjunctival SCC and *adenosquamous carcinoma* (formerly called *mucoepidermoid carcinoma*), may demonstrate aggressive behavior, with higher rates of recurrence when compared with conventional SCC, intraocular spread, and orbital invasion. Although regional lymph node metastasis and distant metastasis are less common with conjunctival SCC than with squamous carcinomas of the skin or other sites, dissemination and death occur in a small percentage of cases.

UV light exposure is a known risk factor for OSSN, especially in individuals with light skin pigmentation. Therefore, prevalence is increased in equatorial regions of the world. Some reports have shown disease-causing variants in tumor suppressor genes such as *p53* secondary to UV light exposure. A hereditary impairment of DNA repair, as in xeroderma pigmentosum, also increases risk. Other risk factors include immunosuppression, such as in posttransplant patients; individuals with ocular surface HPV infection, particularly subtypes 16 and 18; and in those with HIV infection/AIDS. In fact, OSSN is commonly the first presenting sign of HIV/AIDS in regions where HIV infection is endemic. HIV-associated OSSN may exhibit rapid growth and aggressive behavior, and HIV infection should be suspected in any patient with OSSN younger than 50 years.

OSSN typically arises in the interpalpebral limbal zone. It usually presents as a unilateral vascularized, gray, gelatinous limbal mass located medially or laterally in the sun-exposed interpalpebral fissure and may extend onto the peripheral cornea. Features such as tortuous dilated "corkscrew" feeder vessels and overlying leukoplakia (white plaque) may be present. Clinical features overlap with those of other ocular surface lesions, making the histopathologic diagnosis of CIN/SCC based solely on clinical assessment difficult. Clinical differential diagnosis for OSSN includes pannus, benign papilloma, pinguecula, pterygium, vitamin A deficiency, benign intraepithelial dyskeratosis, nevus, and amelanotic melanoma.

Clinical Pearl OSSN is a clinical term, while CIN, SCC in situ (CIS), and SCC are histopathologic terms that are used to denote specific pathophysiologic findings.

Histologically, the epithelium in individuals with CIN often exhibits an abrupt transition from normal epithelium to an area of hyperplasia with loss of goblet cells, loss of polarity (loss of normal maturation from basal to superficial layers), nuclear hyperchromatism and pleomorphism, and mitotic figures in superficial epithelium, including atypical mitoses. Dyskeratosis, including surface keratinization (resulting in the clinical appearance of leukoplakia) may be present, and keratin pearls may form within the epithelium. Often, there is chronic inflammation and increased vascularity in the underlying superficial stroma. Elastotic degeneration is also often present in the stroma.

Lesions are graded as mild, moderate, or severe according to the degree of cellular atypia; in particular, by how much of the thickness of the epithelium has been replaced by

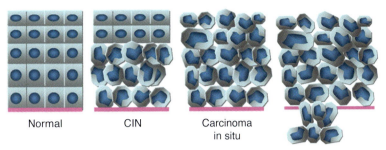

Normal   CIN   Carcinoma in situ   Invasive carcinoma

Figure 4-14 Schematic representation of the degrees of atypia in conjunctival intraepithelial neoplasia (CIN). The first panel represents normal epithelium with a basement membrane *(pink line)*. In CIN, the deeper layers of the epithelium are replaced with disorganized, often atypical cells that do not mature normally (dysplasia). Carcinoma in situ is characterized by full-thickness replacement of epithelium by dysplastic cells, with the basement membrane still intact. In invasive squamous cell carcinoma, neoplastic cells invade through the basement membrane into the stroma. *(Courtesy of Patricia Chévez-Barrios, MD.)*

atypical cells (Fig 4-14). The most important histologic assessment of CIN is determining whether the epithelial basement membrane is intact (CIN or SCC in situ) or breached (SCC), allowing for invasion of the tumor into the stroma. For full-thickness dysplastic lesions, the term *squamous carcinoma in situ* is used (Fig 4-15A, B). Invasion of the stroma by neoplastic cells is diagnostic of *invasive SCC* (Fig 4-15C, D). Invasion of the sclera or cornea with intraocular spread is an uncommon complication of invasive SCC (Fig 4-15E, F) that typically occurs at the site of a previous surgical procedure or in immunocompromised patients. Squamous eddies, dyskeratosis, keratin whorls, or pearls may be present in all cases but are most common in invasive SCC (Fig 4-15D).

Less invasive methods that can assist with diagnosis include anterior segment optical coherence tomography (AS-OCT), ultrasound biomicroscopy (UBM), and impression cytology (IC). AS-OCT imaging has been reported to correlate with histologic findings in distinguishing noninvasive CIN from invasive SCC (Fig 4-16). Classic AS-OCT findings include thickened hyperreflective epithelium with an abrupt transition zone from normal epithelium. However, these diagnostic techniques may not be universally available, and therefore biopsies are still commonly performed for diagnosis.

Conjunctival biopsy and handling of these specimens require special care and attention not only for accurate diagnosis of CIN/SCC but for the evaluation of surgical margins as well (see Chapter 2 for more information on specimen preparation).

> Conway RM, Graue GF, Pelayes DE, et al. Conjunctival carcinoma. In: American Joint Committee on Cancer (AJCC). *AJCC Cancer Staging Manual.* 8th ed. Springer; 2017: 795–802.
> Polski A, Sibug Saber M, Kim JW, Berry JL. Extending far and wide: the role of biopsy and staging in the management of ocular surface squamous neoplasia. *Clin Exp Ophthalmol.* 2019;47(2):193–200.
> Rathi SG, Kapoor AG, Kaliki S. Ocular surface squamous neoplasia in HIV-infected patients: current perspectives. *HIV AIDS (Auckl).* 2018;10:33–45. doi:10.2147/HIV.S120517

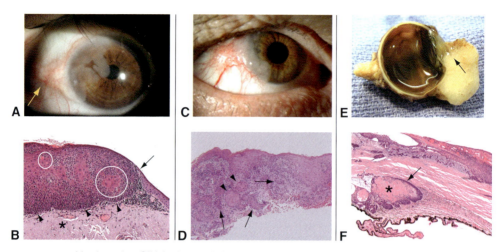

Figure 4-15 Noninvasive CIN (column 1), invasive conjunctival squamous cell carcinoma (SCC) (column 2), and invasive conjunctival SCC with anterior orbital and intraocular extension (column 3). **A,** Slit-lamp photograph of a grayish-white semitransparent slightly elevated conjunctival lesion *(arrow)* extending into the cornea. **B,** Histology of noninvasive CIN from a different patient, demonstrating an abrupt transition *(arrow)* from the normal epithelium on the right of the arrow to the acanthotic, dyskeratotic *(circles)*, and severely dysplastic epithelium on the left. The basement membrane *(arrowheads)* is intact. Note the gray amorphous stroma demonstrating actinic elastotic changes *(asterisk)*. **C,** Slit-lamp photograph of a temporal limbal gelatinous lesion with large feeder vessels and extension onto the cornea. **D,** Histology of the lesion depicted in part C demonstrates bands and nests of superficially invasive SCC *(arrows)* with focal pink dyskeratosis *(arrowheads)*. **E,** Gross photograph of large SCC invading the anterior orbit, corneoscleral limbus, and anterior chamber angle through a previous surgical incision *(arrow)*. **F,** Histology of lesion depicted in part E reveals intraocular invasion by SCC *(arrow)* with central dyskeratosis/keratin *(asterisk)*. *(Part A courtesy of Taher K. Eleiwa, MD, PhD, and Abdelrahman M. Elhusseiny, MD, MSc; parts B and F courtesy of Tatyana Milman, MD; part C reproduced with permission from Polski A, Sibug Saber M, Kim JW, Berry JL. Extending far and wide: the role of biopsy and staging in the management of ocular surface squamous neoplasia.* Clin Exp Ophthalmol. *2019;47(2):193–200; parts D and E courtesy of George J. Harocopos, MD.)*

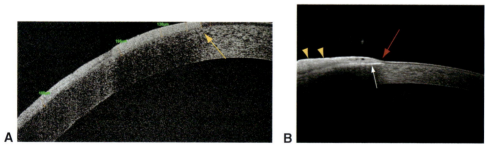

Figure 4-16 Anterior segment optical coherence tomography (AS-OCT) features of CIN and SCC. **A,** AS-OCT image of the noninvasive CIN depicted in Figure 4-15A demonstrates an abrupt epithelial thickening (to the left of the *arrow*) and hyperreflectivity. **B,** AS-OCT image of the superficially invasive SCC depicted in Figure 4-15E. Red arrow denotes an abrupt transition between the unremarkable corneal epithelium to the right and a thickened hyperreflective dysplastic epithelium on the left *(arrowheads)* as well as prominent subepithelial hyperreflectivity *(white arrow)*, suggestive of stromal invasion. *(Part A courtesy of Taher K. Eleiwa, MD, PhD, and Abdelrahman M. Elhusseiny, MD, MSc; part B reproduced with permission from Polski A, Sibug Saber M, Kim JW, Berry JL. Extending far and wide: the role of biopsy and staging in the management of ocular surface squamous neoplasia.* Clin Exp Ophthalmol. *2019;47(2):193–200.)*

Melanocytic Lesions

About half of all conjunctival lesions in adults are pigmented and/or melanocytic. Conjunctival melanocytes are normally dendritic and located exclusively in the epithelial basal layer alongside basal squamous cells that also contain melanin. The melanocytes produce melanin, which is taken up by the adjacent epithelium, providing them with protection from UV light. However, the amount of conjunctival melanin in the epithelium is usually insufficient to be visible to the naked eye. Therefore, the presence of clinically apparent pigmentation of the conjunctiva may necessitate further investigation. Although not all entities discussed in this section are neoplasms, they are covered here because they involve ocular surface pigmentation.

Pigmented conjunctival epithelial lesions, melanocytic neoplasms of the conjunctiva and caruncle, and other pigmented lesions of the ocular surface include the following:

- conjunctival junctional, compound, and stromal nevi, including
  - inflamed juvenile conjunctival nevus (inflamed juvenile nevus of childhood and adolescence)
  - blue nevus of the conjunctiva
- congenital ocular or oculodermal melanocytosis (nevus of Ota)
- secondary acquired melanosis or reactive melanosis of the conjunctiva
- complexion-associated melanosis (benign epithelial melanosis of the conjunctiva)
- primary acquired melanosis (PAM) with or without atypia (conjunctival melanocytic intraepithelial neoplasia [C-MIN], conjunctival melanocytic intraepithelial lesion [C-MIL])
- conjunctival melanoma

Table 4-1 summarizes the clinical features of common nonmalignant intraepithelial melanocytic conjunctival lesions. See also Activity 4-1.

 ACTIVITY 4-1 Comprehensive catalogue of non-nevoid intraepithelial pigmented lesions of the conjunctiva. *Developed by Vivian Lee, MD, and Tatyana Milman, MD. Available at: aao.org/bcscactivity_section04*

Melanocytic nevi

Melanocytic nevi (also called *nevocellular nevi, nevus cell nevi*) are benign proliferations of specialized melanocytes known as a nevus cells. They can be classified as hamartomas or neoplasms depending on whether they are congenital or acquired. Nevi usually become clinically apparent in childhood and/or adolescence, and they commonly evolve during this period of time. They are typically unilateral, circumscribed pigmented lesions on the perilimbal interpalpebral bulbar conjunctiva. Frequently, small, clear epithelial cysts are visible within the lesion (Fig 4-17A). Melanocytic nevi are also common in the caruncle but are found in the palpebral conjunctiva only in rare cases. Pigmented lesions in this area are highly suspicious for intraepithelial acquired melanosis or melanoma.

Amelanotic nevi of the conjunctiva are nevi that do not contain any pigment. They often have a pinkish hue, which can make clinical diagnosis challenging. The pigmentation and size of a nevus may increase during puberty, at which point the lesion may become more noticeable.

Table 4-1 Clinical Comparison of Nonmalignant Intraepithelial Melanocytic Lesions of the Conjunctiva

Lesion (Alternative Terminology)	Onset	Characteristics	Location	Malignant Potential
Nevus	Childhood or adolescence	Circumscribed brown or pink patch with small cysts; usually unilateral	Bulbar conjunctiva Caruncle	Yes, for conjunctival melanoma, but low
Ocular and oculodermal melanocytosis	Congenital	Patchy or diffuse slate-gray patches; usually unilateral	Episclera/sclera (deep to the conjunctiva)	Yes, for uveal and primary orbital melanoma
Complexion-associated melanosis (benign epithelial melanosis, racial melanosis, primary conjunctival melanosis)	Young adulthood, often increases with age	Flat brown patches with irregular margins; usually bilateral but not symmetric	Conjunctiva, typically bulbar	None
Primary acquired melanosis (PAM) (conjunctival melanocytic intraepithelial neoplasia [C-MIN], conjunctival melanocytic intraepithelial lesion [C-MIL])	Middle age	Flat, brown, sometimes granular patches with irregular margins; usually unilateral	Anywhere on the conjunctiva	Yes, for conjunctival melanoma when atypia is present

Table adapted with permission from Tatyana Milman, MD.

Histologically, conventional melanocytic nevi are composed of nests or sheets of nevus cells with benign features that include round to oval, uniformly staining nuclei with a moderate amount of cytoplasm. Epithelial cysts are often present in the stroma; these cysts are typically, but not always, indicative of a benign lesion (Fig 4-17B).

Like conventional cutaneous melanocytic nevi, conjunctival nevi evolve with age. In individuals in the first and second decades of life, nevus cells are typically arranged in nests at the interface (junction) between the epithelium and stroma (see Fig 4-17B). Nevus cells residing exclusively at the epithelial–stromal junction are called *junctional nevi*. With increasing age, the nests start to descend into the stroma. Nevi located exclusively in the stroma with no junctional component are termed *subepithelial* or *stromal nevi*. Nevi with both junctional and subepithelial components are referred to as *compound nevi*. A junctional component

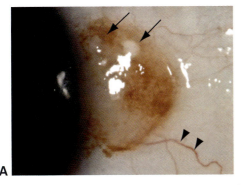 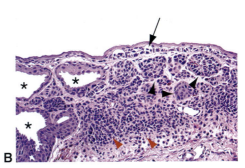

Figure 4-17 Conjunctival melanocytic nevus. **A,** Clinical appearance with characteristic cystic areas *(arrows)* in a circumscribed elevated pigmented conjunctival lesion, associated with a feeder vessel *(arrowheads)*. **B,** Histologically, the nevus cells are present at the epithelial–stromal junction *(arrow)* and in the underlying substantia propria; hence, this is a compound nevus. Nevus cells are mostly arranged in nests *(black arrowheads)*, which become confluent as the cells go deeper into the stroma *(red arrowheads)*. Note the epithelial inclusion cysts *(asterisks)* within the lesion, correlating with the clinical appearance. *(Part A courtesy of Tatyana Milman, MD; part B courtesy of George J. Harocopos, MD.)*

may be typically observed in younger patients; however, the presence of an extensive junctional component in an older individual is suspicious for malignant transformation.

Clinical Pearl A junctional nevus in an adult can be assumed to be PAM with atypia until proven otherwise.

An *inflamed juvenile conjunctival nevus* is a compound nevus that typically becomes apparent in childhood or adolescence and clinically appears to grow rapidly, suggestive of malignancy. Histologically, the aggregates of nevus cells are surrounded and invaded by lymphocytes, plasma cells, and often eosinophils. This lesion may be misinterpreted histologically as malignant if the pathologist is not familiar with it.

Another form of melanocytic nevi that may occur in the conjunctiva is a *blue nevus*. Clinically, it appears as a dark blue–gray to blue-black nodule. The melanocytes have a spindle-cell morphology, similar to that of nevus cells seen in the uveal tract, and they tend to contain a large amount of cytoplasmic melanin. *Ocular* and *oculodermal melanocytosis,* which is more often seen in individuals with darker skin tones, occurs beneath the conjunctiva in the episclera and sclera, and consists of aggregates of dendritic melanocytes (Fig 4-18).

Intraepithelial melanosis

Intraepithelial melanosis is a clinical term for localized or diffuse acquired pigmentation of the conjunctival epithelium. Histologically, the term *melanosis* can be confusing because it does not distinguish between increased melanin in epithelial cells and proliferation of melanocytes. The term *intraepithelial nonproliferative melanocytic pigmentation* may be more accurate, referring to lesions in which there is no increase in the number of melanocytes

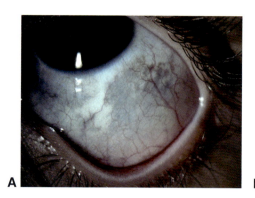 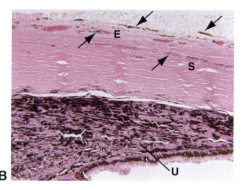

Figure 4-18 Ocular melanocytosis. **A,** Clinical photograph illustrates slate-gray patches of pigmentation of the scleral surface. **B,** Histologic examination shows an increased population of intensely pigmented spindle and dendritic melanocytes *(arrows)* in the episclera (E), sclera (S), and uvea (U). *(Part A courtesy of Gabriela M. Espinoza, MD; part B courtesy of George J. Harocopos, MD.)*

but instead there is an increase in pigmentation from increased melanin in surrounding basal epithelial cells transferred from the melanocytes. *Intraepithelial melanocytic proliferation without atypia* refers to lesions with increased numbers of unremarkable dendritic melanocytes from hyperplasia or early neoplasia; these melanocytes are predominantly confined to the basal epithelial layer, usually in a linear arrangement.

The classification of and terminology used for various forms of melanosis are subjects of debate. In general, conjunctival melanosis can be divided into 3 forms: primary, secondary, and complexion-associated (Fig 4-19). *Secondary* and *complexion-associated melanoses* generally do not involve atypical melanocytic proliferation. *Primary acquired melanosis (PAM)* can involve atypical melanocytic proliferation and thus carries a risk of progression to malignancy. An understanding of the nomenclature and processes that underlie the diagnosis is important when considering management of these lesions. Equally important is communicating the suspected clinical diagnosis to the pathologist; proper interpretation of histologic findings is greatly enhanced by this knowledge.

Secondary acquired melanosis Secondary acquired melanosis (also called *reactive melanosis of the conjunctiva*) refers to pigmentation derived from a small increase in normal-appearing dendritic melanocytes. This increase may be triggered by another conjunctival lesion (eg, squamous papilloma or carcinoma) or by underlying conjunctival inflammation or prior trauma.

Complexion-associated melanosis Complexion-associated melanosis (CAM) (also called *benign epithelial melanosis, racial melanosis, primary conjunctival melanosis*) appears as bilateral flat patches of brown pigmentation with irregular margins, typically involving the bulbar conjunctiva in individuals with dark skin pigmentation (Fig 4-20A). Streaks and whorls of melanotic pigmentation may extend onto the peripheral cornea, a condition called *striate melanokeratosis*. The caruncle and palpebral conjunctiva may also be involved. Histologically, pigmentation is primarily limited to increased melanin in the

CHAPTER 4: Conjunctiva • 79

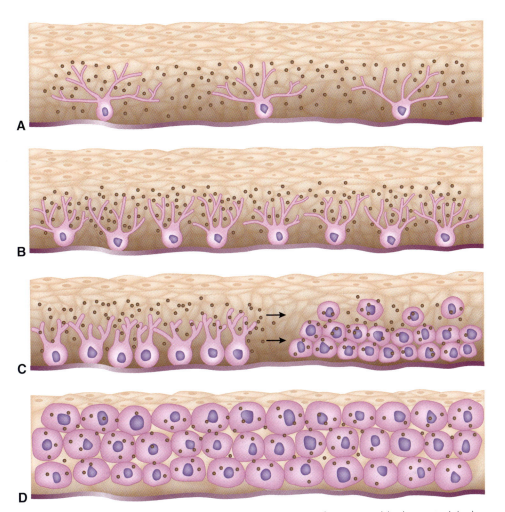

Figure 4-19 Schematic representation of the spectrum of non-nevoid pigmented lesions of the conjunctiva. Small brown dots denote melanin. **A,** Complexion-associated melanosis (CAM) represents a mostly nonproliferative melanocytic process in which a normal or mildly increased number of morphologically normal dendritic melanocytes produce an increased amount of melanin that is transferred to the surrounding basal epithelial cells. **B,** Primary acquired melanosis (PAM) without atypia or with mild atypia (conjunctival melanocytic intraepithelial neoplasia [C-MIN] 1, 2; low-grade conjunctival melanocytic intraepithelial lesion [C-MIL]) refers to low-grade lesions in which there is both increased pigment production and an increased number of melanocytes but no change or a very mild change in melanocyte morphology. Proliferating melanocytes are predominantly arranged along the basal epithelium. **C,** PAM with moderate to severe atypia (C-MIN 5–10; high-grade C-MIL). Pigment production and the number of melanocytes have increased, and melanocytes have migrated into the more superficial epithelial layers. Melanocytes acquire atypical morphology, such as an epithelioid shape with loss of dendritic processes. **D,** Melanoma in situ (C-MIN >5) with full-thickness replacement of the epithelium by morphologically atypical melanocytes. *(Illustration by Cyndie C. H. Wooley.)*

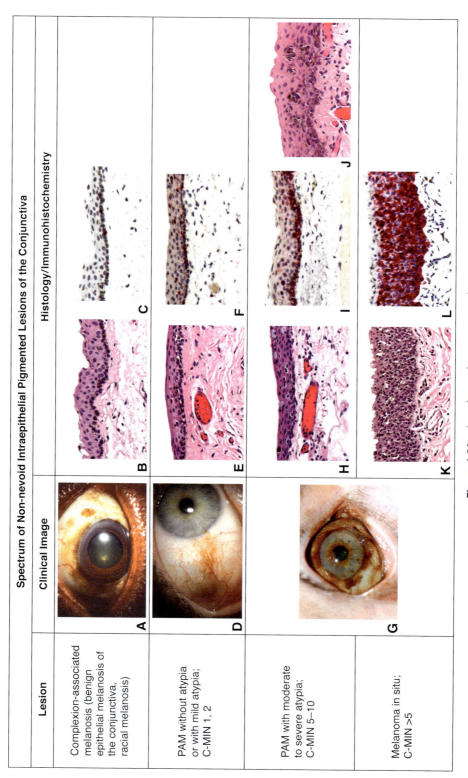

Figure 4-20 (see legend on next page)

Figure 4-20 Spectrum of non-nevoid intraepithelial pigmented lesions of the conjunctiva. **A,** Clinical appearance of CAM (benign acquired melanosis). **B,** Histology of CAM with morphologically unremarkable melanocytes confined to the basal epithelial layer. **C,** Immunohistochemical (IHC) staining for SOX-10, a neural crest and melanocyte marker, demonstrates a normal number of melanocytes. **D,** Clinical photograph of PAM without atypia (C-MIN 0–1) or with mild atypia (C-MIN 1–2; low-grade C-MIL). **E,** Histology of PAM without atypia demonstrates a linear pattern of proliferating morphologically unremarkable pigmented melanocytes in the basal layer of the epithelium. **F,** SOX-10 IHC stain demonstrates an increase in the number of melanocytes restricted to the basal epithelial layer. **G,** Clinical photograph demonstrates the appearance of PAM with moderate to severe atypia (C-MIN 5–10; high-grade C-MIL) involving 12 clock-hours and/or melanoma in situ (C-MIN >5; high-grade C-MIL/melanoma in situ [MIS]). These 2 degrees of atypical melanoses cannot be distinguished clinically. **H,** Histology of PAM with moderate atypia (C-MIN 5–10; high grade C-MIL). Note the cells with dark nuclei in the more superficial epithelial layers. **I,** MITF-1 IHC stain, another marker of melanocytes, stains melanocytes red and highlights the atypical pattern of melanocytic growth. **J,** Histology of PAM with severe atypia (C-MIN 5–10; high-grade C-MIL) with nests of atypical, pigmented melanocytes in the more superficial layers of the epithelium. **K,** Histology of melanoma in situ (C-MIN >5; high-grade C-MIL/MIS). Note the full-thickness replacement of conjunctival epithelium with atypical, largely nonpigmented melanocytes with small, dark nuclei. **L,** Melan-A IHC stain, also a marker for melanocytes, demonstrates full-thickness replacement of conjunctival epithelium with atypical melanocytes (red-staining cells). *Note:* The clinical appearance of PAM (C-MIN or C-MIL) of various stages can be indistinguishable; thus, these lesions usually require biopsy for a definitive diagnosis. *(Parts A and D courtesy of George J. Harocopos, MD; part G courtesy of Vahid Feiz, MD; all other parts courtesy of Tatyana Milman, MD.)*

basal epithelial cells; the epithelial melanocytes are normal or mildly increased in number and appear morphologically normal (Fig 4-20B, C).

Primary acquired melanosis *Primary acquired melanosis (PAM)* characteristically presents as a unilateral melanotic macule or patch in middle-aged individuals with lighter skin tones. The lesion may remain stable, or it may wax and wane over several years. The recommendations regarding when to observe PAM versus when to perform a biopsy are controversial. In general, clinical findings such as larger size (3 clock-hours or more) and a caruncular, forniceal, or palpebral location portend a worse prognosis. Management of PAM is also discussed in BCSC Section 8, *External Disease and Cornea*.

The terminology and classification used for non-nevoid intraepithelial melanocytic proliferations are unique to the conjunctiva and have been subjects of ongoing debate. PAM has historically been divided into PAM without atypia and PAM with atypia; however, this terminology is not used to describe analogous lesions at other body sites. In addition, the grading of mild, moderate, and severe atypia is somewhat subjective. To unify terminology across various organ systems and perhaps more accurately predict prognosis, several other classification schemes have been proposed, including the adaption of terminology used for cutaneous lesions. One alternative classification scheme is the conjunctival melanocytic intraepithelial neoplasia (C-MIN) scoring system. The purpose of the C-MIN classification schema is to improve objectivity and reproducibility by assigning each lesion a score of 1–10 based on a complex matrix of histologic findings that includes the horizontal and vertical extent of epithelial involvement and degree of cellular atypia. Currently, PAM with atypia and C-MIN are considered synonymous terms for describing intraepithelial melanocytic neoplasia. The recently published World Health Organization (WHO) Classification of Tumours of the Eye proposes an alternative, simplified classification that grades conjunctival intraepithelial melanocytic lesions (C-MIL) as low-grade, high-grade, or melanoma in situ.

Nevertheless, the PAM with/without atypia classification is familiar to most ophthalmologists and has generated more published information linked to prognosis and risk of metastasis than have other classification systems. Therefore, despite the histologic ambiguity of the term *melanosis,* this classification is still the most used system for grading and prognostication of intraepithelial melanocytic proliferations and is described here (see Fig 4-20). Table 4-2 provides equivalent staging using the C-MIN and C-MIL classifications as a reference.

It is impossible to clinically distinguish PAM without atypia from PAM with atypia; this distinction can only be made histologically. *PAM without atypia* is characterized by an increased number of cytologically unremarkable melanocytes arranged linearly along the basal epithelial layer, with pigment localized mainly to the epithelial cells (see Fig 4-20D–F). In *PAM with atypia,* melanocytes are increased in number and are cytologically atypical with a bloated appearance or pleomorphic nuclei. The atypical melanocytes may migrate into the superficial layers of the epithelium (see Fig 4-20G–J) as individual cells (ie, pagetoid spread) or as small clusters, forming discohesive intraepithelial nests. Atypical melanocytes may completely replace the epithelium (ie, melanoma in situ). Migration of melanocytes into the more superficial layers of the epithelium and cytologic atypia

Table 4-2 Non-nevoid Intraepithelial Pigmented Conjunctival Lesions

Nomenclature	Alternative Terminologies	Histology	Risk of Association With or Progression to Invasive Melanoma
Non-neoplastic Lesions			
Secondary melanosis of the conjunctiva	Benign acquired melanosis	Depends on specific etiology (ie, related to systemic disease or reactive)	None
CAM	Benign acquired melanosis Racial melanosis	Increased *melanin production* by melanocytes that is transferred and localized to the basal epithelial cells *without increase in number or change in the morphology of melanocytes*	None
	Constitutional melanosis	*Occasionally: slight or focal melanocytic hyperplasia without atypia*	
Neoplastic Lesions			
PAM without atypia	C-MIN score = 0–1	Increased *melanin production* by melanocytes that is transferred and localized to the basal epithelial cells *without increase in number or change in the morphology of melanocytes* OR Increase in pigment production and proliferation of *normal-appearing melanocytes* (hyperplasia) arranged in a linear fashion and *localized* to the basal epithelial layer	None
PAM with mild atypia	C-MIN score = 2–4 Low-grade C-MIL	Proliferation of melanocytes with *low-grade cytologic atypia* and predominantly basilar spread	Lower
PAM with moderate to severe atypia	C-MIN score = 5–10 High-grade C-MIL	More confluent basilar and significant nonbasilar proliferation, including nested and/or pagetoid growth; melanocytes with epithelioid cytomorphology	Higher
Conjunctival melanoma in situ	High-grade C-MIL/MIS	*Full-thickness* or close to full-thickness intraepithelial proliferation of melanocytes with *severe cytologic atypia*	Highest
Invasive conjunctival melanoma		*Violation of the epithelial basement membrane by* atypical melanocytes and invasion into the stroma	

CAM = complexion-associated melanosis; C-MIL = conjunctival melanocytic intraepithelial lesion; C-MIN = conjunctival melanocytic intraepithelial neoplasia; MIS = melanoma in situ; PAM = primary acquired melanosis.

occur to varying degrees and, as previously mentioned, are graded by the pathologist as mild, moderate, or severe (see Fig 4-20). Features of moderate-to-severe atypia include mitotic activity, nesting, extensive pagetoid spread, epithelioid cell morphology, enlarged pleomorphic hyperchromatic nuclei, and prominent nucleoli. IHC stains for melanocytes (eg, Melan A, HMB-45, MITF, SOX-10) often highlight the presence and extent of melanocytic proliferation. IHC stains complexed with a red chromogen are preferred over the standard brown chromogen to differentiate positive IHC staining from native pigment in the tissue (see Fig 4-20C, F, I, L).

Clinical Pearl The clinical appearance of PAM (C-MIN or C-MIL) of various stages can be indistinguishable; thus, these lesions usually require biopsy for a definitive diagnosis.

PAM without atypia carries no risk of malignant transformation. *PAM with mild atypia* carries a low risk of malignant transformation. In contrast, *PAM with moderate* or *severe atypia* (see Fig 4-20G–J) and *melanoma in situ* (see Fig 4-20G, K, L) carry a high risk of progression to melanoma.

Clinical Pearl Clinical correlation is extremely important in interpreting conjunctival melanocytic intraepithelial lesions. For example, PAM without atypia and PAM with mild atypia can be histologically indistinguishable from complexion-associated and secondary melanosis. The patient's skin tone, whether the lesion is bilateral or unilateral, the location and extent of the lesion, and the patient's relevant medical and ocular history can help establish an accurate diagnosis.

Table 4-2 summarizes the histology of non-nevoid intraepithelial pigmented conjunctival lesions with correlations of the clinical nomenclature to the histologic classification schemes. See also BCSC Section 8, *External Disease and Cornea*.

Coupland SE, Brouwer NJ, Milman T, Verdijk RM. Conjunctival melanocytic intraepithelial lesions. In: *WHO Classification of Tumours of the Eye*. 5th ed. International Agency for Research on Cancer; 2023. WHO Classification of Tumours Series; vol. 13. Accessed April 7, 2023. https://tumourclassification.iarc.who.int/chapters/44

Milman T, Eiger-Moscovich M, Henry RK, et al. Validation of the newly proposed World Health Organization classification system for conjunctival melanocytic intraepithelial lesions: a comparison with the C-MIN and PAM classification schemes. *Am J Ophthalmol.* 2021;223:60–74.

Conjunctival melanoma

Approximately 50%–70% of conjunctival melanomas arise from PAM with atypia (Fig 4-21), while the remainder develop from a nevus or are de novo. Melanomas are usually nodular, can be pigmented or amelanotic (15%–25% of conjunctival melanomas), and can involve any portion of the conjunctiva. In 25% of patients, conjunctival melanomas metastasize to regional lymph nodes, as well as to the lungs, liver, brain, bone, and skin.

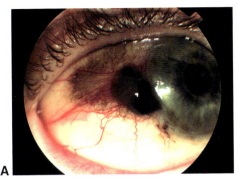
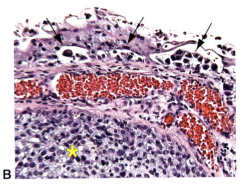

Figure 4-21 Melanoma arising from PAM with atypia. **A,** Clinical photograph. Note the elevated melanoma nodule adjacent to the limbus, arising from a background of PAM (diffuse, flat, brown pigmentation). Also note the prominent vascularity. **B,** Histologic examination shows melanoma *(asterisk)* arising from PAM *(arrows)*. *(Part A courtesy of Morton E. Smith, MD; part B courtesy of Tatyana Milman, MD.)*

The overall mortality rate in these cases ranges from 15% to 30%. Features associated with a worse prognosis include

- nonbulbar conjunctival location (ie, plica semilunaris/caruncle, forniceal or palpebral conjunctiva)
- increased tumor thickness (>1.8 mm)
- involvement of the eyelid margin

When clinical suspicion for melanoma is high, referral to a surgeon with extensive experience in excision and treatment of ocular surface tumors should be considered because an incomplete excision portends a worse outcome for the patient.

Occasionally, extrascleral extension of an anterior uveal melanoma can present as an episcleral/conjunctival mass that mimics a primary conjunctival melanoma. Extrascleral extension of an anterior uveal melanoma should be included in the differential diagnosis, particularly in cases of a nonmobile pigmented or amelanotic episcleral nodule overlying the ciliary body with sentinel vessels but without surrounding PAM (Fig 4-22). A complete eye examination, including gonioscopy and dilated ophthalmoscopy, is warranted in any patient with a conjunctival mass. In individuals with darker skin tones, conjunctival SCC is occasionally associated with reactive pigmentation (secondary melanosis) masquerading as melanoma.

On histologic examination, the atypical melanocytes in melanoma range from spindle to polyhedral to epithelioid. The atypical cells may replace the entire thickness of the epithelium with an intact basement membrane *(melanoma in situ, C-MIN >5)*, involve both the epithelium and the stroma, and/or involve just the stroma *(invasive melanoma)*. Mitotic figures may be present and are more often present in more aggressive lesions. The morphological cell types present in conjunctival melanoma do not have the same prognostic significance as they have in uveal melanoma. Rather, as in cutaneous melanoma, depth of invasion has a stronger correlation with prognosis.

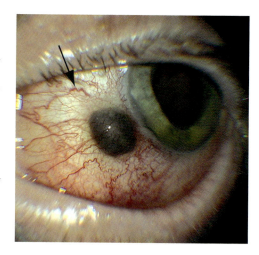

Figure 4-22 Melanoma of the ciliary body with extrascleral extension, presenting as an ocular surface mass. Note that there is no PAM surrounding the nodule, a clue that the lesion might have an intraocular origin. Also note that the lesion is associated with deep episcleral/scleral vessels (sentinel vessels; *arrow*) and does not obscure the overlying conjunctival vessels. This indicates that the lesion is deep to the conjunctiva. *(Courtesy of J. William Harbour, MD.)*

Use of IHC stains for melanocytes (eg, Melan A, HMB-45, MITF, S100, SOX-10) may be helpful in diagnostically challenging cases. Preferentially expressed antigen in melanoma (PRAME) IHC stain can help distinguish melanoma from nevi (this marker is frequently positive in cases of melanoma and is generally negative in nevi). In addition, identification of tumor-specific biomarkers, such as *BRAF, NRAS, NF1,* and *ATRX* pathogenic variants, has enhanced the assessment of conjunctival melanoma. Identification of melanoma biomarkers is critical in treating disease that has spread beyond the ocular surface, because targeted therapies are available for many of these disease-causing variants. See also BCSC Section 8, *External Disease and Cornea.*

> Cisarova K, Folcher M, El Zaoui I, et al. Genomic and transcriptomic landscape of conjunctival melanoma. *PLoS Genet.* 2020;16(12):e1009201. doi:10.1371/journal.pgen.1009201
>
> Conway RM, Graue GF, Pelayes DE, et al. Conjunctival melanoma. In: American Joint Committee on Cancer (AJCC). *AJCC Cancer Staging Manual.* 8th ed. Springer; 2017: 803–812.
>
> Lally SE, Milman T, Orloff M, et al. Mutational landscape and outcomes of conjunctival melanoma in 101 patients. *Ophthalmology.* 2022;129(6):679–693.

Lymphoid Lesions

Both benign and malignant lymphoid proliferations can occur in the conjunctiva. Normal conjunctiva contains mucosa-associated lymphoid tissue (MALT), including a few small lymphoid follicles that are often visible clinically in the normal inferior fornix. However, lymphoid tissue may proliferate abnormally in the conjunctiva, often in the absence of inflammatory signs. This type of lymphoid hyperplasia may be benign (reactive) or malignant. Clinically, both benign and malignant lymphoid conjunctival lesions appear as soft, mobile, salmon-pink masses with a smooth surface, characteristically localized to the forniceal and bulbar conjunctivae (Fig 4-23A, B). The condition may be unilateral (more common) or bilateral, and an orbital component may also be present.

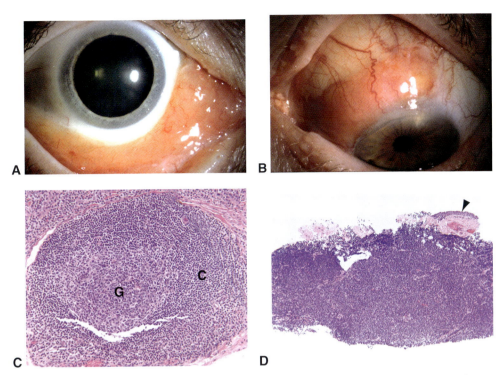

Figure 4-23 Lymphoid proliferations of the conjunctiva. Clinical photographs show a salmon-pink mass in the inferior fornix **(A)** and in the bulbar conjunctiva **(B)**. **C,** Histologic examination of benign lymphoid hyperplasia reveals normal follicular architecture with a well-defined germinal center (G) and corona (C). **D,** Histologic examination of lymphoma shows a monotonous sheet of lymphocytes infiltrating the stroma, without well-defined follicles. Note the conjunctival epithelium *(arrowhead)*. *(Part A courtesy of Anthony J. Lubniewski, MD; part B courtesy of Anjali K. Pathak, MD; parts C and D courtesy of George J. Harocopos, MD.)*

Benign lymphoid hyperplasia (reactive lymphoid hyperplasia) consists of a polyclonal proliferation of lymphocytes, often with a follicular pattern demonstrating germinal centers. *Lymphoma* is a malignant neoplasm derived from a monoclonal proliferation of B or T lymphocytes and, less frequently, natural killer cells (NK cells). It is divided into 2 major groups: Hodgkin lymphoma and non-Hodgkin lymphoma (NHL). The NHLs form a large heterogeneous group of neoplasms that can be divided into those originating from B lymphocytes and those developing from their precursors, T cells, and NK cells. Non-Hodgkin B-cell lymphoma is the most common type of lymphoma observed in the ocular adnexa.

A biopsy of conjunctival lymphoid lesions is required to determine the nature of the neoplasm (ie, benign vs malignant). Because the pathologic evaluation of these lesions is limited by the size of the biopsy specimen obtained, communication with the pathologist regarding optimal specimen submission (including handling and fixation) is essential. Histologic examination and IHC stains are routinely used. IHC analysis includes staining for a variety of lymphocyte antigens. When the submitted tissue is sufficient for additional studies, flow cytometry and molecular genetic studies can also be performed. Flow cytometry can be especially useful in identifying clonality, which is typical of lymphoid malignancies. Also see Chapter 2 in this volume.

On routine hematoxylin and eosin (H&E) sections, histologic features that indicate a diagnosis of benign lymphoid hyperplasia include the presence of normal-appearing lymphoid follicles with distinct germinal centers and small, mature coronal lymphocytes (Fig 4-23C; see also Fig 13-10C, D). In contrast, characteristic features of lymphoma often include a diffuse monomorphic sheet of lymphocytes in the stroma without well-defined follicles (Fig 4-23D). IHC staining of conjunctival lymphoma typically show a predominance of B lymphocytes that are often kappa or lambda light-chain restricted. The most common type of lymphoma involving the conjunctiva is extranodal marginal zone lymphoma of mucosa-associated lymphoid tissue (EMZL), also known as MALT lymphoma (Fig 4-24).

Of all ocular adnexal sites, a conjunctival lymphoma has the most favorable prognosis, because only 25%–30% of cases are associated with systemic disease. When a conjunctival lymphoma is diagnosed, systemic evaluation is necessary to exclude other sites of involvement (tumor staging). See Chapter 13 for additional information on periocular

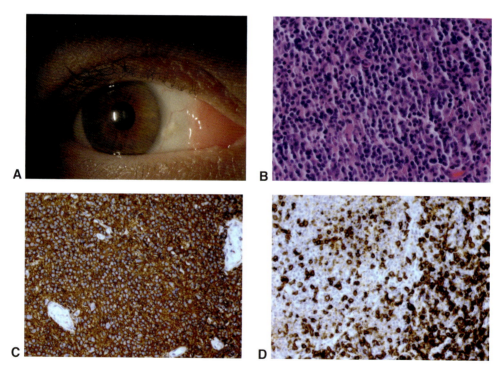

Figure 4-24 Conjunctival extranodal marginal zone lymphoma of mucosa-associated lymphoid tissue (EMZL), also known as mucosa-associated lymphoid tissue (MALT) lymphoma. **A,** Clinical photograph of a salmon patch–like conjunctival lesion. **B,** H&E-stained preparation demonstrates a diffuse proliferation of small lymphocytes with mildly irregular nuclear contours, inconspicuous nucleoli, and scant cytoplasm. **C,** IHC staining shows that nearly all lymphocytes are CD20+, which is a B-cell marker. **D,** Scattered reactive CD3+T cells are present. *(Courtesy of Hans E. Grossniklaus, MD.)*

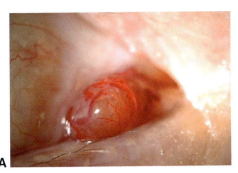 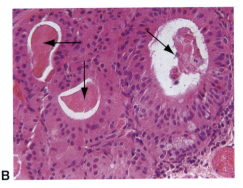

Figure 4-25 Oncocytoma. **A,** Clinical photograph of a circumscribed reddish mass in the caruncle. **B,** Histology shows cystadenomatous proliferation of large polygonal epithelial cells with abundant, intensely eosinophilic, granular cytoplasm. Some of the cells surround protein-filled lumina *(arrows)*. *(Part A courtesy of Mark J. Mannis, MD; part B courtesy of George J. Harocopos, MD.)*

lymphoproliferative lesions. See BCSC Section 8, *External Disease and Cornea,* and Section 7, *Oculofacial Plastic and Orbital Surgery,* for additional discussion.

> Tanenbaum RE, Galor A, Dubovy SR, Karp CL. Classification, diagnosis, and management of conjunctival lymphoma. *Eye Vis (Lond).* 2019;6:22.
> WHO Classification of Tumours Editorial Board. *Haematolymphoid Tumours.* 5th ed. International Agency for Research on Cancer; 2023. *WHO Classification of Tumours Series;* vol. 13. Accessed April 7, 2023. https://tumourclassification.iarc.who.int

Glandular Neoplasms

Oncocytoma (oxyphilic adenoma) is a benign neoplasm that typically arises in the accessory lacrimal glands of the caruncle but can occasionally occur elsewhere on the conjunctiva. Oncocytoma most commonly occurs in women with a median age of 73 years. Clinically, this tumor appears as a tan to reddish vascularized nodule (Fig 4-25A). Histologically, the lesion shows a cystadenomatous proliferation of enlarged polygonal, somewhat columnar, epithelial cells with abundant, intensely eosinophilic granular cytoplasm (reflecting the presence of numerous mitochondria) and granular eosinophilic, periodic acid–Schiff–positive material in the lumen (Fig 4-25B).

Other Neoplasms

Virtually any neoplasm that can occur in the orbit and eyelid skin can occur in the conjunctiva, albeit less frequently. These include sebaceous, neural, muscular, vascular, and fibrous/fibroblastic tumors. Metastasis to the conjunctiva is rare. Orbital neoplasms are discussed in Chapter 13. See also BCSC Section 8, *External Disease and Cornea,* and Section 7, *Oculofacial Plastic and Orbital Surgery.*

CHAPTER 5

Cornea

 Indicates that supplemental case studies are available in the Pathology Atlas *(aao.org/education/resident-course/pathology-atlas).*

Highlights

- The precise structure and normal function of each of the 5 corneal layers are essential for maintaining its transparency. Disruption of any of these layers may result in vision loss due to loss of corneal clarity or refractive capacity.
- Infectious keratitis can be caused by a variety of organisms and may result in significant scarring, ulceration, and even perforation of the cornea.
- Degeneration of corneal structures and stromal ectasias may be primary or may be secondary to other ocular conditions.
- Corneal dystrophies are bilateral, typically progressive, inherited conditions that often interfere with visual function.

Topography

The normal cornea is avascular and composed of 5 layers (Fig 5-1):

- epithelium
- Bowman layer
- stroma
- Descemet membrane
- endothelium

The corneal *epithelium* is a nonkeratinized stratified squamous epithelium that is 5 to 8 cell layers thick. Unlike the conjunctival epithelium, the corneal epithelium contains no goblet cells. Corneal epithelial cells are self-renewing, turning over completely every 10 days. Studies have shown that epithelial stem cells reside at the corneoscleral limbus in special niches referred to as palisades of Vogt. These niches are most pronounced along the vertical corneal axis. The basement membrane laid down by the epithelial cells is thin and indistinct and is therefore best visualized with periodic acid–Schiff (PAS) stain.

Clinical Pearl   The presence of goblet cells in the corneal epithelium is generally indicative of a limbal stem cell deficiency.

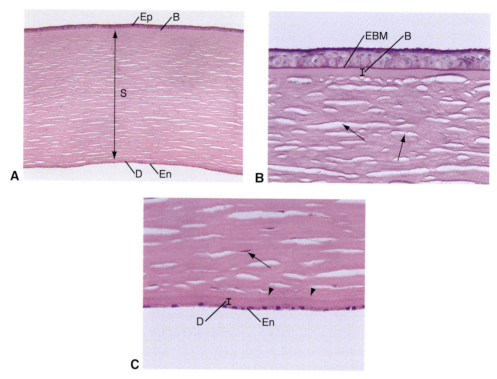

Figure 5-1 Normal cornea. **A,** The cornea is composed of epithelium (Ep), Bowman layer (B), stroma (S), Descemet membrane (D), and endothelium (En). **B,** On higher magnification, periodic acid–Schiff (PAS) stain highlights the epithelial basement membrane (EBM), distinguishing it from Bowman layer (B). Because of dehydration of the tissue during processing for paraffin embedding, multiple areas of separation (clefts) between the stromal lamellae are evident on normal histology *(arrows)*. If the stromal clefts are absent, corneal edema or scarring is likely. This is an example of a meaningful artifact. **C,** Higher magnification (hematoxylin and eosin [H&E] stain) also delineates Descemet membrane (D), endothelium (En), and a thin acellular layer of pre-Descemet stroma *(arrowheads)*. The keratocyte nuclei *(arrow)* are apparent. Descemet membrane is the basement membrane of the endothelium and is best visualized with PAS stain. *(Courtesy of George J. Harocopos, MD.)*

Located immediately beneath the epithelial basement membrane is *Bowman layer,* an acellular segment of the anterior stroma that is composed of densely packed, randomly arranged collagen fibrils.

The corneal *stroma* makes up 90% of the total corneal thickness and consists of collagen-producing keratocytes (fibroblast-like cells), collagenous lamellae, and proteoglycan ground substance. The uniform size and periodicity of the collagen lamellae, along with the water content of the corneal stroma, result in corneal transparency. The anterior stroma is denser than the posterior stroma, which facilitates the placement of refractive corneal implants posteriorly. The difference in density between the anterior and posterior stroma also enables easier separation of the stroma in procedures such as deep anterior lamellar keratoplasty (DALK). The most posterior section of the stroma is acellular and strongly adherent to the underlying Descemet membrane, resulting in a surgical cleavage plane between the posterior-most stroma and the remaining stroma (pre-Descemet *Dua layer*); this plane can be exploited in deep lamellar keratoplasty.

Descemet membrane is a PAS-positive true basement membrane that is produced by the corneal endothelium. The anterior portion of Descemet membrane (known ultrastructurally as the *anterior banded layer*) is formed during embryogenesis. The membrane increases in thickness throughout life due to the continuous production of basement membrane material by the endothelial cells. This postembryonic layer, referred to as the *posterior unbanded layer*, becomes thicker over time than the anterior banded layer.

The corneal *endothelium* is composed of a single layer of cells that are hexagonal *en face* (eg, on confocal microscopy). A histological cross section of the cornea reveals that the endothelial cells have a slightly flattened cuboidal appearance. The endothelium is primarily responsible for corneal deturgescence. See BCSC Section 2, *Fundamentals and Principles of Ophthalmology*, and Section 8, *External Disease and Cornea*, for discussion of the embryology, structure, and physiology of the cornea.

Developmental Anomalies

Dermoid

Dermoid, a type of choristoma that may involve the cornea, is discussed in Chapter 4 (see Fig 4-2). See also BCSC Section 6, *Pediatric Ophthalmology and Strabismus*.

Peters Anomaly

Peters anomaly represents the severe end of the spectrum of *anterior segment dysgenesis* syndromes, in which neural crest cells do not properly migrate or differentiate during embryologic development. This disrupts anterior segment development and, in severe cases, prevents cleavage of the lens from the corneal endothelium. Peters anomaly is typically bilateral and sporadic, but autosomal dominant and recessive modes of inheritance have been reported. Studies suggest that pathogenic variations in genes, including paired box protein 6 *(PAX6)*, paired-like homeodomain transcription factor 2 *(PITX2)*, and forkhead box C1 *(FOXC1)*, can cause anterior segment dysgenesis, including the heritable form of Peters anomaly.

In the mildest form of this condition, only the cornea is involved, with a characteristic localized central or paracentral defect of the endothelium and Descemet membrane, known as *internal ulcer of von Hippel*. At the edges of the defect, iris strands typically adhere to the posterior corneal surface. In the most severe form of Peters anomaly, the lens adheres to the posterior corneal surface. The anterior chamber angle may be malformed, predisposing the eye to congenital glaucoma. Associated findings can include *sclerocornea*, which is characterized by peripheral corneal stromal opacification and vascularization, and *cornea plana*, in which the curvature of the cornea is flattened (Fig 5-2). In vivo confocal microscopy or anterior segment optical coherence tomography (AS-OCT) can be used to distinguish the structures affected, aiding in surgical planning. See BCSC Section 8, *External Disease and Cornea*, and Section 6, *Pediatric Ophthalmology and Strabismus*.

> Takamiya M, Stegmaier J, Kobitski AY, et al. *PAX6 organizes the anterior eye segment by guiding two distinct neural crest waves. PLoS Genet.* 2020;16(6):e1008774. doi:10.1371/journal.pgen.1008774

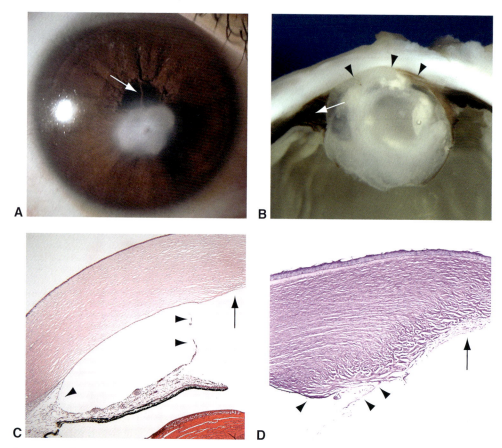

Figure 5-2 Peters anomaly. **A,** Clinical photograph. Note the central corneal opacity (leukoma) with attached iris strands *(arrow)*. The lens is uninvolved. **B,** Gross photograph of a more severe form of Peters anomaly demonstrates attachment of a cataractous lens to the opacified cornea (adherent leukoma) *(arrowheads)*. Note the accompanying peripheral flattening of the corneal curvature (cornea plana) and opacification (sclerocornea). The iris and anterior chamber angle *(arrow)* structures are malformed. **C,** Low-magnification photomicrograph demonstrates internal ulcer of von Hippel *(arrow)* with attached iris strands *(double arrowhead)*. Incomplete cleavage of the anterior chamber angle structures (fetal angle deformity) is also present *(single arrowhead)*. **D,** PAS stain highlights peripheral Descemet membrane *(single arrowhead)*. The central cornea is fibrotic and demonstrates absence of posterior stroma and Descemet membrane *(arrow)*. A fibrotic iris strand *(double arrowhead)* is attached to the edge of the corneal defect. *(Courtesy of Tatyana Milman, MD.)*

Inflammation

Infectious Keratitis

Infectious processes caused by a number of microbial agents may result in inflammation of the cornea. Severe inflammation can lead to corneal necrosis, ulceration, and perforation. See the Corneal Infections Interactive Case Study in the online *Pathology Atlas*.

Bacterial infections

Bacterial infections of the cornea often follow a disruption in corneal epithelial integrity resulting from contact lens wear, trauma, alteration in immunologic defenses (eg, use of topical or systemic immunosuppressive agents), preexisting corneal disease (eg, dry eye disease, exposure keratopathy), and ocular medication toxicity. Bacterial organisms commonly involved in corneal infections include *Pseudomonas aeruginosa, Staphylococcus aureus,* and *Streptococcus pneumoniae,* as well as members of the family Enterobacteriaceae.

Scrapings from infected corneas show collections of neutrophils admixed with necrotic debris. Gram stain may demonstrate the presence of microorganisms (Fig 5-3). A culture is helpful for accurate identification of specific organisms and assessment of antibiotic sensitivities.

Herpes simplex virus keratitis

Herpes simplex virus (HSV) keratitis is usually a self-limited corneal epithelial infection, but it can also be recurrent or chronic. It is particularly prevalent in the pediatric population. HSV epithelial keratitis is characterized by a shallow ulceration that exhibits a linear arborizing pattern with swelling of the epithelial cells, known as a *dendrite* (Fig 5-4A).

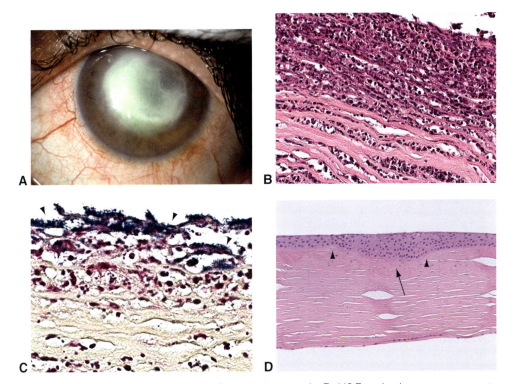

Figure 5-3 Bacterial corneal ulcer. **A,** Clinical photograph. **B,** H&E stain demonstrates acute necrotizing ulcerative keratitis, with necrosis and numerous neutrophils infiltrating the corneal stromal lamellae. **C,** Gram stain shows numerous blue gram-positive cocci *(arrowheads)*. **D,** Keratoplasty specimen shows a scar from healed keratitis. Note the loss of Bowman layer *(between arrowheads)*, stromal thinning with fibrosis *(arrow)*, and compensatory epithelial thickening. *(Part A courtesy of Andrew J. W. Huang, MD; parts B and C courtesy of Tatyana Milman, MD; part D courtesy of George J. Harocopos, MD.)*

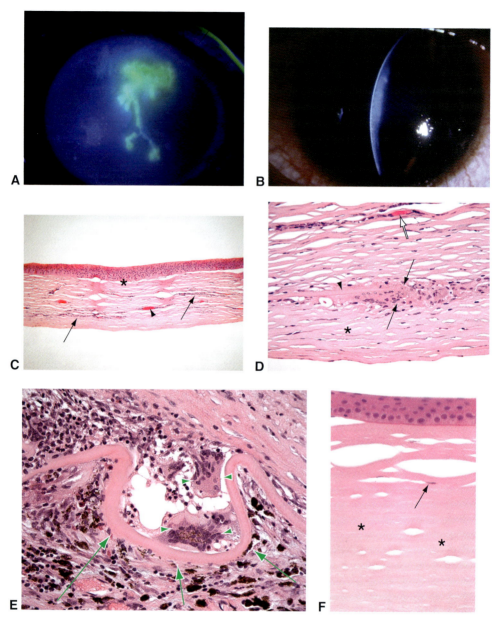

Figure 5-4 Herpes simplex virus keratitis. Clinical photographs depict dendritic **(A)** and stromal (disciform) **(B)** keratitis. Note the central stromal haze and thickening in B. **C,** Histology of a corneal button illustrates stromal keratitis with loss of Bowman layer *(asterisk),* stromal scarring and vascularization *(arrowhead),* and scattered chronic inflammatory cells *(arrows).* **D,** Higher-magnification photomicrograph shows a granulomatous reaction *(area between arrows)* in the region of Descemet membrane *(arrowhead).* Note the fibrous retrocorneal membrane *(asterisk),* scattered chronic inflammatory cells, and blood vessel *(open arrow).* **E,** Multinucleated giant cell *(arrowheads)* located just anterior to Descemet membrane *(arrows).* **F,** Postherpetic neurotrophic keratopathy shows corneal stroma with extensive loss of keratocytes *(asterisks).* There are few residual keratocytes *(arrow).* *(Parts A and B courtesy of Anthony J. Lubniewski, MD; parts C and D courtesy of Tatyana Milman, MD; part E courtesy of Ralph C. Eagle Jr, MD; part F courtesy of Robert H. Rosa Jr, MD.)*

Dendrites are caused by viral reactivation in the corneal nerves and subsequent infection of the epithelial cells. Corneal scrapings obtained from a dendrite and prepared using Giemsa or hematoxylin and eosin (H&E) stain may reveal intranuclear viral inclusions. Viral culture and, especially, polymerase chain reaction (PCR) techniques may be useful for diagnostic confirmation.

Like the dendritic ulcer, a geographic ulcer is caused by replicating virus, but it has a much larger epithelial defect, similar in appearance to a map. Metaherpetic (trophic) ulcer is the only form of epithelial ulceration that does not contain any live virus. These ulcers result from the inability of the epithelium to heal. Stromal and/or disciform keratitis (Fig 5-4B), which may accompany or follow an epithelial infection, is an immune-mediated response directed against viral antigens; active replicating virus may or may not be present in eyes with this condition. Histologically, chronic inflammatory cells and blood vessels may be visible tracking between stromal lamellae, a phenomenon known as *interstitial keratitis (IK)* (Fig 5-4C), which is discussed later in this chapter. In some cases, stromal keratitis may cause significant necrosis, resulting in stromal thinning and even full-thickness perforation. Endotheliitis may also occur, with a granulomatous reaction at the level of Descemet membrane (Fig 5-4D, E). Postherpetic neurotrophic keratopathy may result from corneal hypoesthesia or anesthesia and is characterized histologically by marked loss of stromal keratocytes (Fig 5-4F).

Fungal keratitis

Fungal (mycotic) keratitis is often a complication associated with trauma, especially trauma involving plant or vegetable matter or microtrauma related to contact lens wear. Corticosteroid use, especially topical, is another major risk factor. Unlike most bacteria, some fungi can penetrate the cornea and invade through Descemet membrane into the anterior chamber. The most common organisms in fungal keratitis are the septate, filamentous fungi *Aspergillus* and *Fusarium* and the yeast *Candida*. Cultures, particularly those using Sabouraud agar, are helpful for accurate identification of specific fungi and assessment of antifungal sensitivities. When cultures are negative and the identity of the organism remains elusive, corneal biopsy may be considered. Histologic evaluation can demonstrate the presence of fungal microorganisms with the use of special stains such as Gomori/Grocott methenamine silver (GMS) (Fig 5-5) or PAS. Identification of the exact fungal species solely on the basis of histology is often difficult and is not recommended.

Acanthamoeba *keratitis*

Acanthamoeba protozoa most commonly cause infection in soft contact lens wearers who do not take appropriate precautions in cleaning and disinfecting their lenses or in those whose lenses come into contact with contaminated stagnant water (eg, as found in hot tubs or ponds) or even tap water, which may harbor *Acanthamoeba* in small numbers. Patients presenting with *Acanthamoeba* keratitis usually have severe eye pain caused by radial keratoneuritis. In the late stages of the disease, a corneal ring infiltrate may be present (Fig 5-6A). Special culture techniques and media, including nonnutrient blood agar layered with *Escherichia coli,* are required to grow *Acanthamoeba* but are not widely available. Because the microorganisms can penetrate the deeper layers of the stroma, superficial scrapings may not enable a histologic diagnosis. PCR-based methods for diagnosis

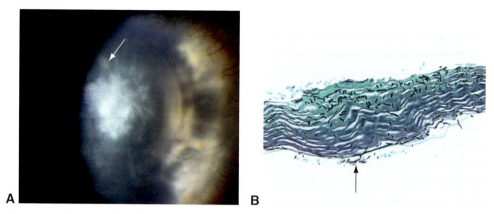

Figure 5-5 *Fusarium* keratitis. **A,** Clinical photograph shows gray-white stromal infiltrate with feathery margins and satellite lesions *(arrow)*. **B,** Grocott methenamine silver (GMS) stain of a corneal button demonstrates frequent fungal hyphae *(black)*. Note that fungal hyphae have penetrated through Descemet membrane *(arrow)*. *(Part A courtesy of Andrew J. W. Huang, MD; part B courtesy of George J. Harocopos, MD.)*

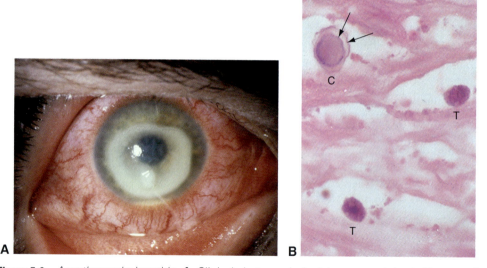

Figure 5-6 *Acanthamoeba* keratitis. **A,** Clinical photograph depicts a corneal ring infiltrate and a small hypopyon. **B,** H&E stain reveals stromal organisms. Note the cyst (C) and trophozoite (T) forms. The cyst has a double wall (ie, endocyst and exocyst) *(arrows)*. *(Part A courtesy of Sander Dubovy, MD.)*

of *Acanthamoeba* keratitis are becoming more widely used. Histologically, corneal epithelial scrapings, biopsy specimens, or corneal buttons may show cysts and trophozoites (Fig 5-6B). The organisms are generally visualized with routine H&E sections but may also be highlighted with PAS and GMS stains. Calcofluor white or acridine orange fluorescent stains may also be used.

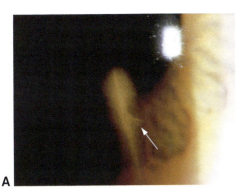 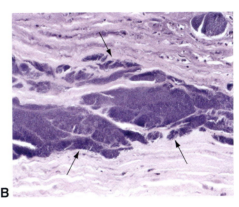

Figure 5-7 Infectious crystalline keratopathy. **A,** Clinical photograph depicts crystalline-appearing, feathery stromal infiltrate *(arrow)*, with intact overlying epithelium. The infection arose along a suture track following repair of a corneal laceration. **B,** Histopathology demonstrates sequestrations of bacteria interposed between stromal collagen lamellae *(arrows)* without an appreciable inflammatory response. *(Part A courtesy of Anthony J. Lubniewski, MD; part B courtesy of Morton E. Smith, MD.)*

Infectious crystalline keratopathy

Infectious crystalline keratopathy (ICK) typically occurs in patients who are on long-term topical corticosteroid therapy, for example, following penetrating keratoplasty (PK). The infection often arises along a suture track or a surgical wound. The most common etiologic microorganism is *Streptococcus viridans* (α-hemolytic strep), but many other causative organisms have been reported, including bacteria, mycobacteria, and fungi. It is thought that in an individual with chronic immunosuppression, growth of the causative organism may be promoted by the properties of the organism's glycocalyx (a glycoprotein and glycolipid covering that surrounds the cell membranes of some bacteria), which can sequester the organism from the suppressed immune system. Despite the name, no true crystals are involved. Rather, this condition derives its name from the crystalloid, feathery clinical appearance of the opacity (Fig 5-7A).

In many cases, the diagnosis is missed clinically and is made histologically after failure of a corneal graft. Histologically, sequestrations of organisms can be observed within the interlamellar spaces of the stroma (with minimal inflammation). The organisms are often apparent on H&E stain but may also be highlighted with Gram, PAS, GMS, or acid-fast stain, depending on the etiologic agent (Fig 5-7B).

Interstitial keratitis

In *interstitial keratitis (IK)*, nonsuppurative inflammatory cells infiltrate the interlamellar spaces of the corneal stroma, often with vascularization. Typically, the overlying epithelium remains intact. The changes observed in IK are thought to result from an immunologic response to infectious microorganisms or their antigens. Transplacental infection of the fetus by *Treponema pallidum* (congenital syphilis) may cause IK (Fig 5-8A). On histologic examination, chronic syphilis-related (luetic) IK is characterized by the presence

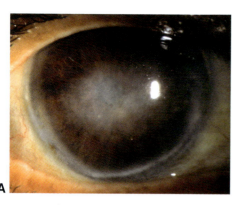 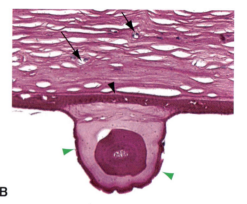

Figure 5-8 Interstitial keratitis caused by congenital syphilis. **A,** Clinical photograph depicts a stromal opacity, with intact overlying epithelium. **B,** PAS stain demonstrates ghost vessels *(arrows)* in the deep stroma, with surrounding fibrosis. Descemet membrane is multilaminated *(black arrowhead)* and demonstrates nodular excrescences *(green arrowheads)*. *(Part A courtesy of Anthony J. Lubniewski, MD; part B courtesy of Tatyana Milman, MD.)*

of stromal ghost vessels devoid of erythrocytes with surrounding stromal fibrosis and a variable degree of chronic inflammation. Bowman layer and Descemet membrane are characteristically intact. In addition, Descemet membrane may demonstrate focal multilaminated excrescences (Fig 5-8B) that are reminiscent of *guttae* observed in eyes with Fuchs endothelial corneal dystrophy (discussed later in this chapter).

Although congenital syphilis represents the "classic" cause of IK, the most common etiologic agent of IK is HSV (see Fig 5-4). Other microorganisms that can cause IK include *Onchocerca volvulus, Mycobacterium tuberculosis, Mycobacterium leprae, Borrelia burgdorferi,* and Epstein-Barr virus.

Noninfectious Keratitis

Corneal inflammation can also result from many noninfectious processes. For example, autoimmune diseases, especially rheumatoid arthritis and graft-vs-host disease, may be associated with sterile corneal ulceration and IK. Topical medication toxicity (eg, as occurs with overuse of topical anesthetics, nonsteroidal anti-inflammatory drugs [NSAIDs], or antiviral drugs) may also result in corneal melting. Histology varies depending on the etiology of the inflammation, but the unifying feature is the absence of organisms.

See also BCSC Section 8, *External Disease and Cornea,* and Section 6, *Pediatric Ophthalmology and Strabismus,* for more discussion of inflammation of the cornea.

Degenerations, Depositions, and Ectasias

Degenerations

Corneal degenerations are secondary changes that occur in previously normal tissue. They are often associated with aging, are not inherited, and are not necessarily bilateral.

Salzmann nodular degeneration

Salzmann nodular degeneration is a slowly progressive degenerative condition of the cornea. Often asymptomatic, it is characterized by the appearance of nodular gray-white to bluish, flat or raised opacities that vary in number and size and are located in the central or paracentral cornea (Fig 5-9A). The condition is usually bilateral, occurring in middle-aged and older individuals, with a female preponderance. It is typically associated with chronic ocular surface inflammation. Although the condition is often idiopathic, underlying causes include (from most to least common)

- meibomian gland dysfunction (MGD)
- exposure keratopathy
- conditions that lead to recurrent erosions
- dry eye disease/keratoconjunctivitis sicca
- contact lens wear (especially hard contact lenses)
- peripheral corneal vascularization
- pterygium
- actinic keratitis
- phlyctenular keratitis, vernal keratoconjunctivitis
- previous IK

Histologic examination reveals nodular, sclerotic subepithelial collagenous tissue and attenuated epithelium. Bowman layer may be disrupted or absent (Fig 5-9B).

Calcific band keratopathy

Calcific band keratopathy presents clinically as a band-shaped calcific plaque in the interpalpebral zone, typically sparing the most peripheral cornea. It is characterized by the deposition of calcium at the level of Bowman layer and anterior stroma. The calcium deposits appear as intensely basophilic (dark purple) granules in H&E-stained sections. The presence of calcium can be further confirmed with the use of special stains such as alizarin red or von Kossa (Fig 5-10).

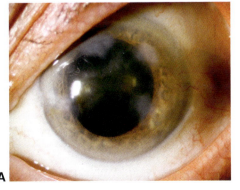
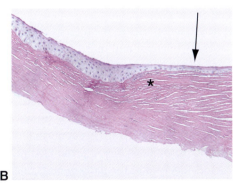

Figure 5-9 Salzmann nodular degeneration. **A,** Clinical photograph demonstrates gray-white to bluish elevated superficial opacities. **B,** Histologic examination of a superficial keratectomy specimen (PAS stain) shows replacement of Bowman layer with disorganized collagenous tissue *(asterisk)* and thinning of the overlying epithelium *(arrow)*. *(Courtesy of George J. Harocopos, MD.)*

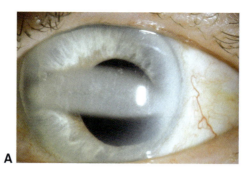
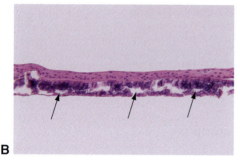
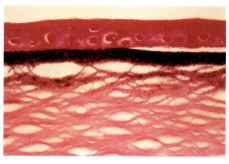

Figure 5-10 Calcific band keratopathy. **A,** Clinical photograph shows a white bandlike opacity extending from 3 o'clock to 9 o'clock, sparing the perilimbal cornea. **B,** The calcium is deposited at the level of Bowman layer *(arrows)*, appearing deeply basophilic *(dark purple)* on H&E stain. **C,** Calcium deposits appear black with von Kossa stain. *(Part A courtesy of Anthony J. Lubniewski, MD; part B courtesy of George J. Harocopos, MD; part C courtesy of Hans E. Grossniklaus, MD.)*

Band keratopathy may develop in chronically inflamed and/or traumatized eyes, following intraocular therapy (eg, intravitreal silicone oil), and, less commonly, in association with systemic hypercalcemic states. The exact pathophysiology is not well understood.

Spheroidal degeneration

Also known as *actinic keratopathy, Labrador keratopathy,* or *climatic droplet keratopathy, spheroidal degeneration* is characterized by aggregates of translucent, golden-brown spheroidal deposits in the interpalpebral superficial cornea (Fig 5-11A). The condition is generally bilateral and more common in males. Smaller spheroidal deposits may mimic calcific band keratopathy, prompting it to be described as "actinic" band keratopathy.

Although the etiology is controversial, cumulative evidence suggests that the deposits may develop from ultraviolet (UV) radiation–induced alteration of preexisting structural connective tissue components or from the synthesis of abnormal extracellular material at the limbal conjunctiva. This abnormal material progressively diffuses into the superficial cornea, precipitates over a prolonged period, and may be further modified by UV light. Factors involved in the pathogenesis of actinic keratopathy include sun exposure and dry climate, as the condition is more prevalent in dry equatorial regions.

Histologic examination reveals irregular, basophilic globules deep to the epithelium in the region of Bowman layer and anterior stroma (Fig 5-11B). Analogous to the actinic degeneration of collagen in pingueculae and pterygia, the deposits stain black with special stains for elastin, such as Verhoeff–van Gieson.

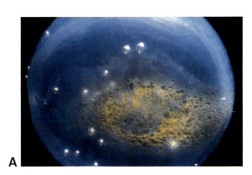
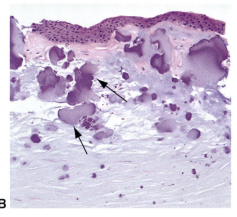

Figure 5-11 Spheroidal degeneration. **A,** Gross appearance of a corneal button shows golden-brown superficial opacities. The air bubbles are artifacts. **B,** Histology shows irregular, pale, basophilic globules *(arrows)* extending from the epithelium into the superficial stroma. *(Part A courtesy of Hans E. Grossniklaus, MD; part B courtesy of Vivian Lee, MD.)*

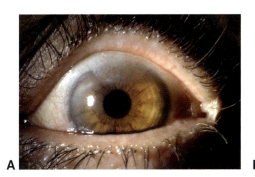
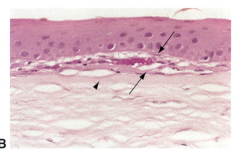

Figure 5-12 Corneal pannus. **A,** Clinical photograph of pannus in the superior cornea. **B,** Fibrovascular degenerative pannus *(area between arrows)* is interposed between the epithelium and an intact Bowman layer *(arrowhead)*. *(Part A courtesy of George J. Harocopos, MD.)*

Pinguecula and pterygium

See Chapter 4 in this volume for discussion of these entities.

Pannus

Pannus refers to the growth of fibrovascular, fibroinflammatory, or fibrous tissue between the corneal epithelium and Bowman layer (Fig 5-12). It is frequently seen in cases of long-term corneal disease. Histologically, the term *inflammatory pannus* is used when Bowman layer is disrupted because inflammation is often required for destruction of this layer. In contrast, the term *degenerative pannus* is used when Bowman layer remains intact under the fibrous or fibrovascular tissue.

Bullous keratopathy

Bullous keratopathy refers to the development of corneal stromal and epithelial edema, leading to irreversible damage. It can occur after cataract surgery (*pseudophakic* or *aphakic bullous keratopathy*) or after other forms of intraocular surgery, as well as endothelial dystrophies such as Fuchs endothelial corneal dystrophy. Bullous keratopathy is the result of widespread endothelial cell loss or dysfunction, causing insufficient endothelial cell function to maintain corneal deturgescence.

Clinically, bullous keratopathy is characterized initially by stromal edema and resulting folds in Descemet membrane, followed by intracellular epithelial edema (hydropic degeneration) and, ultimately, separation of the epithelium from Bowman layer. Small separations called *microcysts* may coalesce to form large separations, known as *bullae*. In advanced cases, secondary epithelial basement membrane changes, loss of stromal keratocytes, and pannus may occur (Fig 5-13).

Corneal graft failure

Corneal graft failure typically results from significant loss of endothelial cells in the grafted donor corneal tissue. It is one of the most common indications for penetrating keratoplasty (PK) or endothelial keratoplasty (EK) (Fig 5-14). Graft failure after PK or EK may occur within a few weeks of surgery (primary graft failure), gradually over time,

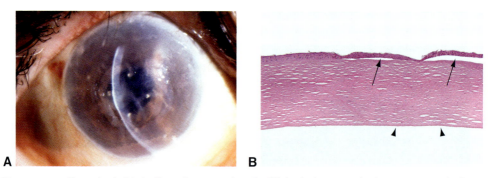

Figure 5-13 Pseudophakic bullous keratopathy. **A,** Clinical photograph shows severe bullous keratopathy associated with an iris clip anterior chamber lens implant. **B,** Corneal button from penetrating keratoplasty (PK). Note the subepithelial bullae *(arrows)*. Also note stromal edema, characterized by focal absence of interlamellar clefts, and diffuse endothelial cell loss without guttae *(arrowheads)*. *(Part A courtesy of Andrew J. W. Huang, MD; part B courtesy of George J. Harocopos, MD.)*

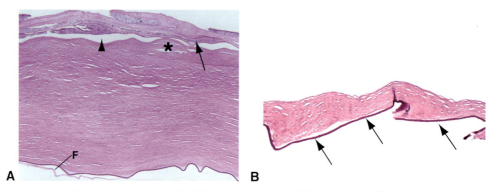

Figure 5-14 Corneal graft failure. **A,** H&E stain of a failed PK graft with diffuse endothelial cell loss, fibrous retrocorneal membrane (F), stromal edema with bullous keratopathy *(arrowhead)* and absence of stromal clefts, epithelial basement membrane thickening *(arrow)*, and focal fibrous pannus *(asterisk)*. **B,** PAS stain of a failed endothelial keratoplasty (EK) donor lenticule. Note the total absence of endothelium *(arrows)*. *(Part A courtesy of George J. Harocopos, MD; part B courtesy of Hans E. Grossniklaus, MD.)*

or following an acute rejection episode. Wound-related complications, such as *fibrous* or *epithelial ingrowth* or *downgrowth,* can also contribute to graft failure and are most common following PK (Fig 5-15). When endothelial failure occurs, bullous keratopathy often develops. For various types of EK, additional important etiologies of graft failure include traumatic intracameral insertion of donor tissue, loss of adherence of the donor lenticule to the posterior stroma, and prolonged presence of the air bubble in the anterior chamber. See also BCSC Section 8, *External Disease and Cornea.*

Depositions

A wide range of deposits may accumulate in the cornea and give rise to focal or diffuse opacities.

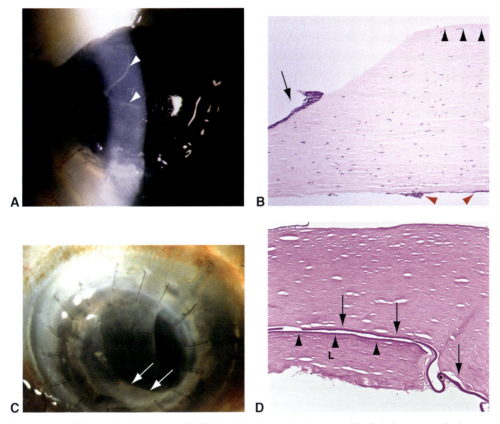

Figure 5-15 Corneal graft failure. **A,** Clinical photograph shows epithelial downgrowth *(arrowheads)* in a PK graft. **B,** Histology of explanted failed EK donor lenticule shows full-thickness cornea with Bowman layer *(black arrowheads)* on the right and partial-thickness cornea on the left indicative of irregular donor cornea trephination. A layer of squamous epithelium is present on the anterior surface of explanted lenticule (epithelial ingrowth) *(arrow)* and on the posterior corneal surface (epithelial downgrowth) *(red arrowheads),* replacing endothelial cells. **C,** Clinical photograph illustrates fibrous downgrowth *(arrows)* in a PK graft. **D,** PAS stain of a failed graft following EK. The donor lenticule is positioned upside down (L) with donor Descemet membrane *(arrowheads)* facing recipient Descemet membrane *(arrows).* Note the loss of corneal endothelium and marked stromal edema in the recipient and donor corneal lenticules. *(Parts A and D courtesy of Tatyana Milman, MD; parts B and C courtesy of Anthony J. Lubniewski, MD.)*

Corneal pigment deposits

Various types of pigment and pigmented chemical compounds can deposit in the corneal epithelium, such as melanin, alkapton (brown color, seen in alkaptonuria), iron, and amiodarone. Amiodarone can result in a clockwise whorl-like pattern of golden-brown or gray deposits in the inferior interpalpebral portion of the cornea, referred to as *cornea verticillata*. Blood staining of the cornea (Fig 5-16A) may complicate a hyphema when intraocular pressure (IOP) is very high for a long duration. However, if the endothelium is compromised, blood staining can occur even at normal or low IOP. Histologically, red blood cell breakdown products (hemoglobin spherules and hemosiderin) are observed in the corneal stroma (Fig 5-16B). Hemosiderin is found in the cytoplasm of keratocytes and may be demonstrated with iron stains such as Perls Prussian blue (Fig 5-16C).

Ectatic Disorders

Keratoectasias (*keratoconus, keratoglobus,* and *pellucid marginal degeneration*) are predominantly sporadic, typically bilateral noninflammatory disorders that share a unifying feature: stromal thinning.

Keratoconus

Keratoconus, which is typically diagnosed during adolescence or young adulthood, is characterized by inferior or inferotemporal corneal stromal ectasia (Fig 5-17A). Although

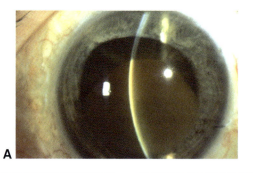

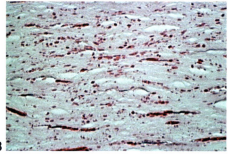
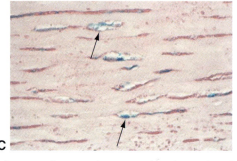

Figure 5-16 Corneal blood staining. **A,** Clinical photograph; note the rust-colored opacity of the central cornea. **B,** Masson trichrome stain. The red particles represent erythrocytic debris and hemoglobin in the corneal stroma. **C,** Perls Prussian blue iron stain (blue staining) demonstrates hemosiderin *(arrows)* within stromal keratocytes. *(Part A courtesy of Anthony J. Lubniewski, MD; parts B and C courtesy of Hans E. Grossniklaus, MD.)*

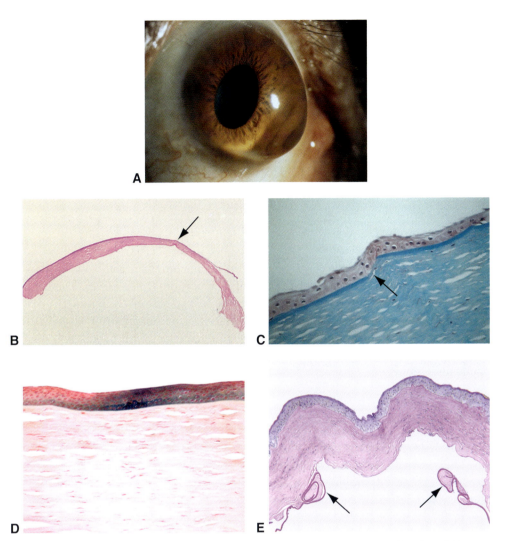

Figure 5-17 Keratoconus. **A,** Clinical photograph shows inferior conical deformity of the cornea. **B,** Low-magnification photomicrograph shows apical stromal thinning *(arrow).* **C,** Masson trichrome stain demonstrates focal disruption of Bowman layer *(arrow).* **D,** Perls Prussian blue stain demonstrates focal intraepithelial iron deposition (Fleischer ring). **E,** In a patient with prior corneal hydrops, PAS stain highlights the rupture of Descemet membrane, with rolled edges on either side *(arrows). (Part A courtesy of Sander Dubovy, MD; part C courtesy of Hans E. Grossniklaus, MD; part D courtesy of Tatyana Milman, MD; part E courtesy of George J. Harocopos, MD.)*

it is frequently sporadic, familial inheritance and association with other ocular and systemic conditions, including atopy, Down syndrome, and Ehlers-Danlos syndrome, have been described. The basic pathophysiologic change is loss of stromal structural integrity, leading to keratoectasia, or stretching and thinning of the corneal stroma.

Histologic findings in keratoconus include central stromal thinning and small focal breaks in Bowman layer. Apical anterior stromal fibrosis is often present (Fig 5-17B, C). Iron deposition in the epithelium at the base of the cone *(Fleischer ring)* can sometimes be demonstrated with Perls Prussian blue stain (Fig 5-17D). In patients with a history of *corneal hydrops,* a focal break in Descemet membrane may be seen (Fig 5-17E).

Alteration in the normal corneal contour produces irregular astigmatism, occasionally requiring DALK. Advanced cases with significant apical scarring are managed with PK. Collagen crosslinking (CXL) using UVA light and topical riboflavin (vitamin B_2) has been used to slow or arrest the progression of the ectasia in keratoconus. Interestingly, crosslinking also occurs in the cornea with age. Histologically, studies have shown that CXL-treated corneas exhibit keratocyte loss, and the remaining keratocytes express surface markers similar to keratocytes in corneal scars. Corneal nerves and endothelial cells appear unaffected by CXL.

> Müller PL, Loeffler KU, Messmer E, et al. Histological corneal alterations in keratoconus after crosslinking—expansion of findings. *Cornea.* 2020;39(3):333–341.

Pellucid marginal degeneration

Pellucid marginal degeneration (PMD) is a rare, bilateral, noninflammatory, ectatic peripheral corneal disorder, usually involving the inferior portion of the cornea. The band of thinning is separated from the limbus by a zone of normal corneal thickness. The cornea protrudes above the thinned area, resulting in high irregular astigmatism. Histologic examination reveals an intact epithelium over the thinned region with microscopic disruptions in Bowman layer similar to those seen in keratoconus. The pathogenesis of PMD is poorly understood.

Dystrophies

Corneal dystrophies are primary, bilateral disorders with an underlying genetic cause. The International Committee for Classification of Corneal Dystrophies (IC3D) categorizes major corneal dystrophies by the predominant corneal layer involved (ie, epithelial, stromal, or endothelial) and underlying genetic alterations. Therefore, the classification system divides major corneal dystrophies into 4 groups:

- epithelial and subepithelial dystrophies
- epithelial–stromal *TGFBI* dystrophies
- stromal dystrophies
- endothelial dystrophies

Although traditional histopathologic methods continue to play an important role in diagnosing corneal dystrophies, clinicians are increasingly relying on ancillary clinical diagnostic modalities, such as confocal microscopy and OCT. These tests offer the clinician information regarding the layers and structures involved, which often guides treatment selection. In addition, molecular genetic studies have started to play a larger role in the categorization of dystrophies by identifying the molecular mechanisms shared by unrelated corneal dystrophies. For example, the discovery of pathogenic variations in the transforming growth factor beta–induced gene *(TGFBI)* in different dystrophies resulted in the classification of these dystrophies under 1 subtype. Studies have also shown that the diverse phenotypes may be caused by different variations in the same gene. Genetic testing for many of these genetic variants are now commercially available and can be performed on peripheral blood.

The following subsections cover only the most common corneal dystrophies. They are described according to a template consisting of clinical, pathologic, and genetic information. See BCSC Section 8, *External Disease and Cornea,* for additional discussion.

See the Corneal Dystrophy Interactive Case Study in the online *Pathology Atlas.*

> Seibelmann S, Scholz P, Sonnenschein S, et al. Anterior segment optical coherence tomography for the diagnosis of corneal dystrophies according to the IC3D classification. *Surv Ophthalmol.* 2018;63(3):355–380.
> Weiss JS, Møller HU, Aldave AJ, et al. IC3D classification of corneal dystrophies—edition 2. *Cornea.* 2015;34(2):117–159.

Epithelial and Subepithelial Dystrophies

Epithelial basement membrane dystrophy

Also called *map-dot-fingerprint dystrophy, epithelial basement membrane dystrophy (EBMD)* is characterized clinically by opacities resembling maps, dots, and fingerprints in the superficial cornea. Focal epithelial basement membrane thickening with deposition of intraepithelial basal laminar material results in large, grayish outlines that look like continents on a map. Intraepithelial pseudocysts containing degenerated epithelial debris appear as dots, while riblike intraepithelial extensions of basal laminar material resemble fingerprints (Fig 5-18). EBMD results in focally impaired adhesion of the epithelial basement membrane to Bowman layer. As a result, patients may experience recurrent epithelial erosions. Management includes superficial and/or phototherapeutic keratectomy and is described in BCSC Section 8, *External Disease and Cornea.*

Clinical Pearl The epithelial changes associated with EBMD are essentially identical to those observed in the epithelium in cases of chronic corneal edema secondary to endothelial decompensation.

Epithelial–Stromal *TGFBI* Dystrophies

Pathogenic variations in the *TGFBI* gene, located at 5q31, result in the most common corneal dystrophies involving both the epithelium and stroma. *TGFBI* encodes for *keratoepithelin,* a protein produced predominantly by the corneal epithelium. These dystrophies, which arise in the epithelium with secondary involvement of the stroma, are inherited in an autosomal dominant fashion.

Reis-Bücklers corneal dystrophy

Reis-Bücklers corneal dystrophy (*RBCD;* formerly known as *corneal dystrophy of Bowman layer type I*) is characterized by confluent irregular, coarse, and angulated geographic-like opacities with varying densities at the level of Bowman layer and superficial stroma (Fig 5-19A). OCT demonstrates a homogeneous, confluent layer of hyperreflective deposits, often with a serrated anterior border, at the level of Bowman layer and anterior stroma.

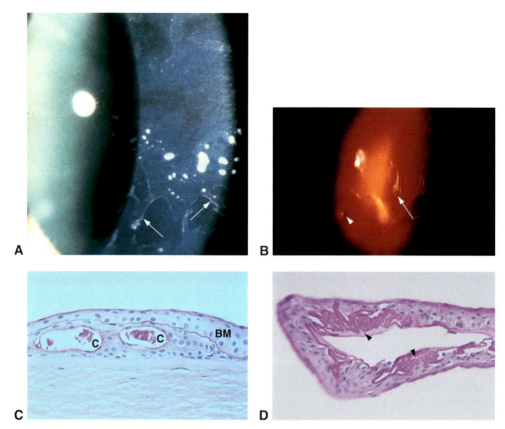

Figure 5-18 Epithelial basement membrane dystrophy (EBMD). **A,** Clinical photograph shows fine, lacy opacities *(arrows)*. **B,** Retroillumination demonstrates wavy lines *(arrow)* and dotlike lesions *(arrowhead)*. **C,** The intraepithelial basement membrane (BM) is highlighted with PAS stain; degenerating epithelial cells are trapped within cystoid spaces (C). **D,** When surgical treatment is required for EBMD, removal of abnormal epithelium (via superficial keratectomy) may be performed, as it was in this case. PAS stain highlights irregular, wavy thickening *(arrowheads)* of the epithelial basement membrane. The changes in primary EBMD are essentially identical to those observed in the epithelium in cases of chronic corneal edema secondary to endothelial decompensation. *(Part A courtesy of Andrew J. W. Huang, MD; part D courtesy of George J. Harocopos, MD.)*

Histologically, Bowman layer is replaced by a multilayered pannus comprising material that stains intensely red with Masson trichrome stain (Fig 5-19B) and immunoreacts with anti-TGFBI antibodies. The thickness of the overlying epithelium is irregular. Ultrastructural studies show crystalloids that stain deeply black with osmium tetroxide, resembling those in granular corneal dystrophy.

Thiel-Behnke corneal dystrophy

Thiel-Behnke corneal dystrophy (TBCD; formerly known as *corneal dystrophy of Bowman layer type II)* manifests clinically as solitary flecks or irregularly shaped, scattered opacities at the level of Bowman layer that progress to symmetric subepithelial honeycomb-shaped opacities (Fig 5-20A). OCT demonstrates prominent hyperreflective material at the level of Bowman layer that extends into the epithelium in a characteristic sawtooth

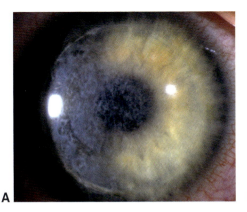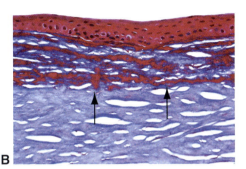

Figure 5-19 Reis-Bücklers corneal dystrophy. **A,** Clinical photograph shows coarse opacities resembling a geographic map in the superficial cornea. Note the circumferential linear scar in the peripheral cornea associated with a lamellar graft, in this case of recurrent corneal dystrophy. **B,** Masson trichrome stain demonstrates diffuse loss of Bowman layer, superficial stromal fibrosis, and numerous red deposits *(arrows)*. *(Part A courtesy of Brandon Ayres, MD; part B courtesy of Tatyana Milman, MD.)*

pattern (Fig 5-20B). Histologic evaluation shows diffuse replacement of Bowman layer by a fibrous pannus that stains variably with Masson trichrome and the sawtooth pattern observed with OCT (Fig 5-20C). Ultrastructurally, the abnormal material in TBCD is composed of curly collagen fibers that are distinctly different from the rod-shaped deposits in RBCD.

Lattice corneal dystrophy type 1

Classic *lattice corneal dystrophy (LCD)*, or *LCD type 1 (LCD1)*, is a stromal dystrophy characterized by branching, refractile (lattice) lines in the central corneal stroma (Fig 5-21A), as well as intervening stromal haze in the later stages of disease. Histologic examination reveals poorly demarcated, fusiform amyloid deposits, most conspicuously in the anterior stroma and Bowman layer (Fig 5-21B). These deposits stain red orange with Congo red stain on standard light microscopy; under polarized light, they exhibit apple-green birefringence and dichroism (ie, 2 different colors that change with the angle of the light) (Fig 5-21C, D).

Granular corneal dystrophy type 1

Granular corneal dystrophy type 1 (GCD1) is a disorder characterized by sharply demarcated (granular) central corneal stromal deposits separated by clear intervening stroma (Fig 5-22A). Histologically, irregularly shaped, well-circumscribed, crumblike deposits of hyaline material, which stain bright red with Masson trichrome, are visible in the stroma (Fig 5-22B,C).

Granular corneal dystrophy type 2

Formerly known as *Avellino corneal dystrophy,* GCD type 2 (GCD2) demonstrates clinical, histologic, and ultrastructural features of both GCD1 and LCD1 (Fig 5-23).

> Nielsen NS, Poulsen ET, Lukassen MV, et al. Biochemical mechanisms of aggregation in *TGFBI*-linked corneal dystrophies. *Prog Retin Eye Res.* 2020;77:100843.

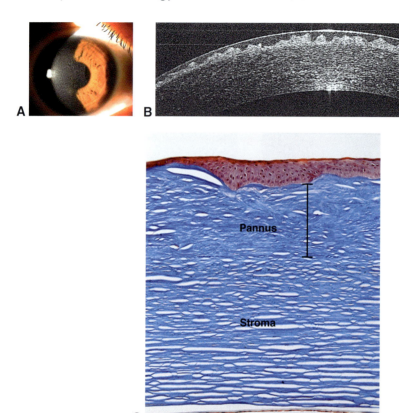

Figure 5-20 Thiel-Behnke corneal dystrophy. **A,** Anterior segment photo demonstrates subepithelial reticular (honeycomb) opacities. **B,** Anterior segment optical coherence tomography (AS-OCT) imaging reveals hyperreflective material *(arrow)* in a sawtooth pattern at Bowman layer. **C,** Masson trichrome stain demonstrates diffuse replacement of Bowman layer by a thick fibrous pannus *(bracket)*. The overlying epithelium exhibits a sawtooth configuration. The underlying stroma appears to be uninvolved. *(Parts A and B reproduced with permission from Vajzovic LM, Karp CL, Haft P, et al. Ultra high–resolution anterior segment optical coherence tomography in the evaluation of anterior corneal dystrophies and degenerations.* Ophthalmology. *2011;118(7):1291–1296. Part C courtesy of Tero Kivelä, MD.)*

Stromal Dystrophies

Macular corneal dystrophy

Macular corneal dystrophy (MCD), an autosomal recessive corneal stromal dystrophy, is caused by variations in the carbohydrate sulfotransferase 6 gene *(CHST6)*, located at 16q22. This dystrophy is characterized by diffuse stromal haze that extends from limbus to limbus and is associated with poorly demarcated focal opacities (macules) (Fig 5-24A). Histologically, H&E staining reveals subtle eosinophilic stromal deposits. Alcian blue and colloidal iron stains highlight nonsulfated glycosaminoglycan deposits, which accumulate intracellularly in the stromal keratocytes, endothelium, and extracellularly in the stroma (Fig 5-24B,C). Pathologic changes in the endothelium are frequently accompanied by guttae in Descemet membrane (Fig 5-24D). Table 5-1 compares the histologic characteristics of select corneal dystrophies.

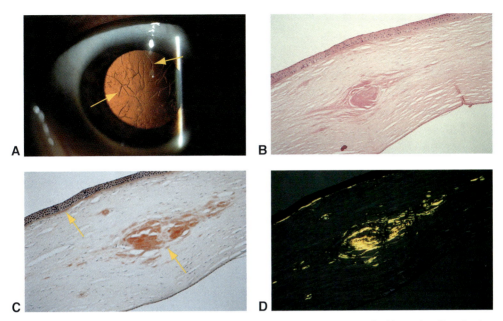

Figure 5-21 Lattice corneal dystrophy type 1. **A,** Clinical photograph. Note the fine lattice lines *(arrows)*. **B,** H&E stain shows scattered fusiform, eosinophilic deposits in the anterior and midstroma. **C,** Congo red stain (red orange) highlights fusiform stromal amyloid deposits and subepithelial deposits *(arrows)*. **D,** With Congo red stain, under polarized light, amyloid deposits exhibit apple-green birefringence and dichroism. *(Parts B–D courtesy of Hans E. Grossniklaus, MD.)*

Aggarwal S, Peck T, Golen J, Karcioglu ZA. Macular corneal dystrophy: a review. *Surv Ophthalmol*. 2018;63(5):609–717.

Descemet Membrane and Endothelial Dystrophies

Fuchs endothelial corneal dystrophy

Although *Fuchs endothelial corneal dystrophy (FECD)* can be inherited in an autosomal dominant fashion, the mode of inheritance is unknown in most cases. In the early stages of FECD, guttae, which are anvil-shaped or droplike excrescences (*guttae* is the Latin word for *drops*), are present along Descemet membrane (Fig 5-25A). When confluent, they give the appearance of "beaten metal" clinically. In some cases, progressive endothelial cell loss occurs over time, ultimately resulting in visually significant corneal edema and bullous keratopathy, typically in middle-aged and older individuals. Consequently, FECD is a leading cause of bullous keratopathy (discussed earlier in this chapter). Endothelial cell loss and irregular thickening of Descemet membrane are the major histologic features of FECD. The irregularly thickened Descemet membrane is studded with guttae, which may protrude into the anterior chamber or may be buried within a new layer of basement membrane (Fig 5-25B,C). The epithelium demonstrates changes identical to those of bullous keratopathy resulting from degenerative causes. Ultrastructural studies reveal

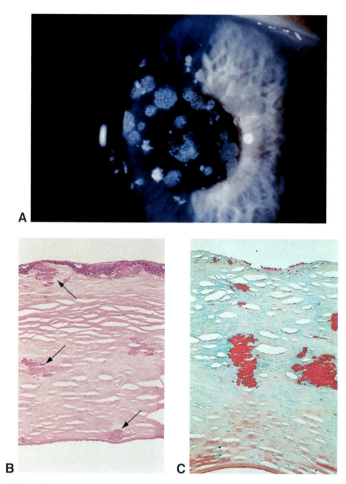

Figure 5-22 Granular corneal dystrophy type 1. **A,** Clinical photograph. Note the well-demarcated stromal opacities with clear intervening stroma. **B,** H&E stain reveals eosinophilic deposits *(arrows)* at all levels of the corneal stroma. **C,** Masson trichrome stain. The stromal collagen stains blue, and the granular hyaline deposits stain brilliant red.

the presence of new wide-spaced collagen, made of collagen type VIII, in the pathologic, posterior collagenous layer of Descemet membrane and in the guttae. Treatment is surgical, with either PK or, more commonly, EK.

Congenital hereditary endothelial dystrophy

Congenital hereditary endothelial dystrophy (CHED) was traditionally classified as either autosomal dominant (CHED1) or autosomal recessive (CHED2). The updated IC3D classification eliminated CHED1; evidence suggests that this entity is part of the posterior polymorphous corneal dystrophy spectrum (see the following section). CHED2, in which a variant in the solute carrier family 4, sodium borate transporter, member 11 (*SLC4A11*) gene, located at 20p13, has been implicated, is now known simply as CHED.

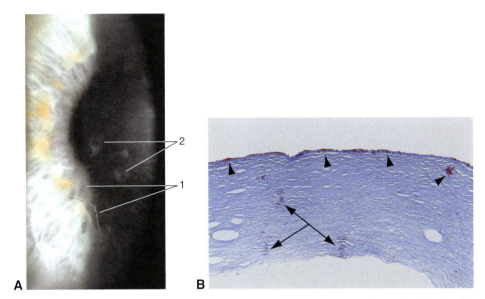

Figure 5-23 Granular corneal dystrophy type 2. **A,** Clinical photograph shows both lattice lines (1) and granular deposits (2). **B,** Masson trichrome stain of deep anterior lamellar keratoplasty (DALK) button highlights hyaline deposits at the level of Bowman layer and the anterior stroma *(arrowheads).* Other deposits at various levels of the stroma stain a darker blue than the stromal background *(triple arrow);* Congo red stain (not shown) confirmed that these deposits were amyloid. The large empty spaces in the posterior stroma were caused by pneumatic dissection. *(Part A modified with permission from Krachmer JH, Palay DA. Cornea Atlas. 2nd ed. Mosby-Elsevier; 2006:163. Part B courtesy of George J. Harocopos, MD.)*

CHED presents early in life with diffuse or ground-glass, milky, and frequently asymmetric corneal clouding associated with marked corneal thickening (Fig 5-26A). The primary abnormality in CHED is thought to be a degeneration of endothelial cells during or after the fifth month of gestation. Histologically, Descemet membrane is diffusely thickened and occasionally multilaminated and there is marked loss of endothelial cells (Fig 5-26B).

Posterior polymorphous corneal dystrophy

Posterior polymorphous corneal dystrophy (PPCD) is an autosomal dominant dystrophy that typically manifests early in life, frequently with asymmetric opacities of various shapes at the level of Descemet membrane, including nummular, vesicular (blisterlike), and "railroad track"–like lesions (Fig 5-27A). The condition can be progressive and may be associated with corneal edema, peripheral iridocorneal adhesions, and IOP elevation. Histologically, although the corneal endothelium is generally atrophic, overlapping or multilayered aggregates of endothelial cells with spindle morphology may be present focally (Fig 5-27B). These transformed endothelial cells demonstrate immunophenotypic and ultrastructural features of epithelial cells (ie, epithelialization of the endothelium) with aberrant expression of cytokeratins (CKs) such as CK19, CK5/6, and CK903.

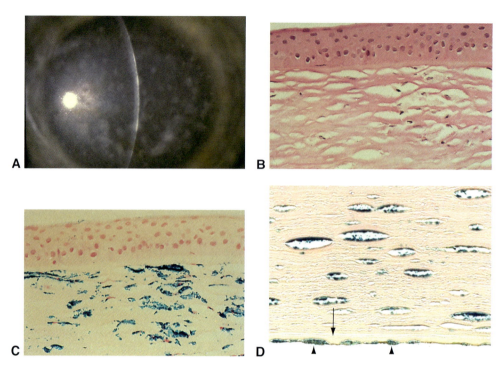

Figure 5-24 Macular corneal dystrophy. **A,** Clinical photograph shows a diffuse limbus-to-limbus corneal haze with scattered dense opacities. **B,** H&E stain demonstrates pale pink, fluffy material within the keratocytes and extracellularly in the stroma. **C,** Colloidal iron stain reveals mucopolysaccharides (nonsulfated glycosaminoglycans) in the keratocytes and stroma. **D,** Colloidal iron stain highlights mucopolysaccharides in the corneal endothelium *(arrowheads)*. Note the Descemet membrane excrescences, or guttae *(arrow)*. *(Part D courtesy of Tatyana Milman, MD.)*

Table 5-1 Histologic Differentiation of Select Anterior Corneal Dystrophies

Dystrophy	Deposit	Stain	Gene involved
Granular, type 1	Hyaline	Masson trichrome (+ in deposits)	*TGBI*[a]
Granular, type 2 (Avellino)	Hyaline and amyloid	Congo red (+ with dichroism) Masson trichrome (+ in deposits) PAS (weakly + in deposits)	*TGBI*[a]
Lattice, type 1	Amyloid	Congo red (+ with dichroism) PAS (weakly + in deposits)	*TGBI*[a]
Macular	Nonsulfated glycosaminoglycan	Alcian blue (+ in deposits) PAS (weakly + in deposits)	*CHST6*
Reis-Bücklers	Hyaline Crystalloid deposits on EM	Masson trichrome (+ in deposits)	*TGBI*[a]
Thiel-Behnke	Curly collagen fibers on EM	Masson trichrome (−/+ in deposits)	*TGBI*[a]

Key: + = positive; − = negative.
EM = electron microscopy.
[a] Differences in clinical presentation are due to different mutations in the same gene.

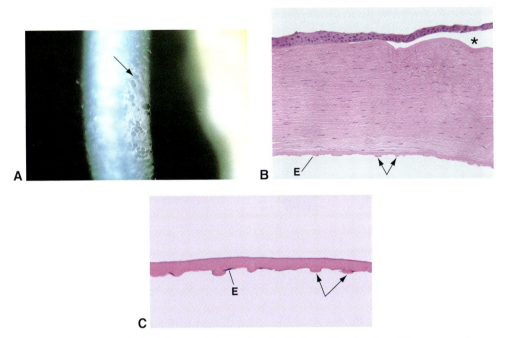

Figure 5-25 Fuchs endothelial corneal dystrophy. **A,** Slit-lamp illumination of the cornea shows the "beaten metal" appearance of Descemet membrane *(arrow)*. **B,** Corneal button from PK shows endothelial cell loss, with only a few surviving endothelial cells (E). Numerous guttae are seen in Descemet membrane *(arrows)*. The result of endothelial decompensation is bullous keratopathy. Note the diffuse stromal edema (loss of interlamellar clefts) and epithelial bulla *(asterisk)*. **C,** Stripped Descemet membrane from EK shows scant endothelial cells (E) and numerous guttae *(arrows)*. *(Part A reproduced from* External Disease and Cornea: A Multimedia Collection. *American Academy of Ophthalmology; 2000. Parts B and C courtesy of George J. Harocopos, MD.)*

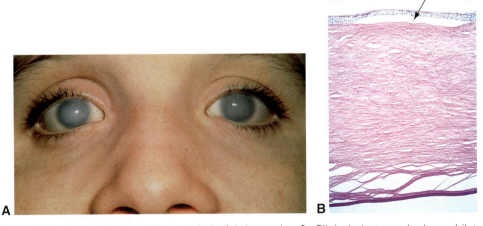

Figure 5-26 Congenital hereditary endothelial dystrophy. **A,** Clinical photograph shows bilateral diffuse, severe corneal clouding. **B,** PAS stain reveals diffuse stromal edema with bullous keratopathy *(arrow)*. Descemet membrane is diffusely thickened, without guttae, and endothelial cells are absent. *(Courtesy of Hans E. Grossniklaus, MD.)*

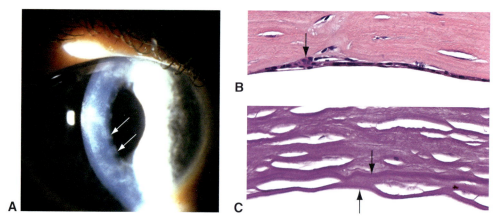

Figure 5-27 Posterior polymorphous corneal dystrophy. **A,** Clinical photograph shows nummular opacities *(arrows)* and linear opacities on the endothelial surface. **B,** Histology image shows overlapping and multilayered aggregates of endothelial cells *(arrow).* **C,** PAS stain highlights multilaminated Descemet membrane *(arrows).* In this region, corneal endothelium is severely atrophic. *(Part A courtesy of Andrew J. W. Huang, MD; parts B and C courtesy of Tatyana Milman, MD.)*

Descemet membrane is thickened and multilaminated with focal nodular and fusiform excrescences (Fig 5-27C).

> Malhotra D, Casey JR. Molecular mechanisms of Fuchs and congenital hereditary endothelial corneal dystrophies. *Rev Physiol Biochem Pharmacol.* 2020;178:41–81.

Neoplasia

Ocular surface squamous neoplasia, melanocytic neoplasms, and sebaceous carcinoma may extend from adjacent structures to involve the cornea. In rare cases, squamous neoplasia may arise primarily in the corneal epithelium. See Chapters 4 and 12 for more information on this topic.

See BCSC Section 8, *External Disease and Cornea,* for additional discussion of the topics in this chapter.

CHAPTER 6

Anterior Chamber and Trabecular Meshwork

 This chapter includes a related activity. Go to aao.org/bcscactivity_section04 or scan the QR code in the text to access this content.

Highlights

- Gonioscopic landmarks of the anterior chamber angle correspond to histologically identifiable structures.
- The term *anterior segment dysgenesis* refers to a spectrum of developmental anomalies.
- Pseudoexfoliation syndrome is a systemic fibrillopathy, the features of which are manifested clinically and histologically in the eye.
- Pigment dispersion may be a primary process, or it may be secondary to inflammation or neoplasia.

Topography

The anterior chamber is bounded anteriorly by the corneal endothelium; posteriorly by the anterior surface of the iris, ciliary body, and pupillary portion of the lens; and peripherally by the trabecular meshwork (Fig 6-1, Activity 6-1). The normal central depth of the anterior chamber is approximately 3.0–3.5 mm. The trabecular meshwork is derived predominantly from the neural crest.

 ACTIVITY 6-1 Anatomy of the anterior chamber and angle. *Courtesy of Amanda C. Maltry, MD.* Available at: aao.org/bcscactivity_section04

The histologic features of the anterior chamber angle correlate with its gonioscopic landmarks (Fig 6-2). For example, the termination of Descemet membrane manifests gonioscopically as the Schwalbe line. The scleral spur, a triangular extension of the sclera that appears gonioscopically as a white band, can be identified histologically by tracing the outermost longitudinal ciliary muscle fibers to its insertion. Anterior to the scleral spur in an internal indentation of the sclera are the trabecular meshwork and Schlemm canal. On gonioscopy, the posterior trabecular meshwork appears more pigmented than the rest

120 • Ophthalmic Pathology and Intraocular Tumors

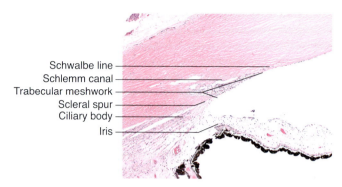

Figure 6-1 The normal anterior chamber angle, the site of drainage for the major portion of the aqueous humor flow, is defined by the anterior border of the iris, the pupillary zone of the anterior lens capsule, the face of the ciliary body, the internal surface of the trabecular meshwork, and the posterior surface of the cornea. *(Courtesy of Amanda C. Maltry, MD.)*

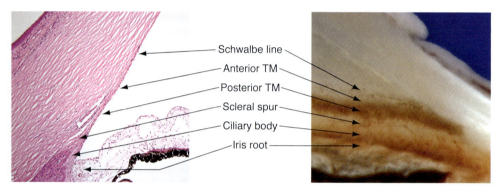

Figure 6-2 Gonioscopic landmarks of a normal anterior chamber angle seen on gross examination *(right)* with histologic correlation *(left)*. TM = trabecular meshwork. *(Courtesy of Tatyana Milman, MD.)*

of the meshwork because of its increased thickness. The meshwork is lined with cells that appear flat and have slender spindle-shaped nuclei known as *trabeculocytes*. These cells phagocytose material from the aqueous humor and have contractile properties.

See BCSC Section 2, *Fundamentals and Principles of Ophthalmology*, which includes additional images and discussion of the structure and physiology of the anterior chamber and trabecular meshwork.

> Abu-Hassan DW, Acott TS, Kelley MJ. The trabecular meshwork: a basic review of form and function. *J Ocul Biol.* 2014;2(1):9. doi:10.13188/2334-2838.1000017

Developmental Anomalies

Primary Congenital Glaucoma

Primary congenital glaucoma (PCG) can be evident at birth or become evident within the first few years of life. The pathogenesis of PCG is likely related to arrested development of

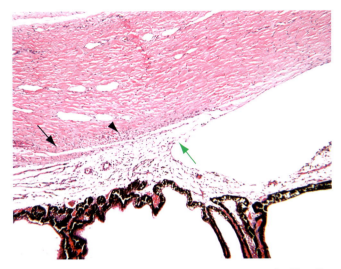

Figure 6-3 Primary congenital glaucoma. This histologic example of a "fetal" anterior chamber angle demonstrates the anterior insertion of the iris root *(green arrow)*, the anteriorly displaced ciliary processes, and a poorly developed scleral spur *(black arrow)* and trabecular meshwork *(arrowhead)*. *(Courtesy of Tatyana Milman, MD.)*

the anterior chamber angle structures. Histologically, the anterior chamber angle retains an "embryonic" or "fetal" conformation, characterized by the following:

- anterior insertion of the iris root
- mesenchymal tissue in the anterior chamber angle
- poorly developed scleral spur, allowing the ciliary muscle to insert directly into the trabecular meshwork (Fig 6-3)

See BCSC Section 6, *Pediatric Ophthalmology and Strabismus,* and Section 10, *Glaucoma,* for further discussion of PCG.

Anterior Segment Dysgenesis

The term *anterior segment dysgenesis* refers to a spectrum of developmental anomalies resulting from abnormalities of neural crest cell migration and differentiation during embryologic development (eg, Axenfeld-Rieger syndrome, Peters anomaly, posterior keratoconus, and iridoschisis). Maldevelopment of the anterior chamber angle is most prominent in *Axenfeld-Rieger syndrome,* most commonly an autosomal dominant disorder, which itself encompasses a spectrum of anomalies, ranging from isolated bilateral ocular defects to a fully manifested systemic disorder.

Ocular manifestations of Axenfeld-Rieger syndrome include posterior embryotoxon (Fig 6-4), iris strands attached to the Schwalbe line, iris hypoplasia and atrophy, corectopia and pseudopolycoria, a maldeveloped or "fetal" anterior chamber angle (discussed in the previous section), and glaucoma in 50% of cases occurring in late childhood or adulthood (Fig 6-5). Posterior embryotoxon is often described as a thickening of Descemet membrane at its termination (Schwalbe line), but it is, in fact, a nodular thickening of

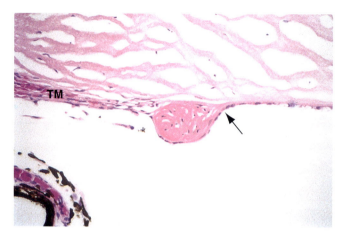

Figure 6-4 Posterior embryotoxon. Light micrograph reveals a nodular, collagenous prominence under the termination of Descemet membrane *(arrow)*. TM = trabecular meshwork. *(Courtesy of Hans E. Grossniklaus, MD.)*

the collagen just under the terminal portion of Descemet membrane. See Chapter 5 for discussion of Peters anomaly. See also BCSC Section 8, *External Disease and Cornea*, for discussion of anterior segment dysgenesis.

Seifi M, Walter MA. Axenfeld-Rieger syndrome. *Clin Genet*. 2018;93(6):1123–1130.

Inflammation

Inflammation in the anterior chamber and angle is typically secondary to inflammation in adjacent structures (Fig 6-6) from infectious (eg, herpesvirus) etiologies or noninfectious (trauma, anterior uveitis) etiologies. Inflammation in the angle structures can result in elevation of intraocular pressure due to obstruction of aqueous outflow. See also BCSC Section 9, *Uveitis and Ocular Inflammation*.

Degenerations

Iridocorneal Endothelial Syndrome

Iridocorneal endothelial (ICE) syndrome is a spectrum of acquired unilateral abnormalities of the corneal endothelium, anterior chamber angle, and iris.

> ICE syndrome comprises 3 recognized clinical variants of ICE (when combined, the first letter of each variant also forms the mnemonic *ICE*):
>
> - **I**ris nevus syndrome (also called Cogan-Reese syndrome)
> - **C**handler syndrome
> - **E**ssential (progressive) iris atrophy

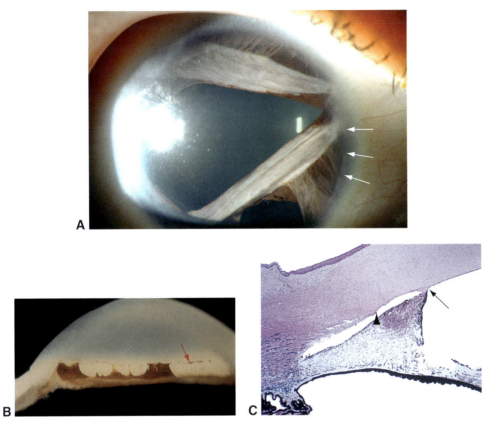

Figure 6-5 Axenfeld-Rieger syndrome. **A,** Clinical photograph of the anterior segment. Iris atrophy, pseudopolycoria, and iris strands in the periphery are present. Posterior embryotoxon is visible laterally *(arrows)*. **B,** Gross photograph shows a prominent Schwalbe line *(arrow)* and the anterior insertion of iris strands (Axenfeld anomaly). **C,** Histology shows the anterior attachment of iris strands *(arrow)* to posterior embryotoxon, which is anteriorly displaced relative to the termination of trabecular meshwork *(arrowhead)*. *(Part A courtesy of Wallace L. M. Alward, MD. Copyright University of Iowa. Part B courtesy of Robert Y. Foos, MD. Part C modified with permission from Yanoff M, Fine BS. Ocular Pathology. 6th ed. Elsevier; 2009.)*

All forms of ICE syndrome, which typically affects young to middle-aged women, have the following 2 features in common: epithelial-like metaplasia of the corneal endothelium and abnormal proliferation of the corneal endothelium. Abnormal endothelial cells migrate over the anterior chamber angle while laying down new basement membrane (Descemet membrane), leading to the formation of peripheral anterior synechiae and subsequent secondary angle-closure glaucoma in approximately half of patients with this condition (Fig 6-7). See BCSC Section 8, *External Disease and Cornea,* and Section 10, *Glaucoma,* for further discussion.

    Silva L, Najafi A, Suwan Y, Teekhasaenee C, Ritch R. The iridocorneal endothelial syndrome. *Surv Ophthalmol.* 2018;63(5):665–676.

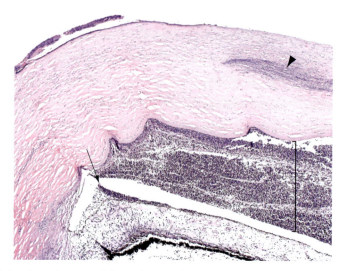

Figure 6-6 Collection of neutrophils and necrotic debris in the anterior chamber (hypopyon) *(bracket)*, resulting from a dense inflammatory infiltrate in the corneal stroma *(arrowhead)*. Inflammation may result in the formation of peripheral anterior synechiae in the angle *(arrow)*, which could lead to secondary angle-closure glaucoma. *(Courtesy of Amanda C. Maltry, MD.)*

Secondary Open-Angle Glaucoma

See BCSC Section 10, *Glaucoma,* and BCSC Section 11, *Lens and Cataract,* for more information on the topics discussed in this section.

Pseudoexfoliation syndrome

Pseudoexfoliation syndrome is the most common cause of secondary open-angle glaucoma. It is a systemic condition characterized by the production and progressive accumulation of a fibrillar material in tissues throughout the anterior segment and in the connective tissue of various visceral organs (eg, lung, heart, liver, and kidney) (Fig 6-8). These deposits help differentiate pseudoexfoliation syndrome from true exfoliation, in which infrared radiation induces splitting of the lens capsule. Pseudoexfoliation syndrome is usually identified in individuals older than 50 years.

Data suggest that the pathogenesis of pseudoexfoliation syndrome is a combination of excessive production and abnormal aggregation of elastic microfibril and extracellular matrix components, as well as abnormal biomechanical properties of the elastic components of the trabecular meshwork and lamina cribrosa. Polymorphisms in the lysyl oxidase–like 1 gene, *LOXL1*, on chromosome 15 (15q24) are markers for pseudoexfoliation syndrome. Lysyl oxidase is a pivotal enzyme in extracellular matrix formation, catalyzing covalent crosslinking of collagen and elastin.

Pseudoexfoliative material is most apparent on the surface of the anterior segment structures, where it exhibits a positive periodic acid–Schiff (PAS) stain reaction; presents as delicate, feathery or brushlike fibrils arranged perpendicular to the surfaces of the intraocular structures; and is easiest to identify on the anterior lens capsule (Fig 6-9A). Pseudoexfoliative material also accumulates in the trabecular meshwork and the wall of Schlemm canal, leading to increased intraocular pressure and secondary glaucoma.

CHAPTER 6: Anterior Chamber and Trabecular Meshwork • 125

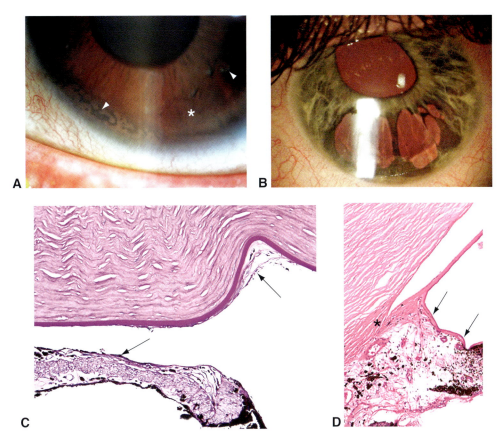

Figure 6-7 Iridocorneal endothelial (ICE) syndrome. **A,** Iris nevus syndrome. The anterior iris architecture is effaced by a membrane growing on the anterior iris surface *(asterisk).* This membrane pinches off islands of normal iris stroma, resulting in a nodular, nevuslike appearance *(arrowheads).* **B,** Essential iris atrophy. Atrophic holes in the iris and a narrow anterior chamber, consistent with peripheral anterior synechiae formation. **C,** Histopathology of ICE syndrome. A membrane composed of spindle cells lines the posterior surface of the cornea and the anterior surface of the atrophic iris *(arrows).* Metaplastic endothelial cells deposit on the iris surface a thin basement membrane that stains with periodic acid–Schiff (PAS) dye and is analogous to Descemet membrane. **D,** Histopathology of ICE syndrome. Descemet membrane lines the anterior surface of the iris *(arrows).* The iris is apposed to the cornea (peripheral anterior synechiae; *asterisk*). *(Part A courtesy of Paul A. Sidoti, MD; parts B and C courtesy of Tatyana Milman, MD.)*

Associated degenerative changes in the iris pigment epithelium manifest histologically as a "sawtooth" configuration (Fig 6-9B). These degenerative changes lead to pigment aggregation in the anterior chamber angle.

> Vazquez LE, Lee RK. Genomic and proteomic pathophysiology of pseudoexfoliation glaucoma. *Int Ophthalmol Clin.* 2014;54(4):1–13.

Phacolytic glaucoma

In cases of phacolytic glaucoma, denatured lens protein leaks from a mature or hypermature cataract through an intact but permeable lens capsule. The trabecular meshwork

126 • Ophthalmic Pathology and Intraocular Tumors

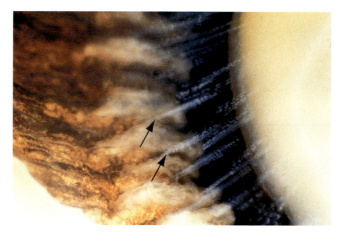

Figure 6-8 Gross photograph shows white fibrillar deposits on the lens zonular fibers *(arrows)* in an eye with pseudoexfoliation syndrome. *(Courtesy of Hans E. Grossniklaus, MD.)*

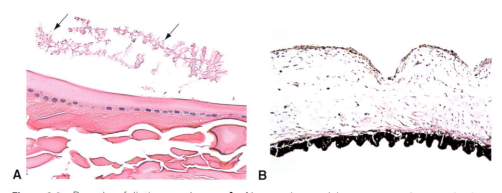

Figure 6-9 Pseudoexfoliation syndrome. **A,** Abnormal material appears on the anterior lens capsule like iron filings on the edge of a magnet *(arrows)*. **B,** The iris pigment epithelium demonstrates a "sawtooth" configuration, consistent with pseudoexfoliation. *(Part A courtesy of Amanda C. Maltry, MD; part B courtesy of Tatyana Milman, MD.)*

becomes occluded by the lens protein and by histiocytes that are engorged with phagocytosed proteinaceous, eosinophilic lens material (Fig 6-10).

Clinical Pearl Lytic glaucomas occur when material released into the anterior chamber is engulfed by histiocytes (macrophages), which then block the trabecular meshwork. These glaucomas are classified by the type of material released:

- *phacolytic:* degenerated lens protein
- *hemolytic:* red blood cell debris and hemosiderin (discussed in the following section)
- *melanomalytic:* melanin pigment released from a melanoma or melanocytoma (see Fig 6-15)

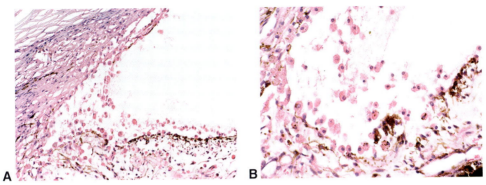

Figure 6-10 Phacolytic glaucoma. **A,** Photomicrograph of histiocytes filled with light pink degenerated lens cortical material in the angle. **B,** Higher magnification of the same image. *(Courtesy of Michele M. Bloomer, MD.)*

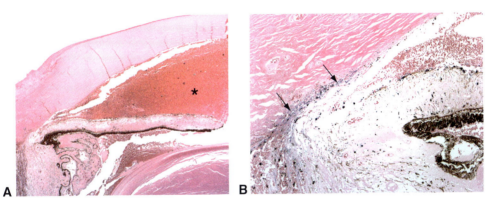

Figure 6-11 Hyphema. **A,** Hemorrhage fills the anterior chamber with blood *(asterisk)*. **B,** Higher magnification of the anterior chamber angle stained with Perls Prussian blue stain highlights blue hemosiderin deposits in the trabecular meshwork *(arrows)*. *(Courtesy of Amanda C. Maltry, MD.)*

Trauma

Blunt trauma may cause injury to the anterior segment that can lead to different types of secondary glaucoma.

Hyphema (Fig 6-11), defined as blood in the anterior chamber, may lead to increased intraocular pressure, peripheral anterior synechiae, hemosiderosis bulbi, and, potentially, vision loss. Following an intraocular hemorrhage, blood breakdown products may accumulate in the trabecular meshwork. The rigidity and spherical shape of hemolyzed erythrocytes (ghost cells) make it difficult for them to escape through the trabecular meshwork (Fig 6-12). The ghost cells obstruct the meshwork and block aqueous outflow, leading to *ghost cell glaucoma,* a type of secondary open-angle glaucoma. Ghost cell glaucoma often occurs following a vitreous hemorrhage, in which blood cells may be retained for prolonged periods, allowing the hemoglobin in erythrocytes to denature.

In *hemolytic glaucoma,* another type of secondary open-angle glaucoma, histiocytes in the anterior chamber phagocytose erythrocytes and their breakdown products, and

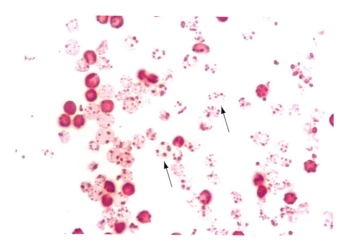

Figure 6-12 Aqueous aspirate demonstrates numerous ghost cells. The degenerating hemoglobin is present as small globules known as *Heinz bodies (arrows)* within the red blood cells. *(Courtesy of Nasreen A. Syed, MD.)*

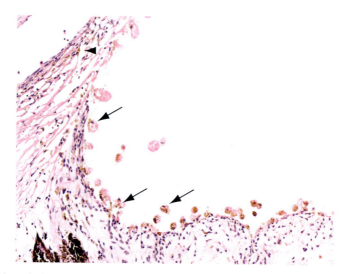

Figure 6-13 Hemolytic glaucoma. The anterior chamber angle contains histiocytes with erythrocyte debris and rust-colored intracytoplasmic hemosiderin *(arrows)*. Hemosiderin is also observed within the trabecular meshwork endothelium *(arrowhead)*. *(Courtesy of Michele M. Bloomer, MD.)*

these hemoglobin- and hemosiderin-laden histiocytes block trabecular outflow channels (Fig 6-13). The histiocytes may be a sign of trabecular obstruction rather than the actual cause of an obstruction.

In other cases of secondary open-angle glaucoma associated with chronic intraocular hemorrhage, histologic examinations have revealed hemosiderin within the trabeculocytes and within many ocular epithelial structures (see Fig 6-13). The hemosiderin likely releases intracellular iron, which results in intracellular toxicity, probably due to oxidative damage. This is the basis of intraocular dysfunction, including glaucoma, in both *siderosis bulbi* and *hemosiderosis bulbi*. Perls Prussian blue staining can demonstrate iron deposition in hemosiderosis bulbi.

Blunt injury to the globe may be associated with *angle recession, cyclodialysis,* and *iridodialysis*. Progressive degenerative changes in the trabecular meshwork can contribute to the development of glaucoma after injury. See the section Types of Ocular Trauma and Their Sequelae in Chapter 3 for further discussion, including images.

Pigment dispersion associations

Pigment dispersion (of melanosomes) may be associated with a variety of other conditions in which pigment epithelium or uveal melanocytes are injured, such as uveitis and uveal melanoma. These conditions are characterized by the presence of pigment within the trabecular meshwork as well as in histiocytes littering the anterior chamber angle (Figs 6-14, 6-15).

Pigment dispersion syndrome can lead to a secondary open-angle glaucoma that is characterized by transillumination defects in the midperipheral iris in addition to pigment in the trabecular meshwork, the corneal endothelium *(Krukenberg spindle)*, and other anterior segment structures, such as the lens capsule (see Fig 6-14). The dispersed pigment is presumed to result from rubbing of the lens zonular fibers against the iris pigment epithelium.

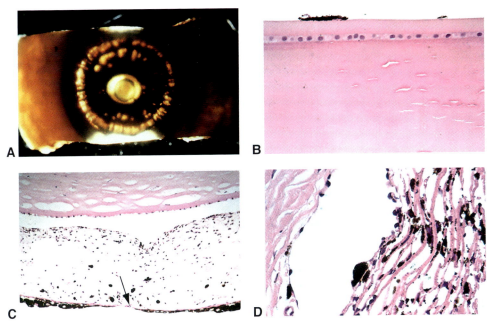

Figure 6-14 Pigment dispersion syndrome. **A,** Gross photograph demonstrates circumferential radial transillumination defects in the iris. **B,** Melanin is present on the anterior surface of the lens. **C,** Note the focal loss of iris pigment epithelium *(arrow)*. Chafing of the zonular fibers against the epithelium may release the pigment that is dispersed in this condition. **D,** Pigment accumulation in the trabecular meshwork.

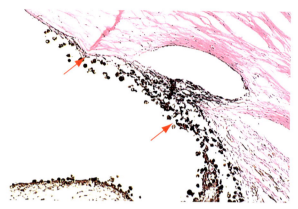

Figure 6-15 Melanomalytic glaucoma. The trabecular meshwork *(between arrows)* is obstructed by histiocytes that have ingested pigment from a necrotic intraocular melanoma.

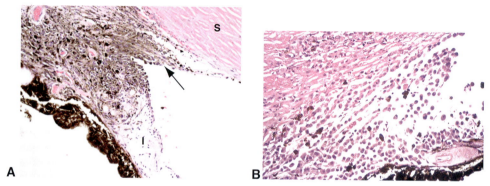

Figure 6-16 Anterior chamber angle melanoma involvement. **A,** Pigmented melanoma cells from a ciliary body melanoma extend anteriorly into the trabecular meshwork *(arrow)* and the adjacent iris root. I = iris; S = sclera. **B,** High-magnification photomicrograph shows discohesive epithelioid melanoma cells filling the anterior chamber angle and obstructing the trabecular meshwork. Iris pigment epithelium is present in the lower right corner. *(Part A courtesy of Michele M. Bloomer, MD; part B courtesy of Hans E. Grossniklaus, MD.)*

Neoplasia

There are no known primary tumors of the angle structures. Melanocytic nevi and melanomas that arise in the iris or extend to the iris from the ciliary body may invade or obstruct the trabecular meshwork (Fig 6-16). See also Chapter 16. In addition, pigment from melanomas and melanocytomas may be shed into the trabecular meshwork, leading to secondary glaucoma *(melanomalytic glaucoma)* (see Fig 6-15). Occasionally, epibulbar tumors such as conjunctival carcinoma can invade the eye through the limbus, resulting in trabecular outflow obstruction and glaucoma. See the section Neoplasia in Chapter 4 for further discussion.

CHAPTER 7

Sclera

Highlights

- The sclera is the tough, relatively avascular outer shell of the eye.
- Inflammation may occur in the sclera either focally or diffusely and is often granulomatous in nature.
- The sclera can thin for a variety of reasons, resulting in staphyloma formation.

Topography

The sclera is the white, nearly opaque portion of the outer wall of the eye that covers most of the eye's surface area. Anteriorly, the sclera is continuous with the corneal stroma at the limbus. Posteriorly, the outer two-thirds of the sclera merge with the dural sheath of the optic nerve; the inner third continues as perforated sclera, known as the *lamina cribrosa*, through which the axonal fibers of the retinal ganglion cells pass and become the retrobulbar optic nerve (see Chapter 14, Fig 14-1). Histologically, the sclera is divided into 3 layers (from outermost inward) (Fig 7-1):

- episclera
- stroma
- lamina fusca

Embryologically, the sclera is derived predominantly from the neural crest. See BCSC Section 2, *Fundamentals and Principles of Ophthalmology*, for further discussion.

The *episclera* is a thin layer of loose fibrovascular tissue that covers the outer surface of the scleral stroma. The bulk of the sclera is made up of the *stroma*, a layer of sparsely vascularized, dense type I collagen fibers. In comparison to the collagen lamellae of the corneal stroma, scleral collagen fibers are thicker and more variable in thickness and orientation, resulting in the opaque appearance of the sclera. Transmural *emissary canals* allow the passage of the ciliary arteries, vortex veins, and ciliary nerves through the scleral stroma (Fig 7-2; see also Fig 7-1). For additional discussion, see BCSC Section 2, *Fundamentals and Principles of Ophthalmology*, Chapter 2.

The *lamina fusca* is a delicate fibrovascular layer containing melanocytes that loosely binds the uveal tract to the sclera. Sclerouveal attachments are strongest surrounding the major emissary canals, at the anterior base of the ciliary body (scleral spur), and surrounding the optic nerve.

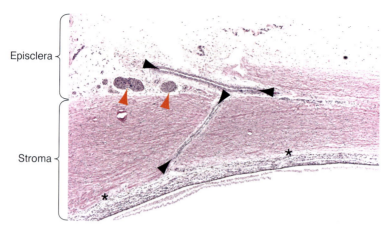

Figure 7-1 The 3 layers of the sclera—episclera, stroma, and lamina fusca *(asterisks)*. Emissary structures, including ciliary arteries *(black arrowheads)* and nerves *(red arrowheads)*, are shown entering and traversing normal sclera (hematoxylin and eosin [H&E] stain). *(Courtesy of Nasreen A. Syed, MD.)*

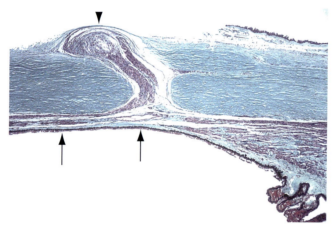

Figure 7-2 An emissary canal through the sclera with Axenfeld nerve loop *(arrowhead)* overlying the pars plana *(arrows)* (Masson trichrome stain). *(Courtesy of Harry H. Brown, MD.)*

Developmental Anomalies

Choristomas and Hamartomas

Epibulbar dermoids and other choristomatous lesions are discussed in Chapter 4.

Nanophthalmos

Nanophthalmos is a rare, usually bilateral, developmental disorder characterized by an eye with short axial length, a normal or slightly enlarged lens, thickened sclera, hyperopia, foveal changes, and a predisposition to uveal effusions and angle-closure glaucoma. The criteria for nanophthalmos differ in various studies, but in most, the size criterion is an axial length less than 20 mm. Nanophthalmos has a strong genetic basis, but sporadic cases (likely representing new pathogenic variations) occur.

Examination of tissue from nanophthalmic eyes has shown disarrangement, fraying, and splitting of scleral collagen fibrils. Abnormalities in the extracellular matrix glycosaminoglycans have also been described. These scleral changes may predispose the nanophthalmic eye to uveal effusion due to reduced protein permeability and impaired venous outflow through the vortex veins.

See BCSC Section 6, *Pediatric Ophthalmology and Strabismus,* and Section 10, *Glaucoma,* for additional discussion of nanophthalmos.

> Carricondo PC, Andrade T, Prasov L, Ayres BM, Moroi SE. Nanophthalmos: a review of the clinical spectrum and genetics. *J Ophthalmol.* 2018;2018:2735465. doi:10.1155/2018/2735465
>
> Rajendrababu S, Shroff S, More S, et al. A report on a series of nanophthalmos with histopathology and immunohistochemistry analyses using light microscopy. *Indian J Ophthalmol.* 2022;70(7):2597–2602.

Microphthalmia

Microphthalmia refers to a smaller than average eye with associated developmental defects (eg, persistent fetal vasculature). Colobomas and scleral defects with cystic outpouchings of intraocular contents (microphthalmia with orbital cyst) are also common, because of failure of the fetal fissure to close completely.

See BCSC Section 6, *Pediatric Ophthalmology and Strabismus,* and Section 7, *Oculofacial Plastic and Orbital Surgery,* for additional discussion of microphthalmia.

Inflammation

See BCSC Section 8, *External Disease and Cornea,* and Section 9, *Uveitis and Ocular Inflammation,* for in-depth discussion of episcleritis and scleritis, including pathogenesis, clinical presentation, laboratory evaluation, and management.

Scleritis

Scleritis may be infectious or noninfectious. Infectious scleritis may be distinguished from noninfectious scleritis by appropriate laboratory testing; special stains may aid in identifying causative organisms (Fig 7-3).

Noninfectious scleritis is typically a painful ocular disease with potentially serious sequelae. Histologic examination of noninfectious scleritis reveals 2 main types: necrotizing and nonnecrotizing inflammation. Either type can occur anteriorly or posteriorly, but anterior scleritis is more common. *Necrotizing scleritis* may be nodular or diffuse (Figs 7-4, 7-5). Both forms demonstrate granulomatous inflammation within the sclera

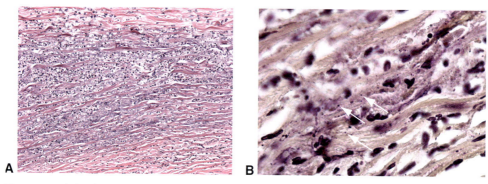

Figure 7-3 Infectious scleritis caused by bacteria. **A,** The sclera is infiltrated with numerous neutrophils, seen as blue dots between the scleral collagen lamellae. The purple areas represent necrobiosis of the sclera (H&E stain). **B,** Gram stain demonstrates the presence of scattered gram-positive cocci *(arrows)*. *(Courtesy of Nasreen A. Syed, MD.)*

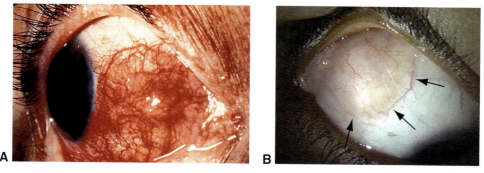

Figure 7-4 Nodular scleritis. **A,** An eye with sectoral nodular anterior scleritis with focal severe episcleral and scleral vascular congestion. **B,** Clinical photograph from a different patient following treatment. The nodule has a tan appearance *(arrows)*. *(Part A courtesy of Harry H. Brown, MD; part B courtesy of Nasreen A. Syed, MD.)*

(Fig 7-6). Lymphocytes and plasma cells are usually present as well. Neutrophils may be present in some cases. Multiple foci may show different stages of evolution. During the healing process, the necrotic stroma is resorbed, leaving a thinned scleral remnant that is prone to staphyloma formation (Fig 7-7). Severe ectasia of the scleral shell predisposes the sclera to herniation of uveal tissue through the defect (staphyloma). In *scleromalacia perforans,* the sclera undergoes focal progressive ectasia without clinical or histologic evidence of an inflammatory infiltrate.

Nonnecrotizing scleritis is characterized by a perivascular lymphocytic and plasmacytic infiltrate, typically without a granulomatous inflammatory component. Vasculitis may be present in the form of fibrinoid necrosis of the vessel walls. When treated, nonnecrotizing scleritis rarely leads to severe vision loss or enucleation.

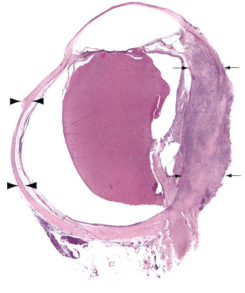

Figure 7-5 Diffuse anterior and posterior scleritis with marked thickening of the sclera *(arrows)* due to a dense inflammatory infiltrate. Compare the thickened sclera with the normal sclera on the opposite side *(arrowheads)*. *(Courtesy of Nasreen A. Syed, MD.)*

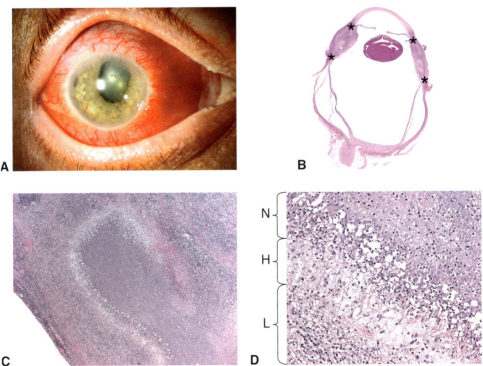

Figure 7-6 Necrotizing granulomatous anterior scleritis in a patient with rheumatoid arthritis. **A,** Clinical photograph of the anterior segment. **B,** Low-magnification photomicrograph illustrates the anterior location of the scleritis *(areas between asterisks)*. **C,** Medium-magnification photomicrograph shows the area of scleritis with central necrosis surrounded by a zonal inflammatory infiltrate. **D,** High-magnification photomicrograph of a zonal granuloma with central neutrophils and necrosis (N), a middle layer of epithelioid histiocytes (H), and an outer layer of lymphocytes (L). *(Courtesy of Nasreen A. Syed, MD.)*

136 • Ophthalmic Pathology and Intraocular Tumors

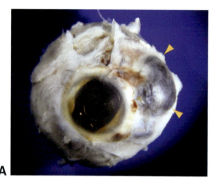 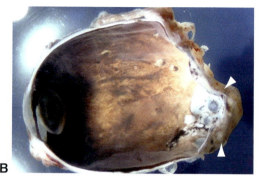

Figure 7-7 Scleral staphyloma. **A,** Anterior staphyloma *(arrowheads)* in an eye with congenital glaucoma. **B,** Posterior staphyloma *(arrowheads)* as a sequela of scleritis. *(Part A courtesy of Ralph C. Eagle Jr, MD; part B courtesy of Hans E. Grossniklaus, MD.)*

Degenerations

Age-Related Calcific Plaque

Age-related calcific plaques commonly occur in individuals older than 70 years. They appear as firm, flat, sharply circumscribed rectangular or ovoid gray scleral patches. The plaques, which appear bilaterally, are typically located anterior to the medial and lateral rectus muscle insertions in the interpalpebral fissure (Fig 7-8A). The etiology of these plaques is unknown; various causes, such as scleral dehydration, actinic damage, and stress on scleral collagen exerted by rectus muscle insertions, have been proposed but not proven.

Histologic sections show that the calcium is present within the midportion of the scleral stroma. The plaque begins as a finely granular deposition but may progress to a confluent plaque involving both superficial and deep sclera (Fig 7-8B). Age-related plaques may be highlighted by special stains for calcium, such as von Kossa and alizarin red.

Scleral Staphyloma

Scleral staphylomas are scleral ectasias that are lined internally by uveal tissue. Staphylomas may develop at points of weakness in the scleral shell, either in inherently thin areas (such as posterior to the rectus muscle insertions; Fig 7-9) or in areas weakened by tissue destruction (as in scleritis; see Fig 7-7B). In children, staphylomas may result from longstanding elevated intraocular pressure or axial myopia, owing to the relative distensibility of the sclera in young eyes. Thus, staphyloma location and age at onset vary according to the underlying etiology. Histologic examination invariably reveals thinned sclera, with or without fibrosis and scarring, depending on the cause.

Melanoma-Associated Spongiform Scleropathy

The sclera may undergo degeneration at the base of a uveal melanoma. This change is typically not apparent clinically, but histologically, it appears as a feathery separation and

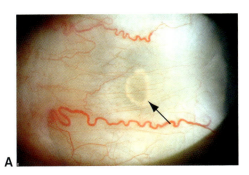
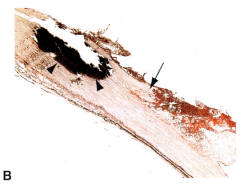

Figure 7-8 A calcific plaque of the sclera. **A,** Calcific plaques *(arrow)* are typically located just anterior to the insertion of the medial and lateral rectus muscles. **B,** Purple calcific deposits are noted in the sclera *(arrowheads)* anterior to the rectus muscle insertion *(arrow)* (H&E stain). *(Part A courtesy of Vinay A. Shah, MBBS; part B courtesy of Tatyana Milman, MD.)*

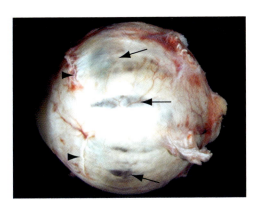

Figure 7-9 Regions of scleral thinning *(arrows)*, which appear blue because of the underlying uveal tissue, are present posterior to the rectus muscle insertions *(arrowheads)* and radially in the equatorial sclera. *(Courtesy of Nasreen A. Syed, MD.)*

fragmentation of the scleral collagen fibers. Studies have shown increased amounts of glycosaminoglycans in these areas. The change is postulated to result from activation of proteinases such as matrix metalloproteinase 2 in the sclera and may facilitate scleral extension of uveal melanoma.

Neoplasia

Neoplasms of the sclera are exceedingly rare. Tumors originate predominantly in the conjunctiva or uveal tract with secondary scleral involvement.

CHAPTER 8

Lens

Highlights

- Understanding the anatomical structure of the crystalline lens is essential for performing cataract surgery and for selecting appropriate surgical techniques to achieve optimal outcomes for the patient.
- Developmental anomalies of the lens must be recognized early to prevent the development of amblyopia.
- Chronic postoperative endophthalmitis presents slowly because causative microorganisms are sequestered between the posterior capsule and the intraocular lens implant.
- Inflammation due to degeneration of the crystalline lens can cause various forms of glaucoma.

Topography

The crystalline lens is an avascular, elastic, disc-shaped biconvex structure located posterior to the iris and anterior to the vitreous body. The lens and zonular fibers (zonules) separate the posterior chamber (the space between the iris and lens) from the vitreous cavity (Fig 8-1). In the adult eye, the lens measures approximately 9–10 mm in diameter equatorially and 5–6 mm anteroposteriorly. It is derived from surface ectoderm. See BCSC Section 11, *Lens and Cataract*, for in-depth discussion of the structure, embryology, and pathology of the lens.

Capsule

The capsule, which surrounds the lens, is a thick basement membrane elaborated by lens epithelial cells and composed partly of type IV collagen fibers (Fig 8-2). The lens capsule is thickest anteriorly (12–21 µm) and peripherally near the equator and thinnest posteriorly (2–9 µm) (Fig 8-3).

Clinical Pearl During surgical removal of a cataract, the extremely thin posterior capsule is at risk for rupture or tear. The posterior capsule serves as a barrier from the vitreous; if it is broken, vitreous may be pulled forward into the anterior segment.

140 • Ophthalmic Pathology and Intraocular Tumors

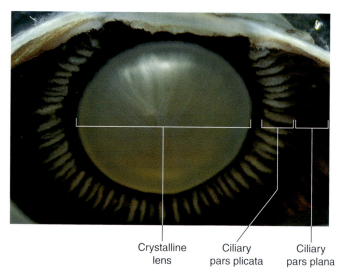

Figure 8-1 Posterior aspect of the crystalline lens, depicting its relationship to the peripheral iris and ciliary body. The zonular fibers are translucent and therefore are not visible. *(Courtesy of Hans E. Grossniklaus, MD.)*

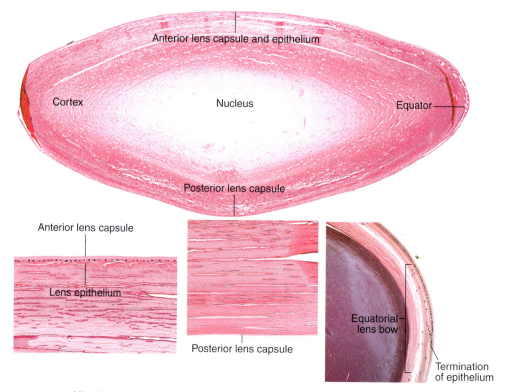

Figure 8-2 Histologic appearance and structure of the adult lens. *(Courtesy of Tatyana Milman, MD, except for lower right image, courtesy of Nasreen A. Syed, MD.)*

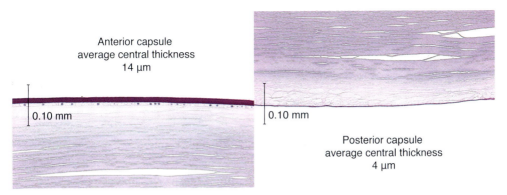

Figure 8-3 A side-by-side comparison of the anterior and posterior lens capsules, periodic acid–Schiff (PAS) stain. The anterior capsule *(left)* is thicker than the posterior capsule *(right)*. Calibration bar = 0.10 mm. *(Courtesy of Nasreen A. Syed, MD.)*

Epithelium

Embryologically, the lens epithelium is derived from the cells of the original lens vesicle that did not differentiate into primary lens fibers. The anterior or axial lens epithelium consists of a single layer of cuboidal cells. The basilar surface of the anterior epithelium is oriented toward the anterior lens capsule. The equatorial cells are mitotically active and appear more elongated as they differentiate into lens fibers. Epithelial cells are not typically observed posterior to the lens equator (see Fig 8-2).

Cortex and Nucleus

In the equatorial, or *bow,* region of the lens, the epithelial cells move centrally, elongate, produce crystalline proteins, lose organelles, and transform into lens fibers. As the lens epithelial cells differentiate, new fibers are continuously laid down over existing fibers, compacting them in a lamellar arrangement. Thus, the outermost fibers, derived from postnatally differentiated lens epithelial cells, are the most recently formed and make up the cortex of the lens, while older layers are located toward the center. The center of the lens contains the oldest fibers, the *embryonic and fetal lens nucleus.* Lens fibers are densely compacted in the nucleus. Clinically and histologically, the demarcation between the nucleus and cortex is not well defined (see Fig 8-2).

The overall shape of the lens changes over the first decade of life. With increasing age, the diameter of the lens nucleus and cortex increases from anterior to posterior.

Zonular Fibers

The lens is supported by the zonular fibers, which insert on both the anterior and the posterior lens capsule in the midperiphery (see Chapter 6, Fig 6-8). These fibers hold the lens in place through their attachments to the nonpigmented epithelium of the ciliary pars plana and the valleys of the pars plicata. The zonular fibers are composed of an elastic type of glycoprotein known as *fibrillin* and have an important role in molding the lens shape for accommodation.

See BCSC Section 2, *Fundamentals and Principles of Ophthalmology,* for more information on the structure and development of the crystalline lens.

Developmental Anomalies

Early recognition of developmental anomalies of the lens is important to prevent the development of amblyopia. See BCSC Section 6, *Pediatric Ophthalmology and Strabismus,* and Section 11, *Lens and Cataract,* for discussion of lens coloboma, ectopia lentis, and congenital cataract, as well as for additional information on the topics discussed in the following sections.

Congenital Aphakia

Congenital aphakia, a rare anomaly, can be divided into 2 forms:

- *Primary aphakia:* the lens is absent histologically; caused by failed lens induction from the surface ectoderm during embryogenesis, which results from homozygous pathogenic variants in the *FOXE3* gene. Primary aphakia is associated with severe ocular anomalies, including microphthalmia.
- *Secondary aphakia:* histologic findings depend on the underlying etiology. In this form, the lens is developed but is resorbed or extruded before or during birth. Secondary aphakia is often associated with congenital infections such as rubella.

Lenticonus and Lentiglobus

The anterior or posterior surfaces of the lens can assume an abnormal shape, either conical *(lenticonus)* or spherical *(lentiglobus)* (Fig 8-4). Clinically, abnormalities can be seen in the red reflex, where, by retroillumination, they appear as an "oil droplet."

Lenticonus may be unilateral or bilateral. Bilateral anterior lenticonus is usually associated with *Alport syndrome,* which is most often an X-linked disorder characterized by hemorrhagic nephritis, deafness, anterior polar cataract, and retinal flecks. Pathogenic variants in type IV collagen genes—specifically, *COL4A3, COL4A4,* and *COL4A5*—have

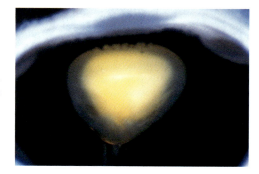

Figure 8-4 Macroscopic image shows posterior lenticonus. *(Courtesy of Hans E. Grossniklaus, MD.)*

been described in some cases of Alport syndrome. Histologic examination reveals thinning of and small defects in the anterior lens capsule, a decrease in the number of anterior lens epithelial cells, and bulging of the anterior cortex.

Posterior lenticonus and lentiglobus are more common than anterior lenticonus and lentiglobus; these deformations usually occur as a sporadic unilateral anomaly and are associated with congenital cataract. Other rare ocular associations include microphthalmia, microcornea, persistent fetal vasculature, and uveal colobomas. Posterior lenticonus may also be a manifestation of Alport syndrome or *oculocerebrorenal syndrome (Lowe syndrome)*, an X-linked disorder characterized by glaucoma, cognitive impairment, and infantile renal tubulopathy (Fanconi type) with resultant aminoaciduria, metabolic acidosis, proteinuria, rickets, and hypotonia. Oculocerebrorenal syndrome is caused by pathogenic variants in the *OCRL* gene. Histologically, the cataracts display focal, internally directed excrescences of the lens capsule.

Inflammation

Cutibacterium acnes Endophthalmitis

Chronic infectious endophthalmitis may develop following cataract surgery. Common causative organisms are *Cutibacterium acnes* (formerly *Propionibacterium acnes*) and *Staphylococcus epidermidis*. Chronic postoperative bacterial endophthalmitis is most commonly caused by *C acnes*; *C acnes* endophthalmitis often has a delayed presentation, usually between 2 months and 2 years following surgery. The organism, a gram-positive coccobacillus that is part of normal skin flora and grows best in anaerobic conditions, may sequester itself between a posterior chamber lens implant and the posterior capsule. In this relatively anaerobic environment, *C acnes* grows and forms colonies. Histologic examination of the lens capsule reveals sequestration of the bacteria within the capsule (Fig 8-5). See BCSC Section 9, *Uveitis and Ocular Inflammation*, Section 11, *Lens and Cataract*, and Section 12, *Retina and Vitreous*, for additional discussion of endophthalmitis.

Phacoantigenic Uveitis

Also known as *lens-induced granulomatous endophthalmitis* and previously called *phacoanaphylactic endophthalmitis*, phacoantigenic uveitis is a type of lens-induced intraocular inflammation. It is thought to be precipitated by the deposition of antigen–antibody complexes in the lens (type III, Arthus-type reaction) following exposure of the immune system to lens antigens after the lens capsule has been violated. The inflammation may develop after accidental or surgical trauma to the lens.

Histologically, an eye with phacoantigenic uveitis shows a central nidus of degenerating lens material surrounded by concentric layers of inflammatory cells *(zonal granuloma)*. Neutrophils are present in the innermost zone of inflammation. The intermediate zone consists primarily of epithelioid histiocytes and multinucleated giant cells. Lymphocytes and plasma cells are present in the outer zone. The inflammatory cells may be surrounded by fibrovascular connective tissue, depending on the duration of the inflammatory response

144 • Ophthalmic Pathology and Intraocular Tumors

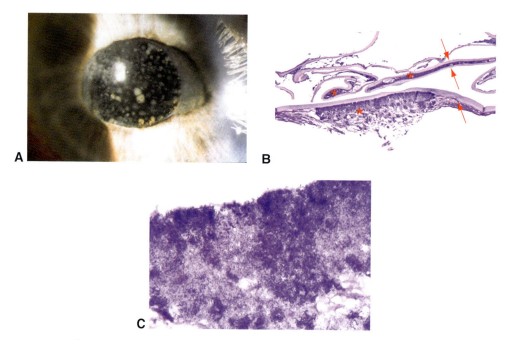

Figure 8-5 *Cutibacterium acnes* endophthalmitis. **A,** Slit-lamp photograph shows white opacities within the lens capsule. **B,** Large aggregates of coccobacilli *(asterisks)* within the fragments of lens capsule *(arrows).* **C,** Higher magnification of the numerous coccobacilli. *(Part A courtesy of Thomas L. Steinemann, MD; parts B and C courtesy of Hans E. Grossniklaus, MD.)*

(Fig 8-6). See also BCSC Section 9, *Uveitis and Ocular Inflammation,* and Section 11, *Lens and Cataract.*

Phacolytic Uveitis

Phacolytic uveitis is an inflammatory condition caused by leakage of lens protein from a hypermature or morgagnian cataract through a grossly intact lens capsule. The proteins are often engulfed by histiocytes. These protein-laden histiocytes may clog the trabecular meshwork or induce an inflammatory response in the angle, leading to a form of glaucoma called *phacolytic glaucoma*. See Chapter 6 in this volume for additional discussion of phacolytic glaucoma. See also BCSC Section 9, *Uveitis and Ocular Inflammation,* and Section 10, *Glaucoma.*

In both phacoantigenic and phacolytic uveitis, an inflammatory response is triggered by lens protein antigens. However, the clinical presentation for each of these conditions is quite different because of the difference in antigen load:

- *phacolytic uveitis:* small amounts of protein leak slowly from an intact capsule, causing mild inflammation
- *phacoantigenic uveitis:* large amounts of lens protein are suddenly released through a broken capsule, causing severe inflammation and endophthalmitis

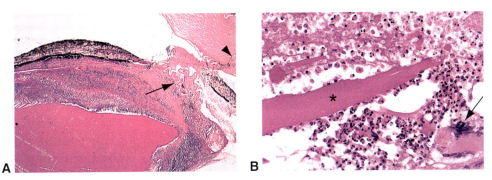

Figure 8-6 Phacoantigenic uveitis. **A,** A zonal inflammatory reaction surrounds the lens *(lower left)*. The torn capsule is visible in the pupillary region *(arrow)*. Note the corneal scar *(arrowhead)*, representing the site of ocular penetration. **B,** Acute and granulomatous inflammation, including giant cells *(arrow)*, surrounds inciting lens fibers *(asterisk)*.

Degenerations

Cataract and Other Lens Abnormalities

Capsule

Mild thickening of the lens capsule can be associated with pathologic proliferation of lens epithelium or with chronic inflammation of the anterior segment. Elements with an affinity for basement membranes, such as copper and silver, can form pigmented deposits in the anterior lens capsule, conditions known as *chalcosis* and *argyrosis,* respectively.

Epithelium

The most common abnormality involving the lens epithelium may be *posterior subcapsular cataract* (Fig 8-7A; see also Fig 8-8A). Histologically, development of this cataract begins with epithelial disarray at the lens equator, followed by posterior migration of the lens epithelial cells along the posterior capsule. As the cells migrate posteriorly, they may enlarge significantly as a result of retention of lens protein in the cytoplasm. These swollen cells, referred to as *Wedl* (or *bladder*) *cells,* can cause significant visual impairment if they involve the axial portion of the lens (Fig 8-7B).

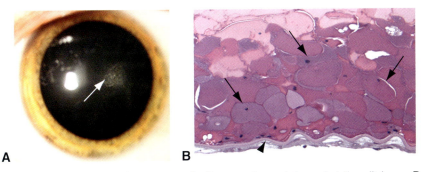

Figure 8-7 Posterior subcapsular cataract. **A,** Cataract *(arrow)* viewed at the slit lamp. **B,** Oval to round nucleated Wedl cells *(arrows)* and smaller lens epithelial cells line the posterior lens capsule *(arrowhead)*. *(Part A courtesy of Arlene V. Drack, MD; part B courtesy of Robert H. Rosa Jr, MD.)*

Inflammation, ischemia, or trauma can result in injury to the lens epithelium, stimulating epithelial metaplasia and the formation of *anterior subcapsular fibrous plaques* (Fig 8-8A). In this condition, the epithelial cells have undergone a metaplastic transformation into fibroblast-like cells that form a plaque just interior to the anterior capsule. Following resolution of the inciting stimulus, the lens epithelium may produce another capsule, thereby completely surrounding the fibrous plaque and creating what is called a *duplication cataract* (Fig 8-8B).

Disruption of the lens capsule often results in proliferation of lens epithelial cells. For example, following extracapsular cataract extraction, remaining epithelial cells can proliferate and cover the inner surface of the posterior lens capsule, resulting in clinically appreciable *posterior capsule opacification*. These accumulations of proliferating epithelial cells may form partially transparent globular masses, referred to as *Elschnig pearls* (Fig 8-9), which are histologically identical to Wedl cells. Sequestration of proliferating lens fibers

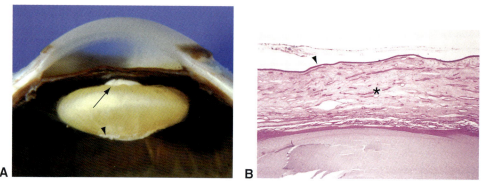

Figure 8-8 Anterior and posterior subcapsular cataracts. **A,** Gross photograph shows white anterior *(arrow)* and posterior *(arrowhead)* subcapsular plaques located centrally. **B,** A fibrous plaque *(asterisk)* is present internal to the original lens capsule *(arrowhead)*. *(Part A courtesy of Tatyana Milman, MD; part B courtesy of Hans E. Grossniklaus, MD.)*

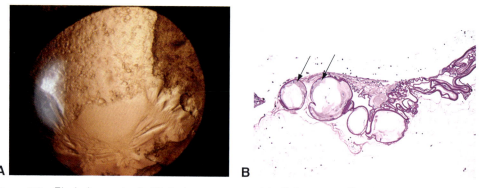

Figure 8-9 Elschnig pearls. **A,** Clinical appearance with slit-lamp retroillumination, demonstrating numerous globular posterior capsule opacities behind the lens implant. **B,** Photomicrograph depicts proliferating lens epithelium *(arrows)* on remnants of the posterior capsule (PAS stain). *(Part A courtesy of Sander Dubovy, MD; part B courtesy of Nasreen A. Syed, MD.)*

in the equatorial region may create a doughnut-shaped remnant, known as a *Soemmering ring secondary cataract* (Fig 8-10).

Severe elevation of intraocular pressure can damage lens epithelial cells, leading to cell degeneration. Clinically, patches of white flecks *(glaukomflecken)* are observed beneath the anterior lens capsule. Histologic examination shows focal areas of necrotic lens epithelial cells, often with associated degenerated cortical material (Fig 8-11). See also BCSC Section 10, *Glaucoma*.

Retention of iron-containing metallic foreign bodies in the eye or long-standing intraocular hemorrhage may result in iron deposition in the lens epithelial cells from siderosis bulbi or hemosiderosis bulbi. The iron is toxic to the epithelial cells. The presence of iron within the epithelial cells can be demonstrated with Perls Prussian blue stain.

Cortex

Clinically, cortical degenerative changes fall into 2 broad categories: (1) generalized discolorations with loss of transparency and (2) focal opacifications. Generalized loss of transparency cannot be reliably diagnosed histologically; the histologic stains used to colorize the lens tissue after it is processed prevent the assessment of lens clarity. The earliest

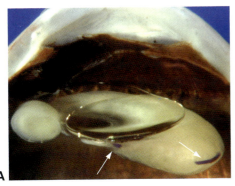
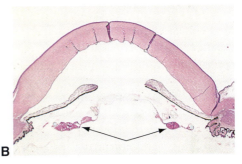

Figure 8-10 Soemmering ring secondary cataract. **A,** Doughnut-shaped white cataractous material is present in the equatorial region of the lens capsule and surrounds a lens haptic *(arrows)*. The lens optic and a second haptic are positioned in front of the lens capsular bag, in the sulcus. **B,** Photomicrograph shows accumulation of lens protein in the residual equatorial lens capsule *(arrows)*. *(Part A courtesy of Tatyana Milman, MD.)*

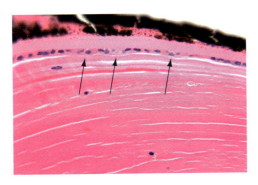

Figure 8-11 Histologic appearance of glaukomflecken. Acute elevation of intraocular pressure and aqueous stasis result in foci of necrotic anterior lens epithelial cells *(arrows)*. *(Courtesy of Tatyana Milman, MD.)*

sign of focal cortical degeneration is hydropic swelling of the lens fibers with decreased intensity of eosinophilic staining. Focal cortical opacities become more apparent when fiber degeneration is advanced enough to cause liquefactive change. Light microscopy shows the accumulation of eosinophilic globules (morgagnian globules) in slitlike spaces between the lens fibers (Fig 8-12; see also Fig 8-13C). As focal cortical lesions progress, these spaces become confluent and form globular collections of lens protein. Ultimately, the entire cortex can become liquefied, allowing the nucleus to sink inferiorly and the capsule to wrinkle; this condition is referred to as *morgagnian cataract* (Fig 8-13).

Nucleus

In the adult lens, the continual production of lens fibers subjects the nucleus to the stress of mechanical compression, which causes hardening of the lens nucleus over time. Aging is also associated with alterations in the chemical composition of the nuclear fibers that contribute to changes in color and refractive index. The pathogenesis of nuclear discoloration is poorly understood and probably involves more than one mechanism, including accumulation of urochrome pigment. Clinically, the lens nucleus may appear yellow, brunescent, or dark brown.

Nuclear cataracts are difficult to assess histologically because they take on a subtle homogeneous eosinophilic appearance. Clinically, the loss of laminations (artifactitious clefts) probably correlates better with nuclear firmness than it does with optical opacification (see Fig 8-13C). Occasionally, crystalline deposits, identified as calcium oxalate, may be observed within a nuclear cataract (Fig 8-14). These deposits are birefringent under polarized light. It is postulated that oxidative DNA damage to lens epithelial cells may contribute to age-related nuclear cataract.

Zonular fibers

Deposition of abnormal protein on the lens zonular fibers in *pseudoexfoliation syndrome* can lead to degeneration of these fibers and their eventual dehiscence. See Chapter 6 in this volume for additional discussion of pseudoexfoliation syndrome. See also BCSC Section 11, *Lens and Cataract*.

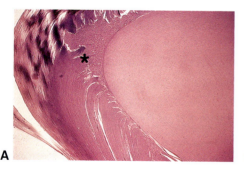 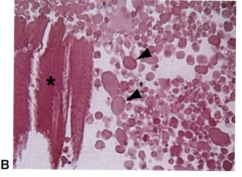

Figure 8-12 Cortical cataract. **A,** Extensive cortical liquefaction is present *(asterisk)*. **B,** Cortical degeneration. Lens cell fibers *(asterisk)* are swollen and fragmented. Note the morgagnian globules *(arrowheads)*. The lenticular fragments, which are opaque, increase osmotic pressure within the capsule. *(Courtesy of Hans E. Grossniklaus, MD.)*

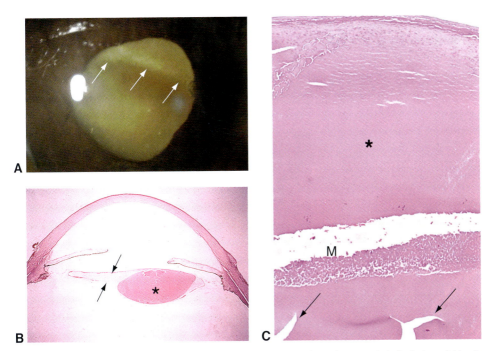

Figure 8-13 Morgagnian cataract. **A,** The brunescent nucleus has sunk inferiorly within the liquefied cortex. *Arrows* mark the superior edge of the nucleus. **B,** The lens cortex has liquefied, leaving the lens nucleus *(asterisk)* floating freely within the capsular bag *(arrows)*. **C,** Loss of artifactitious clefts in nuclear sclerotic cataract *(asterisk)*, signaling lens hardening. Rare artifactitious, sharply angulated clefts *(arrows)* are present. A zone of morgagnian globules (M) is visible. *(Part A courtesy of Bradford Tannen, MD; part B courtesy of Debra J. Shetlar, MD.)*

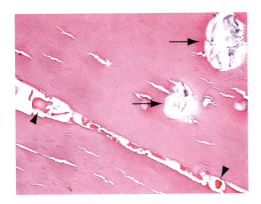

Figure 8-14 Crystalline deposits of calcium oxalate *(arrows)* are visible within the lens. Also apparent is a cortical cleft with morgagnian globules *(arrowheads)*. *(Courtesy of Tatyana Milman, MD.)*

Neoplasia and Associations With Systemic Disorders

There are no reported cases of neoplasms arising in the human lens. Premature opacification of the lens has been observed in many systemic disorders. See BCSC Section 11, *Lens and Cataract*.

CHAPTER 9

Vitreous

 This chapter includes a related activity. Go to aao.org/bcscactivity_section04 or scan the QR code in the text to access this content.

Highlights

- A variety of developmental anomalies can occur in the vitreous, including Mittendorf dot, Bergmeister papilla, and persistent fetal vasculature.
- Inflammation in the vitreous body can be a sign of potentially sight-threatening processes.
- Posterior vitreous detachment plays an important role in the development of many retinal conditions.
- Primary vitreoretinal lymphoma (PVRL) generally presents as cells in the vitreous and may be a challenging diagnosis to make with routine cytology. This diagnosis usually requires special pathologic techniques, communication between the surgeon and pathologist regarding specimen handling, and a pathology laboratory experienced with PVRL.

Topography

The vitreous humor makes up most of the volume of the globe and plays a role in many diseases that affect the eye. The vitreous body is divided into 2 main topographic areas: the central, or core, vitreous; and the peripheral, or cortical, vitreous (Fig 9-1). The strength of vitreoretinal adhesion or attachment is important in the pathogenesis of retinal tears and detachment, macular hole formation, and vitreous hemorrhage from neovascularization. Although the vitreous cavity typically appears empty on routine histologic sections, the hyaluronic acid molecules stain with Alcian blue. The few cells present in the secondary vitreous are called *hyalocytes*.

The embryologic development of the vitreous is generally divided into 3 stages:

- *Primary:* The *primary vitreous* consists of fibrillar material, mesenchymal cells, and vascular components (hyaloid artery, vasa hyaloidea propria, and tunica vasculosa lentis. During formation of the secondary vitreous, the primary vitreous atrophies, leaving only a clear central zone through the vitreous (called the *hyaloid canal,* or *Cloquet canal*) and its anterior extension, the hyaloideocapsular ligament (also known as *Wieger ligament*) (see Fig 9-1).

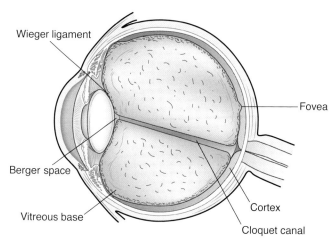

Figure 9-1 Schematic of the topography of the vitreous body demonstrates the distribution of the collagen fibrils *(lines)* at the vitreous base, at the cortex, in the macular region, and at the optic nerve head. *(Illustration by Cyndie C. H. Wooley.)*

- *Secondary:* The *secondary vitreous* begins to form at approximately the ninth week of gestation; in the postnatal and adult eye, it becomes the main portion of the vitreous. The secondary vitreous is relatively acellular and completely avascular. It is composed of thin collagen fibrils and hyaluronic acid (hyaluronan), which is extremely hydrophilic.
- *Tertiary:* The lens zonular fibers (also referred to as the *zonule of Zinn*) develop from the *tertiary vitreous.*

See BCSC Section 2, *Fundamentals and Principles of Ophthalmology,* and Section 12, *Retina and Vitreous,* for discussion of the anatomy of the vitreous.

Developmental Anomalies

Persistent Fetal Vasculature

Persistent fetal vasculature (PFV; previously known as *persistent hyperplastic primary vitreous*) is characterized by the persistence of variable components of the primary vitreous and is most often unilateral. In most cases of clinically significant PFV, a fibrovascular plaque in the retrolental space extends laterally to involve the ciliary processes, which may be pulled toward the visual axis by traction from the fibrovascular tissue. The clinical and gross appearance of elongated ciliary processes results. The anterior fibrovascular plaque is generally contiguous posteriorly with a remnant of the hyaloid artery that may attach to the optic nerve head (optic disc) (Fig 9-2). Involvement of the posterior structures may be more extensive, with detachment of the peripapillary retina resulting from traction caused by preretinal membranes. The lens is often cataractous, and the posterior capsule may be discontinuous. Eyes affected by the more severe forms of PFV are often microphthalmic. See also Chapter 18 in this volume and BCSC Section 12, *Retina and Vitreous.*

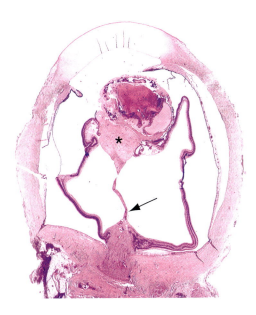

Figure 9-2 Persistent fetal vasculature. The photomicrograph shows a prominent anterior fibrovascular plaque adherent to the lens *(asterisk)*. The lens is distorted, and the peripheral retina is adherent to the plaque. The persistent remnant of the hyaloid artery is visible as a stalk that traverses the vitreous cavity and attaches to the optic nerve head posteriorly *(arrow)*. *(Courtesy of Nasreen A. Syed, MD.)*

Bergmeister Papilla

The persistence of a small part of the posterior portion of the hyaloid artery is referred to as *Bergmeister papilla*. This anomaly generally takes the form of a veil-like structure or a fingerlike projection extending anteriorly from the surface of the optic nerve head (Fig 9-3). Retinal vessels may grow into a Bergmeister papilla and then return to the optic nerve head, creating prepapillary vascular loops (see BCSC Section 12, *Retina and Vitreous*).

Mittendorf Dot

The hyaloid artery connects with the tunica vasculosa lentis just inferior and nasal to the center of the fetal lens. With regression of these vascular structures, a nodular mass or a macule may remain on the posterior lens capsule and appear as a focal posterior lens opacity at this site. This nodule is referred to as *Mittendorf dot* (see BCSC Section 11, *Lens and Cataract*).

Vitreous Cysts

Vitreous cysts generally occur in eyes with no other pathologic findings, but they have been noted in eyes with retinitis pigmentosa and uveitis, as well as in eyes with remnants of the hyaloid system. The exact origin of the cysts is not known. These cysts may be clear, or they may be pigmented owing to the presence of pigment epithelium. Histologic studies have suggested the presence of hyaloid remnants in vitreous cysts.

Inflammation

As a relatively acellular and completely avascular structure, the vitreous is generally not a primary site for the initiation of inflammatory disorders; however, it can become involved secondarily in inflammatory conditions of adjacent tissues. Inflammation in the vitreous

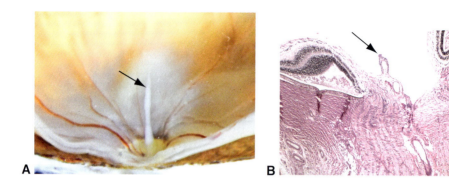
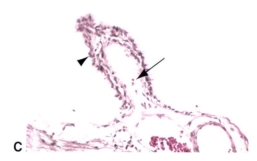

Figure 9-3 Bergmeister papilla. **A,** Gross photograph of an eye shows a fingerlike projection of whitish tissue *(arrow)* from the surface of the optic nerve head. **B,** Low-magnification photomicrograph shows fibroglial tissue *(arrow)* projecting into the vitreous cavity from the optic nerve head. **C,** High-magnification photomicrograph of Bergmeister papilla demonstrates loose fibrous connective tissue with a small capillary *(arrow)*, surrounded by a thin layer of astrocyte-like cells *(arrowhead)*. *(Part A courtesy of Ralph C. Eagle Jr, MD; parts B and C courtesy of Robert H. Rosa Jr, MD.)*

body can be a sign of potentially sight-threatening processes. The term *vitritis* is used to denote the presence of benign or malignant white blood cells in the vitreous.

Vitreous inflammation associated with infectious agents, particularly bacteria and fungi, is clinically referred to as *infectious endophthalmitis*. Bacterial endophthalmitis and fungal endophthalmitis (Fig 9-4) are characterized by neutrophilic infiltration of the vitreous that leads to liquefaction of the vitreous, with subsequent posterior vitreous detachment. Fungal endophthalmitis may have a granulomatous component, manifesting as vitreous "snowballs" clinically. Severe inflammation may be accompanied by formation of fibrocellular membranes, typically in the retrolental space; these may exert traction on the peripheral retina.

The vitreous infiltrate in noninfectious uveitis is typically composed of chronic inflammatory cells, including T and B lymphocytes and histiocytes (Fig 9-5). See also BCSC Section 9, *Uveitis and Ocular Inflammation*. Activity 9-1 shows common patterns of ocular inflammation.

 ACTIVITY 9-1 Patterns of ocular inflammation.
Courtesy of Tatyana Milman, MD.
Available at aao.org/bcscactivity_section04

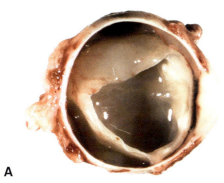
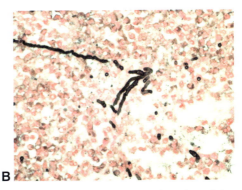

Figure 9-4 Endophthalmitis. **A,** Gross photograph shows opacification and infiltration of the vitreous by inflammatory cells as a result of fungal endophthalmitis. **B,** Photomicrograph shows fungal organisms and cellular infiltration of the vitreous in endophthalmitis. *(Courtesy of Steffen Heegaard, MD.)*

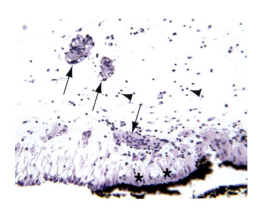

Figure 9-5 Noninfectious uveitis. Aggregates of epithelioid histiocytes *(arrows)* and scattered lymphocytes *(arrowheads)* in the vitreous base overlie the pigmented and nonpigmented ciliary epithelium of the pars plana *(asterisks)*. *(Courtesy of Tatyana Milman, MD.)*

Degenerations

Synchysis, Syneresis, and Aging

Synchysis of the vitreous refers to liquefaction and collapse of the gel; *syneresis* refers to disruption of the collagen fibers of the gel. Synchysis and syneresis of the central vitreous are a nearly universal consequence of aging. They also occur as a result of vitreous inflammation and hemorrhage and in eyes with significant axial myopia. The prominent lamellae and strands that develop in the aging eye or following inflammation or hemorrhage are the result of abnormally aggregated collagenous vitreous fibrils around syneretic pockets of hyaluronate (Fig 9-6). Synchysis and syneresis can lead to vitreous detachment.

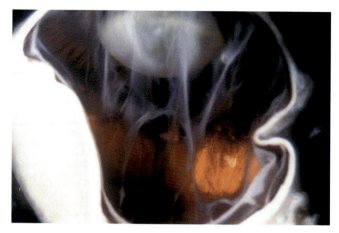

Figure 9-6 Gross photograph demonstrates vitreous condensations outlining syneretic cavities. *(Courtesy of Hans E. Grossniklaus, MD.)*

Posterior Vitreous Detachment

Posterior vitreous detachment (PVD) occurs when a dehiscence in the vitreous cortex allows fluid from a syneretic cavity to enter the potential subhyaloid space, causing the remaining hyaloid face to be stripped from the internal limiting membrane (ILM) of the retina (Fig 9-7). As fluid drains out of the syneretic cavities under the newly formed posterior hyaloid, the vitreous body collapses anteriorly, remaining attached at its base. Vitreous detachment generally occurs rapidly over the course of a few hours to days. Occasionally, traction may occur on the peripheral retina, perifoveal macula, or retinal blood vessels as a PVD occurs.

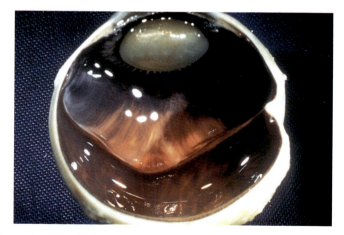

Figure 9-7 Gross photograph shows a posterior vitreous detachment. Retraction of the vitreous from the posterior retina is visible. *(Courtesy of Hans E. Grossniklaus, MD.)*

Age-related weakening of the adherence of the cortical vitreous to the ILM plays a role in the occurrence of PVDs. The prevalence of PVD in individuals aged 70 years and older has been reported as 50% or higher in clinical and pathologic studies. The incidence of PVD is increased in persons with intraocular inflammation, aphakia or pseudophakia, trauma, myopia, or vitreoretinal diseases. PVD is associated with the pathogenesis of many conditions, including retinal tears and detachment, macular hole formation, and vitreous hemorrhage. See BCSC Section 12, *Retina and Vitreous,* for additional discussion of these conditions.

Retinal tears and potential sequelae

Retinal tears (breaks) are often the result of vitreous traction on the retina in association with a PVD or secondary to ocular trauma. Tears are most likely to occur at sites of greatest vitreoretinal adhesion, such as the vitreous base (Fig 9-8) or the margin of lattice degeneration. The vitreous base extends approximately 2 mm anteriorly from the ora serrata over the pars plana of the ciliary body and 4 mm posteriorly over the peripheral retina. Histologic examination of retinal tears reveals that the vitreous adheres to the retina along the flap of the tear. The area of retina separated from the underlying retinal pigment epithelium (RPE) shows loss of photoreceptors.

Rhegmatogenous retinal detachment (RRD) is the most common type of retinal detachment; RRD occurs when vitreous traction and fluid currents resulting from eye movements combine to overcome the forces maintaining retinal adhesion to the RPE. With an RRD, cellular membranes may form on either surface (anterior or posterior) of the retina (Fig 9-9). Clinically, this process is referred to as *proliferative vitreoretinopathy (PVR).* These membranes, which often have a contractile component, form due to proliferation of RPE cells and other cellular elements. The cell biology of PVR is complex and involves the interaction of various growth factors and integrins, as well as cellular proliferation. Studies have shown a significant association between clinical grades of PVR and the expression levels of specific cytokines and/or growth factors in the vitreous fluid. See also Chapter 3 in this volume.

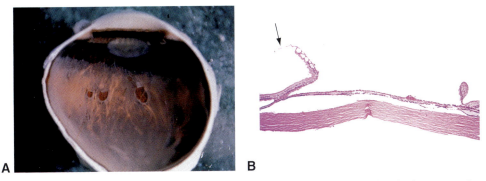

Figure 9-8 Peripheral retinal tears. **A,** Gross photograph shows several retinal tears at the vitreous base. **B,** Photomicrograph demonstrates condensed vitreous *(arrow)* attached to the anterior flap of the retinal tear. Vitreous traction on retinal tears is the underlying etiology of many retinal detachments. *(Courtesy of W. Richard Green, MD.)*

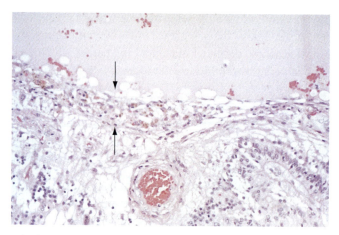

Figure 9-9 Preretinal membrane *(area between arrows)* on the surface of the retina, secondary to proliferative vitreoretinopathy. *(Courtesy of David J. Wilson, MD.)*

Shahlaee A, Woeller CF, Philip NJ, Kuriyan AE. Translational and clinical advancement in management of proliferative vitreoretinopathy. *Curr Opin Ophthalmol.* 2022;33(3): 219–227.

Macular holes

Idiopathic macular holes most likely form as the result of degenerative changes in the vitreous via a focal vitreomacular traction mechanism. Localized perifoveal vitreous detachment (an early stage of age-related PVD) appears to be the primary pathogenetic event in idiopathic macular hole formation (Fig 9-10). Detachment of the posterior hyaloid from the pericentral retina exerts anterior traction on the foveola and localizes the dynamic vitreous traction associated with ocular rotations into the perifoveolar region.

Investigations using OCT have clarified the pathogenesis of macular holes, particularly the early stages:

- *Stage 0:* A premacular hole occurs when a PVD with persistent foveal attachment (ie, vitreomacular adhesion) develops. Subtle loss of foveal depression can be observed.
- *Stage 1:* A foveal pseudocyst (stage 1A) is typically followed by disruption of the outer retina (stage 1B).
- *Stage 2:* In this stage, the macular hole progresses to a full-thickness dehiscence. Histologically, full-thickness macular holes are similar to holes in other locations.
- *Stage 3:* A full-thickness retinal defect with rounded tissue margins is accompanied by loss of the photoreceptor outer segments in adjacent retina, which is separated from the RPE by subretinal fluid (see Fig 9-10C). An epiretinal membrane composed of Müller cells, fibrous astrocytes, and myofibroblasts is often present on the surface of the retina adjacent to the macular hole. Cystoid macular edema in the parafoveal retina adjacent to the full-thickness macular hole is relatively common.

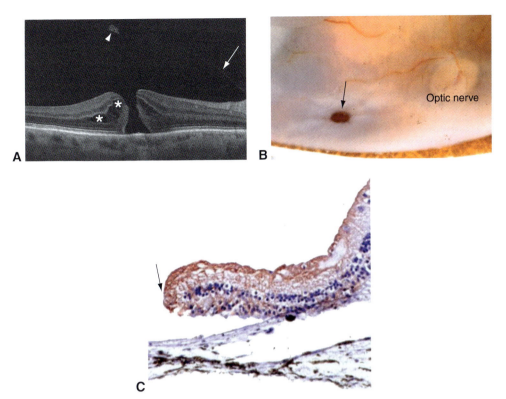

Figure 9-10 Macular holes. **A,** Spectral-domain optical coherence tomography (SD-OCT) image shows a stage 3 macular hole with full-thickness retinal defect, rounded margins, cystoid macular edema *(asterisks)*, and an operculum *(arrowhead)*. Note the posterior hyaloid face *(arrow)* tethered to the peripapillary retina near the optic nerve head. **B,** Gross photograph demonstrates a full-thickness macular hole *(arrow)*. **C,** Photomicrograph of the edge of a full-thickness macular hole shows a rounded gliotic margin *(arrow)* with positive brown staining for glial fibrillary acidic protein (GFAP), highlighting the Müller cells and astrocytes. *(Part A courtesy of Robert H. Rosa Jr, MD; parts B and C courtesy of Patricia Chévez-Barrios, MD.)*

Following surgical repair of macular holes, closer apposition of the remaining photoreceptors and variable glial scarring close the macular defect. See BCSC Section 12, *Retina and Vitreous,* for further discussion.

> Smiddy WE, Flynn HW Jr. Pathogenesis of macular holes and therapeutic implications. *Am J Ophthalmol.* 2004;137(3):525–537.
>
> Steel DHW, Lotery AJ. Idiopathic vitreomacular traction and macular hole: a comprehensive review of pathophysiology, diagnosis, and treatment. *Eye (Lond).* 2013;27(Suppl 1):S1–S21.

Hemorrhage

Following vitreous hemorrhage, a constellation of pathologic features may develop in the vitreous. After 3–10 days, red blood cell clots undergo fibrinolysis, and red blood cells may diffuse throughout the vitreous cavity. Denaturation of hemoglobin in the red blood cells produces ghost cells (see Chapter 6, Fig 6-12) and hemoglobin spherules. Obstruction of the trabecular meshwork by these cells may lead to *ghost cell glaucoma*. See also BCSC Section 10, *Glaucoma*.

The process of red blood cell dissolution attracts histiocytes, which phagocytose the degenerate red blood cells. Ferric iron (Fe^{3+}) is released during hemoglobin breakdown. This can occur intracellularly in histiocytes with iron storage as ferritin or hemosiderin, or extracellularly with iron binding to vitreous proteins such as lactoferrin and transferrin. In massive hemorrhages, cholesterol may deposit in the vitreous in the form of cholesterol crystals, which result from the breakdown of red blood cell membranes. Clinically, cholesterol appears as refractile crystals in the vitreous cavity (synchysis scintillans); the crystals are typically not attached to vitreous fibrils. Syneresis of the vitreous and PVD are common after vitreous hemorrhage.

Asteroid Hyalosis

Asteroid hyalosis is a condition with a dramatic clinical appearance but little clinical significance. Histologically, asteroid bodies are rounded structures measuring 10–100 nm, typically attached to vitreous fibrils (Fig 9-11). The bodies are basophilic with hematoxylin and eosin stain and are usually positive for calcium with stains such as alizarin red and von Kossa. Occasionally, they will be surrounded by a foreign body giant cell reaction, but the condition is not generally associated with vitreous inflammation.

Studies have shown that asteroid bodies are composed of complex lipids and also have a component with structural and elemental similarity to hydroxyapatite, a calcium phosphate complex.

Khoshnevis M, Rosen S, Sebag J. Asteroid hyalosis—a comprehensive review. *Surv Ophthalmol*. 2019;64(4):452–462.

Amyloidosis

Amyloidosis comprises a group of diseases characterized by extracellular deposition of amyloid in various tissues and organs. Amyloid deposits may be composed of many different types of proteins, all of which have a characteristic ultrastructural appearance of nonbranching fibrils with variable length and a diameter of 7–10 nm. The proteins forming amyloid can form a tertiary structure known as a *β-pleated sheet,* which enables the proteins to bind with Congo red stain and show birefringence under polarized light (Fig 9-12).

The type of amyloid protein that is deposited and the location of the deposition depend on the etiology of the underlying condition. The most common amyloid protein that forms deposits in the vitreous is *transthyretin*. Multiple types of genetic pathogenic variations can result in various amino acid substitutions in the transthyretin protein and allow for a conformational change to a β-pleated sheet. The most common variants are associated with *familial amyloid polyneuropathy (FAP)*. Systemic manifestations in patients with FAP include vitreous opacities and perivascular infiltrates (Fig 9-13),

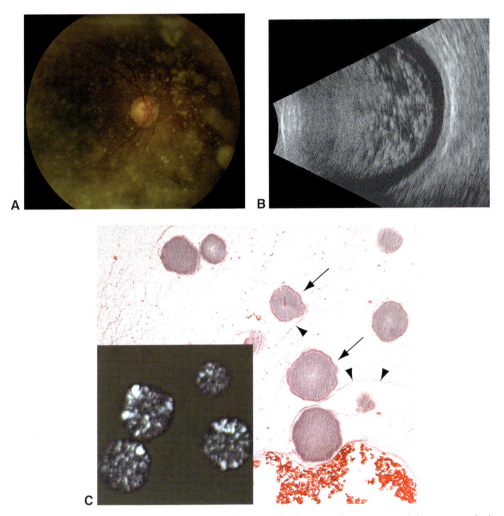

Figure 9-11 Asteroid hyalosis. **A,** Fundus photograph shows yellow-gray particles suspended in the vitreous. **B,** B-scan ultrasonography of asteroid hyalosis shows hyperechoic globular vitreous opacities separated from the retinal surface by a clear band of uninvolved vitreous. **C,** Asteroid bodies *(arrows)* attach to vitreous collagen fibrils *(arrowheads)* and erythrocytic debris from vitreous hemorrhage within the vitreous. *Inset:* Asteroid bodies show characteristic "Maltese-cross" birefringence with polarization microscopy. *(Parts A and B courtesy of Elaine M. Binkley, MD; part C courtesy of Tatyana Milman, MD.)*

peripheral neuropathy, cardiomyopathy, and carpal tunnel syndrome. If amyloid protein is identified in the vitreous, a referral to evaluate for systemic disease should be considered.

The mechanism by which the vitreous becomes involved is not known. Because amyloid deposits are found within the walls of retinal vessels and in the RPE and ciliary body, amyloid may gain access to the vitreous through these tissues. In addition, because transthyretin is a blood protein, it may gain access to the vitreous by crossing the blood–aqueous barrier or blood–retina barrier.

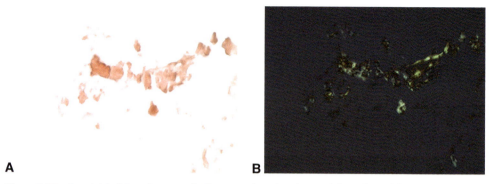

Figure 9-12 Amyloid of the vitreous. **A,** Congo red–stained material, aspirated from the vitreous, shows red-orange staining. **B,** Photomicrograph of the material shown in part A under polarized light; the material exhibits apple-green birefringence (dichroism). *(Courtesy of Nasreen A. Syed, MD.)*

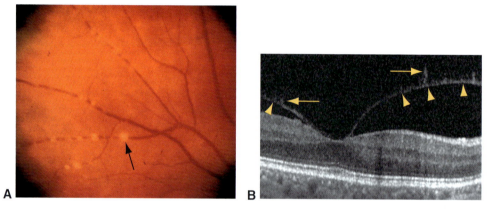

Figure 9-13 Vitreous amyloidosis. **A,** Perivascular sheathing of retinal vessels *(arrow)* associated with vitreous amyloidosis. **B,** OCT demonstrates needlelike amyloid deposits *(arrows)* arranged perpendicular to the partially detached posterior hyaloid face of the vitreous *(arrowheads).* *(Part A courtesy of Hans E. Grossniklaus, MD; part B courtesy of Tatyana Milman, MD.)*

Neoplasia

Intraocular Lymphoma

Primary neoplastic involvement of the vitreous is uncommon because of the relatively acellular nature of the vitreous. However, the vitreous can be the site of primary involvement in cases of large cell lymphoma, which has been referred to as *primary vitreoretinal lymphoma (PVRL)*. Immunohistochemical and molecular genetic studies have confirmed that this entity is typically a B-cell lymphoma; however, T-cell lymphomas may occur in rare instances.

Clinically, PVRL presents most commonly as a vitritis. Some patients have sub-RPE infiltrates with a characteristic speckled pigmentation overlying tumor detachments of the RPE (Fig 9-14). Evidence suggests that the lymphoma cells may be attracted to the

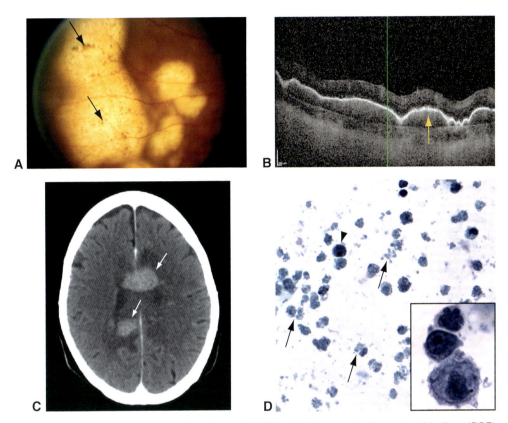

Figure 9-14 Primary vitreoretinal lymphoma (PVRL). **A,** Sub–retinal pigment epithelium (RPE) infiltrates in a patient with PVRL. Note the vitreous debris and subretinal deposits *(arrows)*. **B,** OCT image shows typical sub-RPE infiltrates *(arrow)*. **C,** Axial computed tomography (CT) scan of the brain shows lymphomatous infiltrates *(arrows)*. **D,** Cytologic appearance of PVRL. Note the atypical cells with hyperchromatic nuclei, prominent nucleoli, and scant cytoplasm *(arrowhead)*. Numerous necrotic, smudgy cells *(arrows)* are present. *Inset:* Atypical lymphoid cells with irregular nuclear contours are shown (Papanicolaou [Pap] stain). *(Parts A and D courtesy of Robert H. Rosa Jr, MD; part B courtesy of Elaine M. Binkley, MD; part C courtesy of Steffen Heegaard, MD.)*

RPE by B-cell chemokines and subsequently migrate from the sub-RPE space into the vitreous. In more than half of patients presenting with ocular findings, central nervous system involvement will develop. Neuroimaging of the brain is essential in the workup of patients with PVRL (see Fig 9-14C). See Chapter 19 for more information on the clinical aspects of PVRL.

Diagnosis of PVRL can be challenging and relies primarily on cytologic analysis of vitreous and/or subretinal specimens (for additional information, see BCSC Section 12, *Retina and Vitreous*). Cytologically, the vitreous infiltrate in PVRL is heterogeneous. The atypical cells are large lymphoid cells, frequently with a convoluted nuclear membrane and multiple, conspicuous nucleoli. An accompanying infiltrate of small lymphocytes is almost always present, and the normal cells may obscure the neoplastic cell population. These small round lymphocytes are mostly reactive T cells. Necrotic cells are usually present; their presence is very suggestive of a diagnosis of PVRL (see Fig 9-14D).

Immunohistochemically, the viable tumor cells typically label with B-cell markers. Flow cytometry may be helpful in demonstrating a monoclonal population. Other laboratory tests that may be useful in the diagnosis of PVRL include a panel of immunohistochemical markers (if the amount of tissue is sufficient) and molecular studies for lymphocyte gene rearrangement, as well as for *MYD88* pathogenic variants (found in approximately 80% of cases of PVRL). An IL-10 to IL-6 ratio that is greater than 1.0 may be a useful indicator in select cases.

Clinical Pearl Close communication between the vitreoretinal surgeon and the pathologist is essential prior to scheduling a biopsy in a patient with suspected PVRL. Each pathology laboratory has its own preferred methods for how a specimen is collected and submitted for pathologic analysis. The biopsy sample is usually small, which can be a limiting factor in establishing a diagnosis. To avoid performing multiple biopsies, it is important to ensure that the pathology laboratory is experienced in handling and diagnosing PVRL. See Chapter 2 for further discussion of sample submission requirements and diagnostic testing.

Histologically, the subretinal/sub-RPE infiltrates are composed of neoplastic lymphoid cells (Fig 9-15). With or without treatment, the subretinal infiltrates may resolve, leaving a focal area of RPE atrophy. Optic nerve and retinal infiltration may also be present. Infiltrates in these locations tend to be perivascular and may lead to ischemic retinal

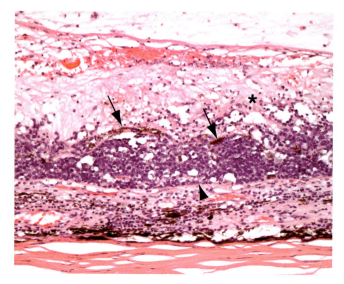

Figure 9-15 Histologic section through retina and choroid shows PVRL. Note the detachment of the inner Bruch membrane and the residual attenuated RPE *(arrows)* by large lymphoid cells, the overlying retinal gliosis *(asterisk),* and the intact outer Bruch membrane *(arrowhead).* Secondary chronic inflammation, composed of small lymphocytes (usually T cells), is present in the underlying choroid. *(Courtesy of Robert H. Rosa Jr, MD.)*

or optic nerve damage. The choroid is typically free of lymphoma cells; however, a secondary reactive population of chronic inflammatory cells, usually small T cells, may be present in the choroid (see Fig 9-15).

In patients with systemic lymphoma with ocular involvement, the choroid (rather than the vitreous, retina, or subretinal space) is usually the primary site of involvement. See Chapter 11 for more information on choroidal lymphoma.

> Soussain C, Malaise D, Cassoux N. Primary vitreoretinal lymphoma: a diagnostic and management challenge. *Blood*. 2021;138(17):1519–1534.

CHAPTER **10**

Retina and Retinal Pigment Epithelium

 This chapter includes related videos. Go to aao.org/bcscvideo_section04 or scan the QR codes in the text to access this content.

 This chapter includes related activities. Go to aao.org/bcscactivity_section04 or scan the QR codes in the text to access this content.

Highlights

- The neurosensory retina has 9 distinct histologic layers; the retinal pigment epithelium lines the outermost of these layers.
- There is a correlation between the clinical appearance and the histologic location of hemorrhage and other deposits in the retina.
- Two vascular sources supply the retina: the retinal circulation supplies the inner layers, and the choroidal circulation supplies the outer layers. Ischemic events involving either vascular source lead to atrophy and thinning of the corresponding retinal layers supplied.
- In many cases of infantile abusive head trauma, histologic abnormalities can be identified in the retina.
- Retinoblastoma is the most common primary intraocular malignancy in children and has characteristic histologic features.

Topography

Two distinct layers form the inner lining of the posterior two-thirds of the globe:

- the neurosensory retina, which is a delicate, transparent layer derived from the inner layer of the optic cup
- the retinal pigment epithelium (RPE), which is a pigmented layer derived from the outer layer of the optic cup

The neurosensory retina is considered part of the central nervous system (CNS). It is continuous anteriorly with the nonpigmented ciliary epithelium, whereas the RPE is continuous with the pigmented ciliary epithelium. The RPE terminates posteriorly at the optic nerve head, along with the underlying Bruch membrane. The nuclear, photoreceptor, and synaptic layers of the neurosensory retina gradually taper at the optic nerve head, and only the nerve fiber layer (NFL) continues to become the optic nerve, making a 90° turn posteriorly as it becomes the optic nerve head (optic disc). See BCSC Section 2, *Fundamentals and Principles of Ophthalmology*, and Section 12, *Retina and Vitreous*, for additional information on the anatomy of the retina and RPE.

Neurosensory Retina

The neurosensory retina has 9 distinct histologic layers (Activity 10-1, Fig 10-1, Video 10-1). An additional layer, the middle limiting membrane (MLM), has been described, but it is not visible as a distinct layer on routine histologic sections of the neurosensory retina.

 ACTIVITY 10-1 Histopathology of the retina.
Developed by Amanda C. Maltry, MD. Photo courtesy of Robert H. Rosa Jr, MD.
Available at: aao.org/bcscactivity_section04

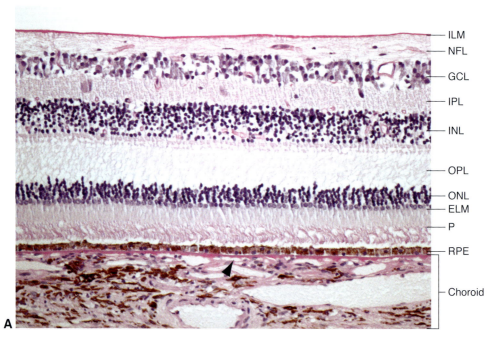

Figure 10-1 Photomicrographs illustrate retinal organization and how it differs depending on location. **A,** Macula, from vitreous *(top of photo)* to choroid *(bottom)*: ILM = internal limiting membrane; NFL = nerve fiber layer; GCL = ganglion cell layer; IPL = inner plexiform layer; INL = inner nuclear layer; OPL = outer plexiform layer; ONL = outer nuclear layer; ELM = external limiting membrane; P = photoreceptors (inner/outer segments) of rods and cones; RPE = retinal pigment epithelium; Bruch membrane *(arrowhead)*. Note that the periodic acid–Schiff (PAS) stain highlights all basement membranes (ILM, basement membrane of retinal capillaries, and Bruch membrane). See also Activity 10-1.

(Continued)

VIDEO 10-1 Histology of the retina and retinal pigment epithelium.
Courtesy of David Hsu, MD, and Vivian Lee, MD. Copyright American Academy of Ophthalmology.
Available at: aao.org/bcscvideo_section04

On optical coherence tomography (OCT), the layers of the neurosensory retina are reminiscent of, but do not exactly correspond with, the 9 layers seen with retinal histopathology (Activity 10-2). The photoreceptor inner segment layer appears as several layers because of its innate optical properties:

- *the myoid zone (MZ):* just external to the external limiting membrane; it contains ribosomes, endoplasmic reticulum, and Golgi bodies
- *the ellipsoid zone (EZ):* closest to the outer segments; it is densely packed with mitochondria of the photoreceptors (Fig 10-2)
- *the interdigitation zone (IZ):* between the outer segments and the RPE

 ACTIVITY 10-2 Optical coherence tomography (OCT) terminology, based on the International Nomenclature for OCT Panel for Normal OCT Terminology.
Reproduced from Staurenghi G, Sadda S, Chakravarthy U, Spaide RF; International Nomenclature for Optical Coherence Tomography (IN·OCT) Panel. Proposed lexicon for anatomic landmarks in normal posterior segment spectral-domain optical coherence tomography: the IN·OCT consensus. Ophthalmology. 2014;121(8):1572–1578. Copyright 2014, with permission from Elsevier.
Available at: aao.org/bcscactivity_section04

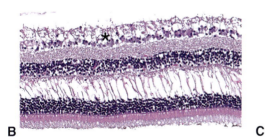

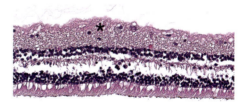

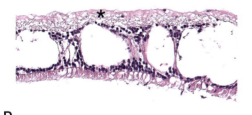

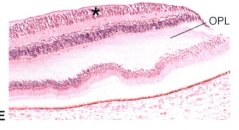

Figure 10-1 *(continued)* **B,** Retina peripheral to the major vascular arcades and posterior to the equator (near-peripheral retina). The *asterisk* denotes the GCL. **C,** Retina in the equatorial region. The *asterisk* denotes the GCL. **D,** Far-peripheral retina near the ora serrata with typical peripheral cystoid degeneration. Note the reduced density of the GCL *(asterisk)* and overall thinning of the inner retinal layers. **E,** In the region of the foveola, the inner cellular layers taper off *(right side of photo)*, with increased density of pigment in the RPE. The incident light falls directly on the photoreceptor outer segments, reducing the potential for distortion of light by overlying tissue elements. Note the multilayered GCL *(asterisk)*, typical of the macula. The OPL fibers travel obliquely in the fovea (Henle fiber layer), and the photoreceptor layer in the fovea consists only of cones.
(Part A courtesy of Robert H. Rosa Jr, MD; parts B–D courtesy of Vivian Lee, MD; part E courtesy of Nasreen A. Syed, MD.)

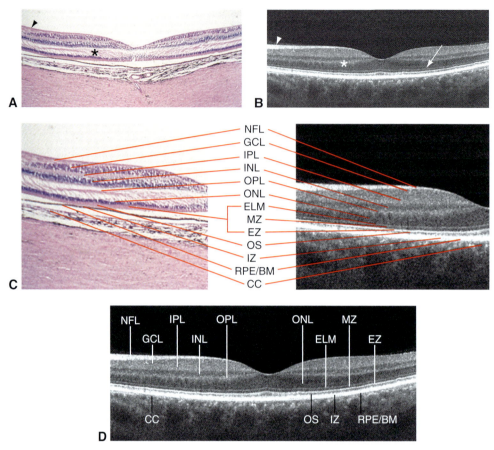

Figure 10-2 Macula. **A,** The normal macula is identified histologically by a thick, multilayered GCL and a central area of focal thinning, the foveola. Note the NFL *(arrowhead)* in the nasal macular region and the oblique orientation of Henle fiber layer (perifoveal OPL) *(asterisk)*. Clinically, the macula lies between the inferior and superior temporal vascular arcades. **B,** Spectral-domain optical coherence tomography (SD-OCT) of the macula shows in vivo imaging with high-resolution details of the lamellar architecture of the retina. Note the NFL *(arrowhead)* in the nasal macular region, Henle fiber layer *(asterisk)*, and the ELM *(arrow)*. **C,** Higher magnification of the photomicrograph shown in part A and the SD-OCT image shown in part B illustrating the corresponding macular layers. **D,** SD-OCT image of the macula. NFL = nerve fiber layer; GCL = ganglion cell layer; IPL = inner plexiform layer; INL = inner nuclear layer; OPL = outer plexiform layer; ONL = outer nuclear layer; ELM = external limiting membrane; MZ = myoid zone; EZ = ellipsoid zone; OS = outer segments; IZ = interdigitation zone between outer segments and RPE; RPE/BM = retinal pigment epithelium/Bruch membrane; CC = choriocapillaris.

(Part B courtesy of Robert H. Rosa Jr, MD; parts C and D adapted from Staurenghi G, Sadda S, Chakravarthy U, Spaide RF; International Nomenclature for Optical Coherence Tomography (IN·OCT) Panel. Proposed lexicon for anatomic landmarks in normal posterior segment spectral-domain optical coherence tomography: the IN·OCT consensus. Ophthalmology. 2014;121(8):1572–1578.)

CHAPTER 10: Retina and Retinal Pigment Epithelium • 171

The morphology of the retina varies depending on the region. For example, histologically, the *macula* is the area of the retina where the ganglion cell layer (GCL) is thicker than a single cell (see Figs 10-1A, 10-2). Clinically, this area corresponds approximately with the area of the retina bounded by the inferior and superior major temporal vascular arcades. The center of the macula is further subdivided into the *fovea*, a central depression in the macula about 1.5 mm in diameter, and the *foveola*, a small pit in the center of the fovea approximately 0.35 mm in diameter. The foveola contains only cone photoreceptor cells (see Fig 10-1E). The concentration of cones is greater in the macula than in the peripheral retina, and only cones are present in the fovea.

In histologic cross sections of the neurosensory retina, the retinal fibers and synaptic processes are arranged perpendicular to the retinal surface, except for the NFL, where the axons bend to run parallel to the retinal surface and converge at the optic nerve head. Consequently, deposits and hemorrhages in the deep retinal layers have a round appearance clinically as they displace the perpendicularly arranged fibers, whereas those in the NFL have a feathery or splinter-shaped appearance (Video 10-2).

 VIDEO 10-2 Appearance of blood in various retinal layers.
Developed by Vivian Lee, MD.
Available at: aao.org/bcscvideo_section04

Clinical Pearl   In the outer plexiform layer (OPL) of the fovea (Henle fiber layer), nerve fibers run obliquely (Video 10-3; see also Figs 10-1E, 10-2A). This morphological feature results in the "flower petal" appearance of cystoid macular edema (CME) on fluorescein angiography (FA), as well as the star-shaped configuration of hard exudates (see Fig 10-18A) observed ophthalmoscopically.

 VIDEO 10-3 Foveal architecture and related pathologies.
Developed by Vivian Lee, MD.
Available at: aao.org/bcscvideo_section04

Xanthophyll pigment gives the macula its yellow appearance clinically and grossly (macula lutea), but the xanthophyll dissolves during tissue processing and is not present in histologic sections. For more on the macula, see BCSC Section 12, *Retina and Vitreous*.

Outside the macula, the GCL consists of a single layer of ganglion cells and astrocytes. The NFL progressively thins moving anteriorly toward the ora serrata from the optic nerve head. In addition, the most peripheral retina near the ora serrata may lack some of the 9 histologic neurosensory layers (see Fig 10-1B–D).

Two vascular sources supply the retina with some overlap (watershed zone) in the inner nuclear layer (INL). The *retinal blood vessels*, branches of the central retinal artery, supply the NFL, GCL, inner plexiform layer (IPL), and inner portion of the INL. The *choroidal vasculature,* specifically the *choriocapillaris,* which is derived from the posterior ciliary arteries, supplies the outer layers of the retina; these include the outer portion of the INL, OPL, outer nuclear layer, photoreceptors, and RPE. The venous network in these layers drains into the vortex veins.

Retinal Pigment Epithelium

The RPE consists of a monolayer of hexagonal cells with apical microvilli. RPE cells appear cuboidal in cross section. The cytoplasm of RPE cells contains numerous melanosomes and lipofuscin. The amount of cytoplasmic lipofuscin increases with age, particularly in the macula. The basement membrane of the RPE forms the inner layer of Bruch membrane. In contrast to the retina, the RPE exhibits more subtle topographic variations. In the macula, the RPE is taller, narrower, and more heavily pigmented than in other regions, and it forms a regular hexagonal array. Anterior to the macula, RPE cells are shorter and larger in diameter. Variability in the diameter of RPE cells increases in the peripheral retina.

Developmental Anomalies

Albinism

The term *albinism* refers to the congenital absence or dilution of the pigment in the skin, eyes, or both. This condition results from genetic pathogenic variations that alter or prevent the biosynthesis of melanin. True albinism is typically divided into *oculocutaneous* and *ocular* forms. Clinically, this distinction is somewhat helpful; however, all cases of ocular albinism have some degree of cutaneous involvement. The 2 types of albinism do have a pathophysiologic difference: in oculocutaneous albinism, transmission is commonly autosomal recessive, and the amount of melanin in each melanosome is reduced; in ocular albinism, transmission is commonly X-linked recessive, and the number of melanosomes is reduced (Fig 10-3). See BCSC Section 6, *Pediatric Ophthalmology and Strabismus,* and Section 12, *Retina and Vitreous,* for further discussion of albinism.

Myelinated Nerve Fibers

Generally, the ganglion cell axonal fibers do not become myelinated until they pass through the lamina cribrosa. However, oligodendroglial cells in the NFL can occasionally produce a myelin sheath around nerve fibers in the retina. Although this type of myelination is usually contiguous with the optic nerve head, it may also occur in isolation, away from the optic nerve head. If large, it can produce a clinically significant scotoma. Myelinated nerve fibers have also been associated with myopia, amblyopia, strabismus, and nystagmus. See BCSC Section 6, *Pediatric Ophthalmology and Strabismus,* for additional discussion of myelinated nerve fibers.

Vascular Anomalies

Numerous developmental anomalies may be observed in the retinal vasculature, including Coats disease and hemangioblastoma. In Coats disease, exudative retinal detachment

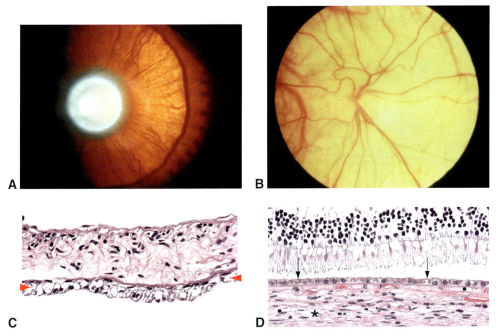

Figure 10-3 Albinism. **A,** Clinical appearance with total iris transillumination. **B,** Fundus photograph illustrating diffuse hypopigmentation. **C,** Photomicrograph illustrates lack of pigment in the iris pigment epithelium *(between arrowheads)*, allowing visualization of the nuclei. No appreciable pigmentation is present in the iris stroma. **D,** Photomicrograph shows the RPE and choroid in an eye with albinism. There is markedly reduced pigment in the RPE cells *(arrows)* and no appreciable pigmentation in the choroid *(asterisk)*. *(Parts A and B courtesy of Robert H. Rosa Jr, MD; parts C and D courtesy of Nasreen A. Syed, MD.)*

is due to leakage from abnormalities in the peripheral retina, which include telangiectatic vessels, aneurysms, and saccular dilatations of the retinal vessels (Fig 10-4). Histologically, retinal detachments secondary to Coats disease are characterized by foamy histiocytes and cholesterol crystals in the subretinal space (see Fig 10-4E).

Retinal hemangioblastoma is a vascular tumor that is often seen in patients with von Hippel–Lindau (VHL) syndrome (retinocerebral angiomatosis) (see Chapter 17). These tumors are composed of many abnormal, capillary-like, fenestrated channels surrounded by vacuolated, foamy stromal cells and reactive glial cells (Fig 10-5). Histologically, retinal and optic nerve hemangioblastomas are similar to hemangioblastomas of the CNS. Loss of heterozygosity of the *VHL* gene has been clearly identified in the vacuolated stromal cells but not in the vascular endothelial or reactive glial cells of retinal and optic nerve hemangioblastomas. Thus, the vacuolated, foamy stromal cells are the actual neoplastic cells of the retinal hemangioblastomas.

See BCSC Section 12, *Retina and Vitreous,* for further discussion of these vascular anomalies and their clinical features.

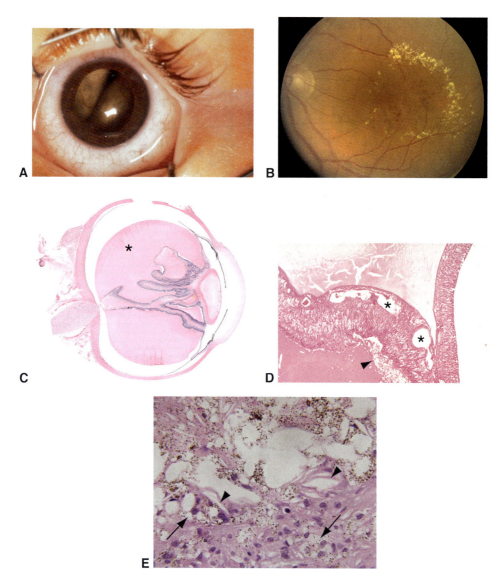

Figure 10-4 Coats disease. **A,** Leukocoria in a patient with Coats disease. **B,** Fundus photograph of mild Coats disease demonstrates multiple retinal macroaneurysms and lipid exudate. **C,** Total exudative retinal detachment in advanced Coats disease with dense subretinal proteinaceous fluid *(asterisk)*. **D,** Telangiectatic retinal vessels *(asterisks)* and foamy histiocytes *(arrowhead)* typical of Coats disease. **E,** High-magnification of subretinal exudate showing lipid-laden and pigment-laden histiocytes *(arrows)* and cholesterol clefts *(arrowheads)*. *(Parts A and D courtesy of Hans E. Grossniklaus, MD; part B courtesy of Benjamin J. Kim, MD; part C courtesy of Amanda C. Maltry, MD; part E courtesy of George J. Harocopos, MD.)*

CHAPTER 10: Retina and Retinal Pigment Epithelium • 175

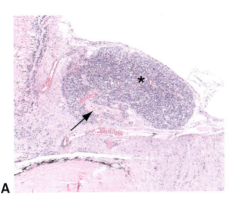 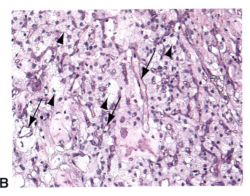

Figure 10-5 Retinal hemangioblastoma in von Hippel–Lindau syndrome (retinocerebral angiomatosis). **A,** Low-magnification photomicrograph shows a retinal tumor *(asterisk)* with a thick-walled feeder vessel *(arrow).* Note the prominent blood vessels and area of dense cellularity composed of stromal cells (PAS stain). **B,** Higher magnification shows the numerous small, capillary-like vascular channels *(arrows).* The vacuolated, foamy stromal cells *(arrowheads)* are the tumor cells that have the pathogenic *VHL* gene variant. *(Part A courtesy of Amanda C. Maltry, MD; part B courtesy of Robert H. Rosa Jr, MD.)*

Congenital Hypertrophy of the RPE

Congenital hypertrophy of the RPE (CHRPE) is a relatively common congenital lesion. It is characterized clinically as a flat, heavily pigmented circumscribed lesion that varies in diameter (see Chapter 16, Fig 16-11). Frequently, with age, central depigmentation may occur in these lesions (lacunae). Histologically, CHRPE is characterized by enlarged RPE cells with densely packed and larger-than-normal melanin granules (Fig 10-6). This

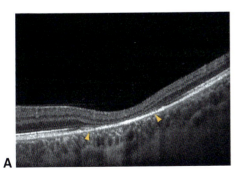 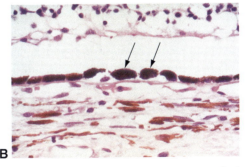

Figure 10-6 Congenital hypertrophy of the RPE (CHRPE). **A,** OCT image shows outer retinal photoreceptor atrophy overlying a CHRPE lesion *(between arrowheads).* **B,** On histopathology, the RPE cells are larger than normal and contain more densely packed melanin granules *(arrows).* There is loss of the overlying photoreceptors correlating with OCT findings (hematoxylin and eosin [H&E] stain). For clinical images of CHRPE, see Chapter 16, Figure 16-11. *(Part A courtesy of Elaine M. Binkley, MD; part B courtesy of Hans E. Grossniklaus, MD.)*

typically benign condition can generally be distinguished from choroidal nevus and melanoma on the basis of ophthalmoscopic features. In rare instances, adenoma and adenocarcinoma of the RPE may develop in eyes with CHRPE.

RPE lesions mimicking CHRPE may be present in *Gardner syndrome,* a subtype of familial adenomatous polyposis. Histologic study reveals that the RPE changes in Gardner syndrome are more consistent with hyperplasia (increase in the number of cells) of the RPE than with hypertrophy. These RPE changes are thus probably more appropriately termed *hamartomas,* consistent with the loss of regulatory control of cell growth that results in other soft-tissue lesions in this syndrome. A germline heterozygous pathogenic variant in the adenomatous polyposis coli gene *(APC)* in individuals with Gardner syndrome confers an increased lifetime risk of developing colorectal polyps and adenocarcinomas and extracolonic benign and malignant neoplasms.

Inflammation

See BCSC Section 9, *Uveitis and Ocular Inflammation,* and Section 12, *Retina and Vitreous,* for further discussion on infectious and noninfectious etiologies of retinitis.

Infectious Etiologies

Bacterial infection
See the discussion of endophthalmitis in Chapter 9 in this volume.

Viral infection
Multiple viruses may cause retinal infections, including rubella virus, measles virus, HIV, herpes simplex virus (HSV), varicella-zoster virus (VZV), and cytomegalovirus (CMV). This section discusses 2 of the most frequent clinical presentations of retinal viral infection, acute retinal necrosis (ARN) and CMV retinitis.

Acute retinal necrosis is a rapidly progressive, necrotizing retinitis caused by infection with HSV types 1 and 2, VZV, or in rare instances, CMV. ARN can occur in healthy or immunocompromised individuals. Histologic findings include moderate to severe inflammation in the vitreous and anterior chamber with prominent obliterative retinal vasculitis and retinal necrosis (Fig 10-7). Inflammatory cells include neutrophils, lymphocytes, plasma cells, and epithelioid histiocytes. Electron microscopy has shown viral inclusions in retinal cells. Polymerase chain reaction analysis of aqueous or vitreous samples is the most sensitive and most rapid method for identifying the presence of virus, reducing the need for viral culture, immunohistochemistry, or other diagnostic techniques.

CMV retinitis is an opportunistic infection that occurs in immunosuppressed patients (Fig 10-8). Histologically, it is characterized by retinal necrosis that heals with a thin fibroglial scar. Acute lesions show enlarged retinal cells (20–30 μm) that contain large eosinophilic intranuclear and/or intracytoplasmic inclusion bodies (see Fig 10-8C, D). At the cellular level, CMV may infect vascular endothelial cells, retinal neurons, glial cells, the RPE, and histiocytes. Because of the immunocompromised status of the infected host, a prominent inflammatory infiltrate is typically not present.

CHAPTER 10: Retina and Retinal Pigment Epithelium • 177

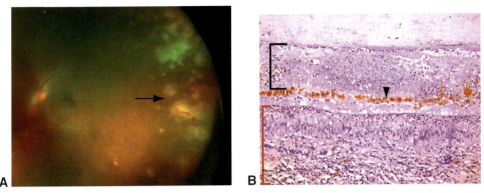

Figure 10-7 Acute retinal necrosis (ARN). **A,** Wide-field fundus photograph reveals areas of retinal necrosis manifesting as white areas and hemorrhage *(arrow)* in the periphery. The hazy appearance is due to vitritis. **B,** Photomicrograph from a different patient reveals full-thickness necrosis of the retina *(black bracket)* above remaining RPE cells *(arrowhead)*. Acute and chronic granulomatous inflammation is present below Bruch membrane *(red bracket)*. Neutrophils, epithelioid histiocytes, lymphocytes, and plasma cells are present with a zonal arrangement from top to bottom. *(Part A courtesy of Benjamin J. Kim, MD; part B courtesy of Vivian Lee, MD.)*

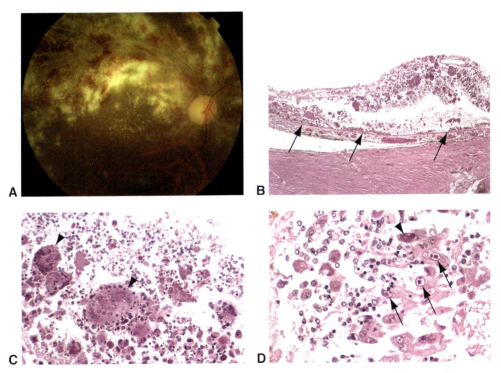

Figure 10-8 Cytomegalovirus (CMV) retinitis. **A,** Retinal hemorrhages and areas of opaque retina are present. Note the white vascular sheathing along the superotemporal arcade and hard exudates in the macular region. **B,** Histologically, full-thickness retinal necrosis is present. Note the loss of the normal lamellar architecture of the retina, including disruption of the RPE above Bruch membrane *(arrows)*. **C,** Large syncytial cells, characteristic of CMV retinitis, form from retinal cells infected with virus *(arrowheads)*. **D,** Intranuclear "owl's eye" inclusions *(arrows)* and intracytoplasmic inclusion bodies *(arrowhead)* are present in CMV-infected cells. *(Courtesy of Robert H. Rosa Jr, MD.)*

Fungal infection

Fungal infections of the retina are uncommon, occurring most often in individuals with endogenous endophthalmitis, in immunosuppressed individuals, and in individuals with fungemia (eg, from parenteral nutrition or intravenous drug use). These infections usually begin as single or multiple small foci in the choroid or retina (Fig 10-9). The most common causative fungi are *Candida* species, particularly *C albicans*, followed by *Aspergillus* species and other less common agents.

Histologically, fungal infections are frequently characterized by necrotizing granulomatous inflammation, comprising a central zone of necrosis surrounded by epithelioid histiocytes and multinucleated giant cells with an outer layer of lymphocytes. Although histologic examination may reveal the causative agent, a culture and/or molecular studies are required for definitive identification of the organism. With treatment, these lesions heal with a fibroglial scar.

Protozoal infection

Toxoplasmic retinochoroiditis (also called *toxoplasmic chorioretinitis, ocular toxoplasmosis*) is the most common type of infectious retinitis. It may be due to reactivation of a congenitally acquired infection or to an acquired *Toxoplasma* infection in healthy or immunocompromised individuals. In patients with reactivated disease, toxoplasmic retinochoroiditis

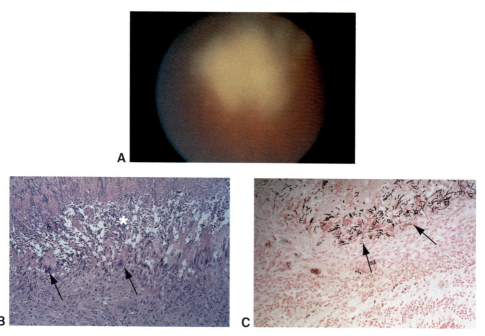

Figure 10-9 Fungal chorioretinitis. **A,** Clinical appearance of vitreous, retinal, and choroidal infiltrates in a patient with fungal chorioretinitis. The vitreous cells give the photograph a hazy appearance. **B,** Granulomatous infiltration surrounds a central area of necrosis *(asterisk)*. Frequent multinucleated giant cells are present *(arrows)*. **C,** Grocott-Gomori methenamine–silver nitrate stain of the section parallel to that shown in part B demonstrates numerous fungal hyphae, which stain black *(arrows)*. *(Courtesy of David J. Wilson, MD.)*

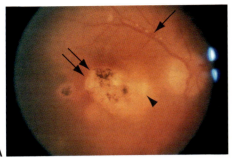 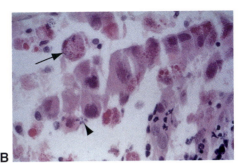

Figure 10-10 Toxoplasmic retinochoroiditis. **A,** Fundus photograph shows chorioretinal scars rimmed with pigment *(double arrow)*, typical of prior infection with *Toxoplasma* species. Active retinitis *(arrowhead)* and perivascular sheathing *(arrow)* are present. **B,** Cysts *(arrow)* and extracellular organisms (tachyzoites; *arrowhead*) in active toxoplasmic retinochoroiditis. *(Courtesy of Hans E. Grossniklaus, MD.)*

typically presents as a posterior uveitis or panuveitis with marked vitritis and focal retinochoroiditis adjacent to a pigmented chorioretinal scar. The absence of a preexisting chorioretinal scar suggests newly acquired disease.

Microscopic examination of active toxoplasmic retinochoroiditis reveals necrosis of the retina, a prominent infiltrate of neutrophils and lymphocytes, and *Toxoplasma* organisms in the form of tissue cysts and tachyzoites (Fig 10-10). There is generally a prominent lymphocytic infiltrate in the vitreous and the anterior segment and granulomatous inflammation in the inner choroid. Healing brings resolution of the inflammatory cell infiltrate with encystment of the organisms in the retina adjacent to the atrophic chorioretinal scar.

Noninfectious Etiologies

Noninfectious inflammation of the retina may be acute with an infiltrate of neutrophils, chronic with an infiltrate of lymphocytes and plasma cells, or granulomatous with the presence of epithelioid histiocytes and/or multinucleated giant cells in the inflammatory infiltrate.

Degenerations

The clinical features of various retinal degenerations are discussed in BCSC Section 12, *Retina and Vitreous*.

Typical and Reticular Peripheral Cystoid Degeneration and Retinoschisis

In *typical peripheral cystoid degeneration (TPCD)*, which is a universal finding in the eyes of individuals older than 20 years, cystoid spaces develop in the outer plexiform layer of the retina. In *reticular peripheral cystoid degeneration (RPCD)*, which is less common than TPCD, cystoid spaces develop in the NFL, posterior to areas of TPCD (Fig 10-11; also see Fig 10-1D). Coalescence of the cystoid spaces of TPCD forms *typical degenerative retinoschisis*, usually in the inferotemporal region. In *reticular degenerative retinoschisis*, the retinal layers split in the NFL.

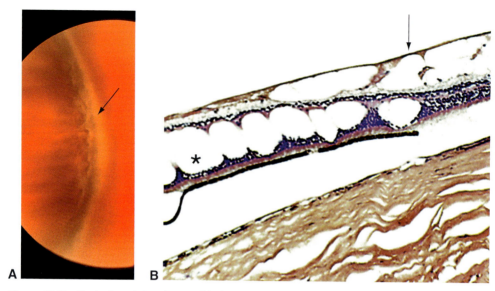

Figure 10-11 Typical peripheral cystoid degeneration (TPCD). **A,** Indented exam of "moth-eaten" appearance at the ora serrata *(arrow)*. The anterior eye is toward the left side of the photograph. **B,** Photomicrograph of cystoid spaces in the OPL *(asterisk)*. Similar to part A, the anterior eye is toward the left side of the photograph. Reticular peripheral cystoid degeneration (RPCD) is posterior to the TPCD *(arrow)* in the NFL. Coalescence of these cystoid spaces results in retinoschisis. *(Part A courtesy of the Retina Image Bank by Norman Byer, MD, from "The Peripheral Retina in Profile." Updated 2012. Image number 1977, © American Society of Retina Specialists.)*

Lattice Degeneration

Although lattice degeneration (Fig 10-12) may be a familial condition, it is found in up to 10% of the general population. Retinal detachment develops in only a small number of individuals with lattice degeneration; on the other hand, lattice degeneration is seen in up to 20%–30% of all patients with rhegmatogenous detachments.

The most important histologic features of lattice degeneration are

- discontinuity of the internal limiting membrane (ILM) of the retina
- an overlying pocket of liquefied vitreous
- focal sclerosis of retinal vessels, which remain physiologically patent
- condensation and adherence of vitreous at the margins of the lesion
- variable degrees of atrophy of the inner layers of the retina

Radial perivascular lattice degeneration has the same histologic features as typical lattice degeneration, but it occurs more posteriorly along the course of retinal vessels.

Clinical Pearl Retinal detachment in individuals with lattice degeneration is caused by vitreous adhesion at the margins of the degeneration, leading to retinal tears. In contrast, atrophic holes that develop in the center of a lattice lesion are rarely the cause of retinal detachment.

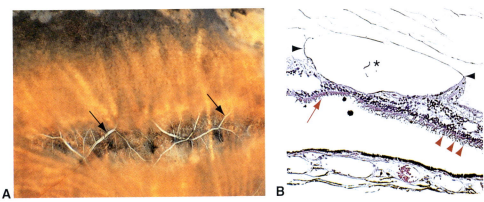

Figure 10-12 Retinal lattice degeneration. **A,** Lattice degeneration appears clinically as prominent sclerotic vessels *(arrows)* in a wicker or lattice pattern. **B,** The vitreous directly over the lattice degeneration is liquefied *(asterisk),* but formed vitreous remains adherent at the margins *(black arrowheads)* of the degenerated area. The inner retinal layers are atrophic and the overlying ILM is disrupted. This disruption is not apparent in this H&E-stained preparation and is best appreciated with PAS stain. The retina shows focal atrophy of photoreceptor outer segments *(arrow)* compatible with a focal chronic retinal detachment from vitreoretinal traction. Elsewhere, the retina shows preservation of photoreceptor outer segments *(red arrowheads),* compatible with artifactitious retinal detachment.

Sequelae of Retinal Detachment

When any type of retinal detachment occurs, loss of the photoreceptor outer segments in the region of the detachment is the earliest change identified. Eventually, if the detachment is not repaired or does not resolve, other degenerative changes can be identified, including loss of the photoreceptor cells, migration of Müller cells, and proliferation and migration of RPE cells. RPE cells, when not in contact with the neurosensory retina, can undergo metaplasia, becoming fibroblast-like cells or even osseous tissue. In addition, the RPE may produce more basement membrane, focally leading to the formation of nodular and calcified drusen. Small cystic spaces develop in the detached retina over time, and in cases of chronic detachment, these cysts may coalesce into large macrocysts (Fig 10-13).

Paving-Stone Degeneration

Focal occlusion of the choriocapillaris can lead to loss of the outer retinal layers and RPE, a condition known as *paving-stone* or *cobblestone degeneration.* This type of atrophy is common in the retinal periphery in older individuals. The well-demarcated, flat, pale lesions seen clinically correspond to circumscribed areas of outer retinal and RPE atrophy and loss of the choriocapillaris, with adherence of the inner retina to Bruch membrane (Fig 10-14). Histologically, these findings are similar to those found in geographic atrophy in age-related macular degeneration and to scarring from application of a thermal laser.

182 • Ophthalmic Pathology and Intraocular Tumors

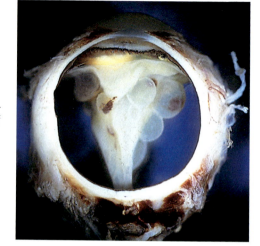

Figure 10-13 Long-standing total retinal detachment with macrocystic degeneration of the retina.

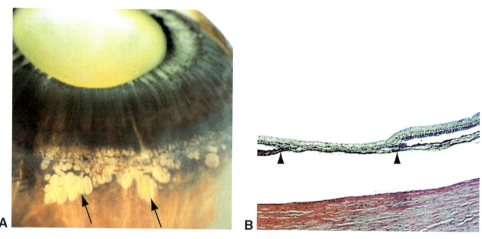

Figure 10-14 Paving-stone degeneration. **A,** Photograph shows the gross appearance of paving-stone degeneration: areas of depigmentation *(arrows)* in the peripheral retina near the ora serrata. **B,** Histologically, paving-stone degeneration shows atrophy of the outer retinal layers and adhesion of the remaining inner retinal elements to Bruch membrane. The sharp boundary *(arrowheads)* between the normal and the atrophic retina corresponds to the clinical appearance of paving-stone degeneration (Masson trichrome stain).

Ischemia

Because the retina has a dual blood supply, the histologic findings associated with ischemic vascular insults vary. Occlusion of the retinal vessels leads to *inner ischemic retinal atrophy* with atrophy of retinal ganglion cells and astrocytes, partial atrophy of the INL, and thinning of the NFL. Occlusion of the choroidal vessels leads to *outer ischemic retinal atrophy,* including loss of the photoreceptor segments and nuclei, loss of the OPL, and sometimes thinning of the INL (Fig 10-15).

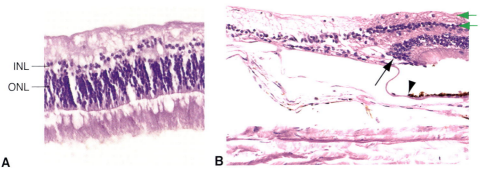

Figure 10-15 Ischemic retinal atrophy. **A,** Inner retinal ischemic atrophy. The photoreceptor nuclei and the outer portion of the INL are normal in appearance. The inner portion of the INL is absent. There are no ganglion cells, and the nerve fiber layer is thin, appearing to merge with the inner plexiform layer. This pattern of ischemia corresponds to the supply of the retinal arteriolar circulation and may be seen after healing from retinal arterial and venous occlusions. **B,** Outer ischemic retinal atrophy. Begin at the right edge of the photograph and trace the ganglion cell and inner nuclear layers *(green arrows).* In this case, there is loss of the nuclei of the photoreceptor layer (ONL) *(arrow),* the photoreceptor inner and outer segments, and the RPE *(arrowhead).* This is the pattern of outer retinal atrophy secondary to interruption in the choroidal blood supply.

Retinal ischemia can be caused by many conditions, including diabetes, retinal artery and vein occlusions, radiation retinopathy, retinopathy of prematurity, sickle cell retinopathy, vasculitis, and carotid occlusive disease (some of these diseases are discussed later in this chapter). Some of these entities result in focal retinal atrophy; others, in diffuse retinal atrophy. The increased use of optical coherence tomography angiography (OCTA), which depicts all capillary layers of the retina, is improving our understanding of vascular pathologies affecting this area. See BCSC Section 12, *Retina and Vitreous,* for further information on OCTA.

Nevertheless, certain histologic findings—both cellular and vascular responses—are common to all disorders that result in retinal ischemia.

Retinal changes

Cellular responses Neurons in the retina are highly active metabolically, requiring large amounts of oxygen for production of adenosine triphosphate (ATP) (see BCSC Section 2, *Fundamentals and Principles of Ophthalmology,* Part IV, Biochemistry and Metabolism). This makes them highly sensitive to interruption of their blood supply. With prolonged oxygen deprivation (>90 minutes in experimental studies), neuronal cell nuclei sustain irreversible damage and are subsequently phagocytosed by microglia. Microglia are involved in the phagocytosis of necrotic cells, as well as of extracellular lipid or blood, that accumulate in areas of ischemia in the CNS. Microglial cells are fairly resistant to ischemia.

Retinal neurons such as ganglion cells, photoreceptors, amacrine cells, horizontal cells, and bipolar cells have no capacity for regeneration after damage. In response to injury, the nerve fibers of the ganglion cells swell, appearing histologically as pseudocells, known as *cytoid bodies* (Fig 10-16). These localized accumulations of axoplasmic material

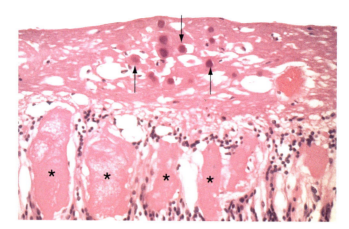

Figure 10-16 NFL infarct. Cytoid bodies *(arrows)* within the NFL represent axoplasmic swelling of ganglion cell axons secondary to ischemia, seen clinically as cotton-wool spots. The cystoid spaces *(asterisks)* in the deeper retina are filled with proteinaceous fluid and represent retinal exudation. Resolution of NFL infarct leads to inner retinal ischemic atrophy (see Fig 10-15A). *(Courtesy of W. Richard Green, MD.)*

are present in ischemic infarcts of the NFL. Cotton-wool spots are the clinical correlate of small infarctions in the NFL. They resolve over 4–12 weeks, leaving an area of inner ischemic retinal atrophy.

Like neurons, glial cells degenerate in areas of infarction. These cells may proliferate adjacent to focal areas of infarction as well as in ischemic areas without infarction, resulting in *gliosis,* a glial scar. The location and extent of atrophic retina resulting from ischemia depend on the size of the occluded vessel and on whether it is a retinal or a choroidal blood vessel.

Vascular responses Ischemia damages the inner blood–retina barrier, resulting in leakage of the retinal vasculature into the extracellular space. Ischemia manifests as *edema* from transudation of fluid and serum components, *exudate* secondary to accumulation of lipid, and *hemorrhage.*

Edema is one of the earliest manifestations of retinal ischemia. Fluid pockets are delimited by the surrounding neurons and glial cells. In the perifoveal region, this results in cystoid macular edema (CME) (Fig 10-17; see also BCSC Section 12, *Retina and Vitreous,* for additional discussion and images of CME). Lipid exudates appear histologically as sharply circumscribed eosinophilic spaces between the retinal fibers (Fig 10-18).

Retinal deposits conform to the surrounding retinal tissue. The pattern of extracellular fluid or blood in the retina is indicative of the retinal area or layer involved (Fig 10-19; see also Videos 10-2 and 10-3):

- *perifoveal outer plexiform layer (Henle layer):* "petaloid" CME, macular star configuration (see Fig 10-18A)
- *NFL:* flame-shaped hemorrhage
- *nuclear or inner plexiform layer:* circular "dot-and-blot" hemorrhage
- *subhyaloid hemorrhage:* boat-shaped configuration

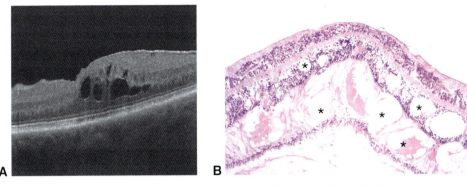

Figure 10-17 Cystoid macular edema (CME). **A,** SD-OCT image of CME. **B,** Histologically, cystoid spaces are present in the INL and OPL *(asterisks)*. *(Part A courtesy of the Retina Image Bank by Theodore Leng, MD, MS. Image number 27394, © American Society of Retina Specialists; part B courtesy of Nasreen A. Syed, MD.)*

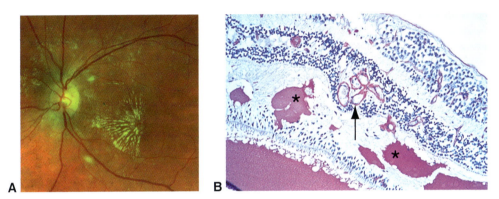

Figure 10-18 Lipid exudates. **A,** Clinical appearance of intraretinal lipid deposits, or hard exudates, in a partial macular star formation. **B,** PAS stain shows intraretinal exudates *(asterisks)* surrounding intraretinal microvascular abnormalities (IRMAs) *(arrow)*. *(Part A courtesy of Amanda C. Maltry, MD; part B courtesy of W. Richard Green, MD.)*

Chronic retinal ischemia leads to architectural changes in the retinal vessels. In the capillary bed, the endothelial cells and pericytes atrophy, and it becomes acellular in an area of vascular occlusion. Adjacent to acellular areas, irregular dilated vascular channels known as *intraretinal microvascular abnormalities (IRMAs)* (Fig 10-20A; also see Fig 10-18B) and microaneurysms often develop. *Microaneurysms* are fusiform or saccular outpouchings of the retinal capillaries; they are best seen clinically with FA and histologically with elastase digest flat mounts stained with periodic acid–Schiff (PAS) stain (Fig 10-20B).

Neovascularization of the retina and the vitreous can occur in cases of retinal ischemia, most commonly in individuals with diabetes and central retinal vein occlusion. Retinal neovascularization arises from existing retinal blood vessels and penetrates the ILM, extending into the vitreous (Fig 10-21). Hemorrhage may develop from retinal neovascularization as the vitreous exerts traction on fragile new vessels.

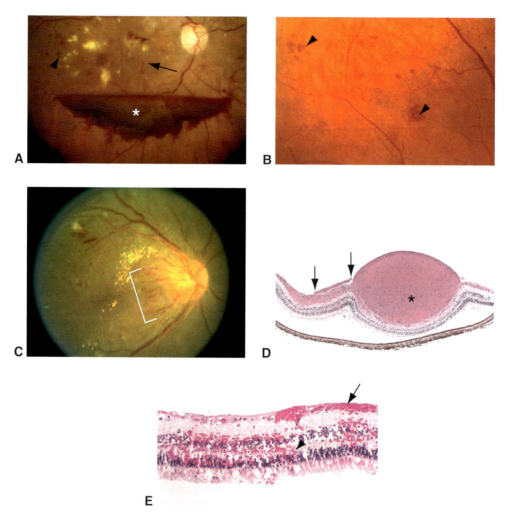

Figure 10-19 Retinal hemorrhage. **A,** Fundus photograph shows dot-and-blot *(arrowhead)* and flame-shaped *(arrow)* intraretinal hemorrhages and boat-shaped preretinal hemorrhage *(asterisk)* in proliferative diabetic retinopathy. **B,** Fundus photograph shows dot-and-blot intraretinal hemorrhages *(arrowheads)*. **C,** Fundus photograph shows multiple flame-shaped hemorrhages *(bracket)* in the retina surrounding the nerve. **D,** Histologically, preretinal hemorrhage may be just inside ILM in the vitreous *(between arrows)* or just outside the ILM, creating a bullous hemorrhage in the innermost retina *(asterisk)*. **E,** Histologically, the dot-and-blot hemorrhage corresponds to blood in the middle layers (INL and OPL) of the retina *(arrowhead)*, whereas flame-shaped hemorrhage corresponds to blood in the NFL *(arrow)*. *(Parts A and E courtesy of Robert H. Rosa Jr, MD; part B courtesy of Benjamin J. Kim, MD; part D courtesy of Nasreen A. Syed, MD.)*

Many of the vascular changes in retinal ischemia are mediated by vascular endothelial growth factor (VEGF), which is a potent stimulus of vascular permeability and angiogenesis. Biologic agents that inhibit VEGF (eg, bevacizumab, ranibizumab, and aflibercept) and intravitreally administered triamcinolone acetonide are used to treat various retinal diseases associated with macular edema and choroidal neovascularization. See BCSC Section 12, *Retina and Vitreous,* for more information on retinal neovascularization.

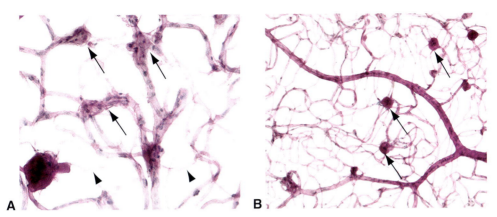

Figure 10-20 Elastase digest preparation of retinal tissue (PAS stain). **A,** Acellular capillaries *(arrowheads)* adjacent to IRMAs *(arrows)*. **B,** Retinal microaneurysms in an individual with diabetic retinopathy *(arrows)*. The density of the endothelial cells that line the IRMAs and microaneurysms frequently varies; the microaneurysms evolve from being thin-walled and hypercellular to being hyalinized and hypocellular. *(Courtesy of Nora V. Laver, MD.)*

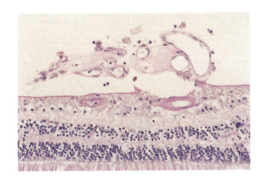

Figure 10-21 Retinal neovascularization. New blood vessels have broken through the ILM into the vitreous (PAS stain). *(Courtesy of Alan Proia, MD, PhD.)*

Laver NM, Robison WG Jr, Pfeffer BA. Novel procedures for isolating intact retinal vascular beds from diabetic humans and animal models. *Invest Ophthalmol Vis Sci.* 1993;34(6):2097–2104.

Specific ischemic retinal disorders

See BCSC Section 12, *Retina and Vitreous,* for additional information on the topics discussed below.

Central and branch retinal artery occlusions *Central retinal artery occlusion (CRAO)* results from localized arteriosclerotic changes, an embolus, and in rare instances, vasculitis (as in giant cell arteritis). As the retina becomes ischemic, it swells and loses its transparency. This swelling is best seen clinically and histologically in the posterior pole, where the NFL and the GCL are thickest (Fig 10-22). In the fovea, where the GCL and the NFL are absent, a cherry-red spot can be appreciated clinically, owing to the stark contrast between the normal color of the choroid and the surrounding swollen white retina.

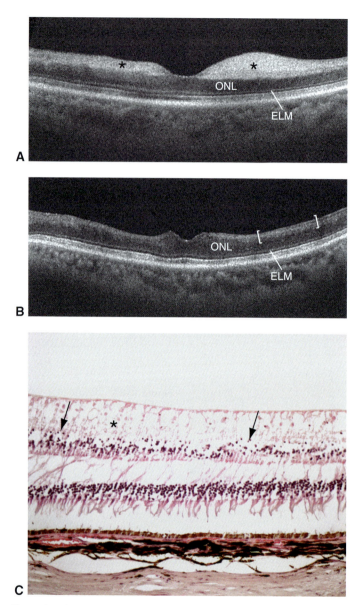

Figure 10-22 Central retinal artery occlusion (CRAO). **A,** SD-OCT reveals increased reflectivity in the area of retinal necrosis *(asterisks).* **B,** SD-OCT performed at a later date in the same patient as in part A reveals thinning of the inner retina *(in brackets)* with loss of the normal lamellar architecture up to the OPL–ONL junction. **C,** Histologically, necrosis occurs in the inner retina *(asterisk),* corresponding to the retinal whitening observed on ophthalmoscopic examination. Note the pyknotic nuclei *(arrows)* in the inner aspect of the inner nuclear layer. ELM = external limiting membrane; ONL = outer nuclear layer. *(Courtesy of Robert H. Rosa Jr, MD.)*

Branch retinal artery occlusion (BRAO) is usually caused by an embolus that lodges at the bifurcation of a retinal arteriole. As in CRAO, this embolic event may be the first or most important indicator of a significant systemic disorder, such as carotid vascular disease (cholesterol emboli or *Hollenhorst plaques*), cardiac valvular disease (calcific emboli), or cardiac thromboembolism (platelet-fibrin emboli). In the acute phase, BRAO is characterized histologically by swelling of the inner retinal layers with early cell death in the distribution of the occluded artery.

As the swelling of the retina eventually clears in eyes with CRAO and BRAO, the classic picture of inner ischemic atrophy emerges, with loss of cells in the NFL, GCL, IPL, and INL (see Figs 10-15, 10-22). Arterial and arteriolar occlusions result in infarcts with subsequent complete atrophy of the affected layers in the distribution of the affected vessel.

> Flaxel CJ, Adelman RA, Bailey ST, et al; American Academy of Ophthalmology Preferred Practice Pattern Retina/Vitreous Committee. Retinal and Ophthalmic Artery Occlusions Preferred Practice Pattern. *Ophthalmology*. 2020;127(2):P259–P287. doi:10.1016/j.ophtha.2019.09.028

Central and branch retinal vein occlusions *Central retinal vein occlusion (CRVO)* usually occurs due to arteriosclerotic changes in the central retinal artery at or posterior to the lamina cribrosa that lead to compression of the central retinal vein where the vessels share a common adventitial sheath. This compression induces turbulent flow and vascular endothelial damage in the vein, leading to thrombosis. The risk factors of CRVO include increasing age, hypertension, diabetes, and glaucoma.

CRVO has 2 forms:

- milder, perfused (nonischemic) type, with <10 disc areas of nonperfusion on FA
- more severe, nonperfused (ischemic) type, with >10 disc areas of nonperfusion on FA

Both forms of CRVO may be recognized clinically by the presence of hemorrhages in all 4 retinal quadrants. Prominent edema of the optic nerve head is typically present, along with dilatation and tortuosity of the retinal veins, variable numbers of cotton-wool spots, and macular edema.

Histologically, acute ischemic CRVO is characterized by marked retinal edema, focal retinal necrosis, and extensive intraretinal hemorrhage. In cases of long-standing CRVO, inner retinal ischemic atrophy develops. The glial cells respond to the insult with proliferation and intracellular deposition of filaments *(gliosis)*. The hemorrhage, disorganization of the retinal architecture, hemosiderosis, and gliosis associated with vein occlusions distinguish the final histologic picture of inner ischemic retinal atrophy in CRVO from that of CRAO (Fig 10-23). After a CRVO, numerous microaneurysms develop in the retinal capillaries, and acellular capillary beds are present to a variable degree. Over time, dilated collateral vessels develop at the optic nerve head. A significant amount of VEGF is often elaborated by oxygen-deprived retinal cells and endothelial cells, with resultant neovascularization of the iris and angle and, less often, the retina.

In *branch retinal vein occlusion (BRVO),* occlusion of a tributary retinal vein occurs at the site of an arteriovenous crossing. At the crossing of a branch retinal artery and vein, the 2 vessels share a common adventitial sheath. With arteriosclerotic changes in the arteriole,

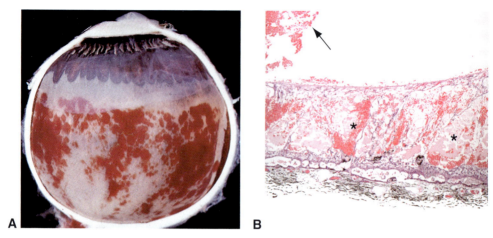

Figure 10-23 Central retinal vein occlusion (CRVO). **A,** Gross appearance of diffuse retinal hemorrhage after CRVO. **B,** Photomicrograph of a long-standing CRVO shows loss of the normal lamellar architecture of the retina, marked edema with cystoid spaces *(asterisks)* containing blood and proteinaceous exudate, and vitreous hemorrhage *(arrow)*. *(Part B courtesy of Robert H. Rosa Jr, MD.)*

the retinal venule may become compressed, leading to turbulent flow and thrombosis similar to that causing CRVO. Systemic arteriosclerosis and hypertension are risk factors for developing BRVO. BRVO leads to sectoral retinal hemorrhages and cotton-wool spots; however, because it does not always result in total inner retinal ischemia, neovascularization is unlikely unless the ischemia is extensive (>5 disc areas). Findings in eyes with permanent vision loss from BRVO include CME, retinal nonperfusion, macular edema with hard lipid exudates, late pigmentary changes in the macula, subretinal fibrosis, and epiretinal membrane formation. Although the histologic picture of BRVO resembles that of CRVO, in eyes with BRVO, the changes are localized to the retinal area in the distribution of the occluded vein.

> Baseline and early natural history report: the Central Vein Occlusion Study. *Arch Ophthalmol.* 1993;111(8):1087–1095.
>
> Flaxel CJ, Adelman RA, Bailey ST, et al; American Academy of Ophthalmology Preferred Practice Pattern Retina/Vitreous Committee. Retinal Vein Occlusions Preferred Practice Pattern. *Ophthalmology.* 2020;127(2):P288–P320. doi:10.1016/j.ophtha.2019.09.029. Published correction appears in *Ophthalmology.* 2020;127(9):1279.

Diabetic retinopathy

Diabetic retinopathy is one of the most common causes of new blindness in the United States and remains the leading cause of blindness among adults aged 25–74 in high-income countries. Early physiologic abnormalities in cases of diabetic retinopathy include

- impaired autoregulation of the retinal vasculature
- alterations in retinal blood flow
- breakdown of the blood–retina barrier

Histologically, the primary changes occur in the retinal microcirculation, including

- thickening of the retinal capillary basement membrane
- selective loss of capillary pericytes
- microaneurysm formation
- retinal capillary closure (histologically recognized as acellular capillary beds)

Dilated intraretinal telangiectatic vessels, or IRMAs, may develop (see Figs 10-18, 10-20), and neovascularization may follow (see Fig 10-21). Intraretinal edema, hemorrhages, exudates, and microinfarcts of the NFL may develop secondary to primary retinal vascular changes. Acutely, microinfarcts of the NFL (see Fig 10-16) manifest clinically as cotton-wool spots. Subsequently, focal inner ischemic atrophy appears (see Fig 10-15).

Laser photocoagulation, used in the treatment of diabetic retinopathy, results in focal destruction of the retina and RPE and occlusion of the choriocapillaris (Fig 10-24). These burns heal by proliferation of the underlying RPE and gliosis, forming a chorioretinal adhesion.

Diabetic choroidopathy

In patients with diabetes, alterations to the choroid are common in addition to retinal findings. Risk factors for diabetic choroidopathy include diabetic retinopathy, poor disease control, and the need for insulin as part of the diabetic treatment regimen. Histologic studies have shown loss of the choriocapillaris, tortuous blood vessels, microaneurysms, drusenoid deposits on Bruch membrane, and choroidal neovascularization. Most of these findings occur at or anterior to the equator.

Lutty GA. Diabetic choroidopathy. *Vision Res.* 2017;139:161–167.

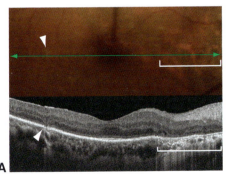
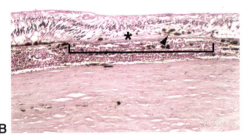

Figure 10-24 Laser photocoagulation scars. **A,** Clinical photograph *(upper panel)* and SD-OCT *(lower panel)* show a focal laser scar *(arrowheads)* and area of peripapillary atrophy *(brackets)*. The *double-headed arrow (upper panel)* indicates the meridian of the SD-OCT scan through the macula *(lower panel)*. In the *lower panel,* note the disruption of the OPL, ONL, EZ, and RPE in the region of the focal laser scar *(bracket)*. **B,** In more intense laser applications, loss of the photoreceptor cell layer and RPE and obliteration of the choriocapillaris *(bracket)* may occur. Note the thin subretinal fibrosis *(asterisk)* in the laser scar. Variable RPE hypertrophy, hyperplasia, and migration into the retina *(arrowhead)*, as well as breaks in Bruch membrane, can occur. *(Courtesy of Robert H. Rosa Jr, MD.)*

Other intraocular changes in diabetes

In diabetes, prolonged hyperglycemia can result in many intraocular changes. The corneal epithelial basement membrane thickens and can result in inadequate adherence of the epithelium to the underlying Bowman layer. This change predisposes patients with diabetes to corneal abrasions and poor corneal epithelial healing. Lacy vacuolation of the iris pigment epithelium (Fig 10-25A) occurs in association with acute hyperglycemia. Histologically, the intraepithelial vacuoles contain glycogen, which is PAS-positive and diastase-sensitive. Thickening of the basement membrane of the pigmented ciliary epithelium (Fig 10-25B) is almost universally present in the eyes of patients with long-standing diabetes. The incidence of cataract formation is also increased.

Abusive Head Trauma

Abusive head trauma (AHT) or nonaccidental trauma (formerly known as *shaken baby syndrome*) is physical abuse that results in traumatic brain injury as well as injury to other structures in the head and neck of a young child. Victims of AHT are usually younger than 5 years and are most commonly younger than 12 months. Though it is not necessarily a degenerative process, AHT induces a variety of changes over time and therefore is included in this section.

Ocular findings in patients with AHT often result from repetitive acceleration-deceleration forces applied to the head with or without direct head trauma. Injuries stem from the complex interactions of ocular and intracranial forces, as well as injuries to other parts of the body. In cases of suspected AHT, the ophthalmologist may elicit critical clinical evidence by performing a thorough dilated fundus examination. On clinical examination, the most frequent ocular finding is retinal hemorrhage, present in up to 90% of cases. However, absence of retinal hemorrhages does not entirely exclude a diagnosis of AHT. Circumferential perimacular folds are considered a specific finding of AHT, but they are not pathognomonic.

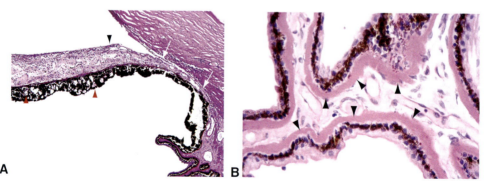

Figure 10-25 Histologic intraocular changes in a patient with diabetes. **A,** PAS stain shows iris neovascularization *(black arrowhead)*, angle closure by peripheral anterior synechiae *(between white arrows)*, and purple glycogen deposits in the lacy vacuolation of the iris pigment epithelium *(red arrowheads)*. **B,** High-magnification photomicrograph shows marked thickening of the basement membrane of the pigmented ciliary epithelium, highlighted with PAS stain *(arrowheads)*. *(Part A courtesy of Tatyana Milman, MD; part B courtesy of Nasreen A. Syed, MD.)*

Because AHT is sometimes fatal, forensic examination of the eyes at autopsy is important. On gross examination of the globe, retinal hemorrhages may be dispersed throughout the fundus (Fig 10-26). Subdural hemorrhage in the optic nerve sheath may also be visible grossly (Fig 10-27; also see Fig 10-26) and can be appreciated macroscopically as a bluish discoloration of the optic nerve sheath.

Histologic findings in the eye may include

- hemorrhages involving any layer of the retina
- hemorrhagic retinal schisis cavities, usually manifesting as hemorrhagic ILM detachment from the neurosensory retina
- retinal hemorrhages that extend from the optic nerve to the ora serrata
- subretinal hemorrhage
- subdural hemorrhage in the optic nerve sheath
- subarachnoid, focal intradural and/or focal epidural hemorrhage of the optic nerve sheath
- perimacular circumferential retinal fold, often associated with sub-ILM hemorrhage
- intrascleral hemorrhage adjacent to the optic nerve (see Fig 10-26)

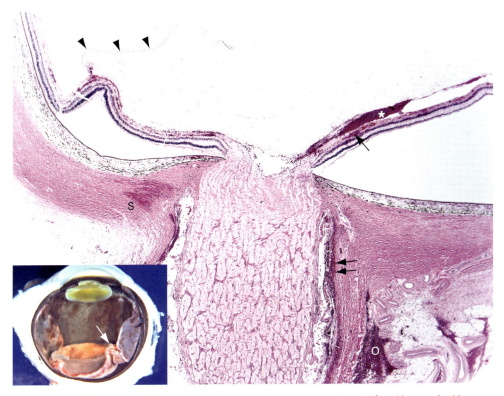

Figure 10-26 Abusive head trauma (AHT). Histopathology reveals multifocal intraretinal hemorrhages *(arrow)*. Vitreous traction results sub-ILM hemorrhages *(asterisk)* and a perimacular fold *(arrowheads)*. Hemorrhage is also seen within the optic nerve sheath *(double arrow)*, the perineural sclera (S), and the orbital tissue (O). *Inset:* Gross examination of the globe reveals diffuse retinal hemorrhages extending to the ora serrata and a perimacular circumferential retinal fold *(white arrow)*. *(Courtesy of Tatyana Milman, MD.)*

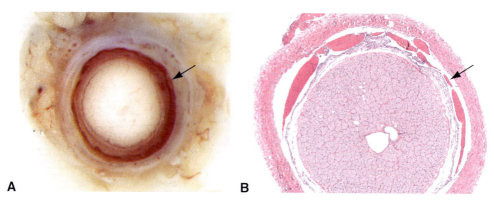

Figure 10-27 AHT. **A,** Cross section of the optic nerve reveals 360° of subdural hemorrhage *(arrow).* **B,** Photomicrograph shows hemorrhage in the subdural optic nerve sheath *(arrow).* *(Part A courtesy of Nasreen A. Syed, MD; part B courtesy of Amanda C. Maltry, MD.)*

Clinical Pearl No clinical or histopathologic findings are pathognomonic for AHT. Each case needs to be interpreted in the context of the clinical history and other clinical and pathologic findings. Whenever AHT is suspected, a physician is required by law in all US states and Canadian provinces to report the incident to a designated government agency.

See BCSC Section 6, *Pediatric Ophthalmology and Strabismus,* for additional information on this topic.

> Breazzano MP, Unkrich KH, Barker-Griffith AE. Clinicopathological findings in abusive head trauma: analysis of 110 infant autopsy eyes. *Am J Ophthalmol.* 2014;158(6):1146–1154.e2.

Age-Related Macular Degeneration

Age-related macular degeneration (AMD) is the leading cause of blindness and vision impairment in adults in the United States aged 60 and older. Although its etiology is poorly understood, evidence suggests that both genetic and environmental factors are involved. Genome-wide and candidate association studies have identified risk loci for AMD and implicated certain genes, particularly *CFH* and *ARMS2/HTRA1*. Older age, tobacco use, positive family history, and cardiovascular disease increase the risk of AMD development. In addition, randomized clinical trials showing the benefit of antioxidant supplementation in AMD suggest that oxidative stress has a role in disease progression.

Several characteristic aging changes occur in the retina, RPE, Bruch membrane, and choroid. The first detectable pathologic change is the appearance of deposits between the basement membrane of the RPE and the elastic portion of Bruch membrane (basal linear deposits) and similar deposits between the plasma membrane and the basement membrane of the RPE (basal laminar deposits). In advanced cases of AMD, the deposits may become confluent and visible with light microscopy without being clinically apparent (Fig 10-28).

The first clinically detectable feature of AMD is the appearance of drusen (Table 10-1). The clinical term *drusen* has been correlated pathologically to large, extracellular PAS-positive

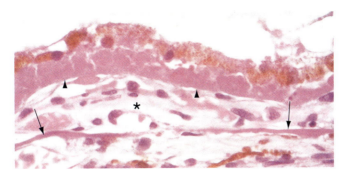

Figure 10-28 Diffuse drusen. Note the diffuse deposition of eosinophilic material *(arrowheads)* beneath the RPE. Choroidal neovascularization *(asterisk)* is present between the diffuse drusen and the elastic portion of Bruch membrane *(arrows)* (PAS stain). *(Courtesy of Hans E. Grossniklaus, MD.)*

Table 10-1 Clinical and Histologic Appearance of Drusen

Type of Drusen	Clinical Appearance	Histologic Appearance
Hard (nodular)	Discrete, yellowish, circumscribed, deep retinal lesions; sometimes have a glistening appearance	PAS-positive deposits composed of hyaline material between the RPE and Bruch membrane or on Bruch membrane (see Fig 10-29)
Soft	Yellow, somewhat amorphous lesions with poorly demarcated edges; usually >63 µm in size; may have appearance of fluid under RPE on OCT	Focal areas of cleavage of the RPE and basal laminar or linear deposits from Bruch membrane that are composed of sub-RPE eosinophilic lipoproteinaceous material (see Fig 10-30)
Basal laminar or cuticular	Small, regular, diffuse nodular deposits that may be difficult to appreciate clinically	Linear deposits of eosinophilic material along the inner surface of Bruch membrane or within the basal portion of RPE cells (see Fig 10-28)
Calcific	Sharply demarcated, glistening, white-to-yellow refractile lesions	Nodular excrescences along the inner surface of Bruch membrane that are deep purple on H&E stain due to calcification
Reticular pseudodrusen	Ill-defined, whitish-yellow lesions in the deep retina with a reticular pattern; usually seen in the superior and temporal macula, with enhanced visibility when viewed with blue light, near-infrared imaging, or fundus autofluorescence	Accumulation of lipid-rich material in the subretinal space between photoreceptor inner/outer segments and RPE (see Fig 10-31)

H&E = hematoxylin and eosin; OCT = optical coherence tomography; PAS = periodic acid–Schiff; RPE = retinal pigment epithelium.

deposits between the RPE and Bruch membrane. Drusen may be transient in their clinical appearance. Table 10-1 lists types of drusen with their clinical and histologic descriptions, and Figures 10-28, 10-29, and 10-30 depict some of these drusen.

Histochemical and molecular/biological analyses have demonstrated that the major constituents of human drusen include albumin, apolipoproteins, complement factors and related proteins, immunoglobulins, lipids, and β-amyloid. *Reticular pseudodrusen (RPD),* also known as *subretinal drusenoid deposits,* are deposits of extracellular material interposed between the photoreceptor inner/outer segments and the RPE that contain

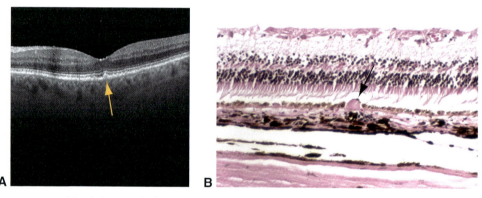

Figure 10-29 Hard drusen. **A,** SD-OCT image of nodular sub-RPE elevation *(arrow).* **B,** Photomicrograph illustrates a dome-shaped, nodular, hard druse *(arrow)* and attenuation of the overlying RPE. *(Part A courtesy of Elaine M. Binkley, MD; part B courtesy of Robert H. Rosa Jr, MD.)*

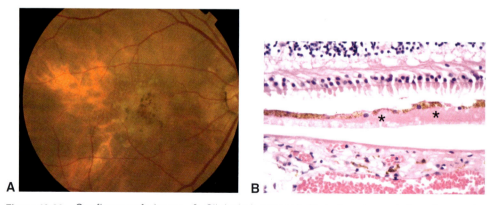

Figure 10-30 Confluent soft drusen. **A,** Clinical photograph. Note the pigment clumping overlying the confluent drusen in the central macula. **B,** Photomicrograph shows thick eosinophilic deposits *(asterisks)* between the RPE and Bruch membrane. The separation between the retina and RPE and the RPE and Bruch membrane is artifact. Note the marked attenuation of the photoreceptor cell nuclei in the ONL and the loss of the outer segments over the confluent drusen. *(Part A courtesy of Robert H. Rosa Jr, MD; part B courtesy of Nasreen A. Syed, MD.)*

membranous debris, unesterified cholesterol, complement factors and related proteins, and apolipoproteins; however, they lack opsins (Fig 10-31). RPD may be associated with progression to advanced AMD (geographic atrophy and choroidal neovascularization). Many eyes with clinically apparent drusen (especially soft drusen) are found to have basal laminar and/or basal linear deposits and diffuse drusen on histologic analysis.

Photoreceptor atrophy occurs to a variable degree in macular degeneration. This atrophy may be a primary abnormality of the photoreceptors or may be secondary to the underlying changes in the RPE, Bruch membrane, and/or choriocapillaris. In addition to

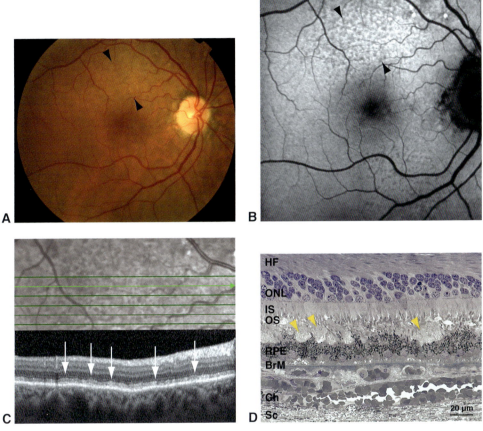

Figure 10-31 Reticular pseudodrusen. **A,** Color photograph shows the ill-defined, yellowish reticular pattern *(between arrowheads)* in the superior macula. **B,** Fundus autofluorescence (FAF) image shows the corresponding region *(between arrowheads)* with dotlike areas of decreased and increased FAF. **C,** Near-infrared image *(upper panel)* shows similar dotlike areas of decreased reflectance that, on SD-OCT *(lower panel)*, correspond to deposits *(arrows)* interposed between the photoreceptor outer segments and the RPE with focal disruption of the EZ. **D,** Subretinal drusenoid deposits *(yellow arrowheads)* are the histologic correlate of reticular pseudodrusen. Note their location in the region of the outer segments. HF = Henle fiber layer; ONL = outer nuclear layer; IS = inner segment; OS = outer segment; RPE = retinal pigment epithelium; BrM = Bruch membrane; Ch = choroid; Sc = sclera. (Toluidine blue stain). *(Parts A–C courtesy of Robert H. Rosa Jr, MD; part D courtesy of Christine A. Curcio, PhD.)*

photoreceptor atrophy, large zones of RPE atrophy may appear. When RPE atrophy occurs in the macular region, it is termed *geographic atrophy* (Fig 10-32). Drusen, photoreceptor atrophy, and RPE atrophy may all be present to varying degrees in *dry,* or *nonneovascular, AMD*. In addition, neovascular buds arising from the choriocapillaris are present in areas adjacent to the atrophic areas and in the peripheral choroid.

In eyes with choroidal neovascularization *(neovascular AMD;* also called *wet,* or *exudative, AMD)*, fibrovascular tissue is present between the inner and outer layers of Bruch membrane, beneath the RPE, and/or in the subretinal space (Fig 10-33; also see Fig 10-28). Excised choroidal neovascular membranes (CNVMs) have demonstrated vascular channels, RPE, and various other components of the RPE–Bruch membrane

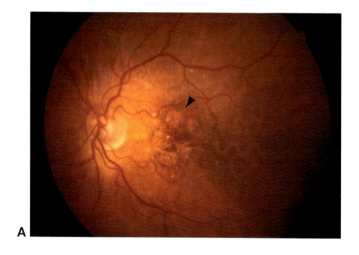

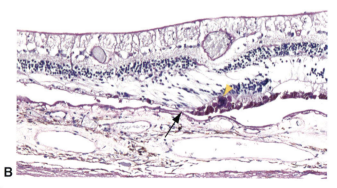

Figure 10-32 Geographic atrophy of the RPE. **A,** Fundus photograph shows focal geographic atrophy of the RPE *(arrowhead)* and drusen in nonneovascular age-related macular degeneration. **B,** Histologically, there is loss of the photoreceptors, RPE, and choriocapillaris *(left of arrow)*. PAS-positive lipofuscin accumulation is seen in the RPE cells adjacent to the atrophy *(arrowhead)*. *(Part A courtesy of Robert H. Rosa Jr, MD; part B courtesy of Tatyana Milman, MD.)*

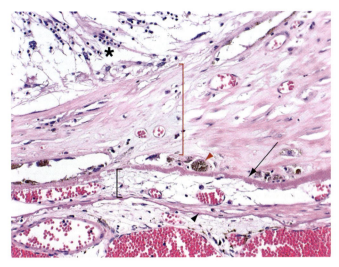

Figure 10-33 Neovascularization within Bruch membrane *(black bracket)*, beneath basal laminar/linear deposit *(arrow)* and above outer Bruch membrane *(black arrowhead)*. Note alternating areas of RPE atrophy and hypertrophy *(red arrowhead)*. Subretinal neovascular membrane *(red bracket)* is also present. Note the loss of retinal photoreceptor inner and outer segments *(asterisk)*. *(Courtesy of Alan Proia, MD, PhD.)*

complex, including photoreceptor outer segments, basal laminar and linear deposits, and inflammatory cells.

The choroidal and subretinal neovascular blood vessels leak fluid and may rupture easily, producing the exudative consequences of neovascular AMD, including macular edema, serous retinal detachment, and subretinal and intraretinal hemorrhages. VEGF inhibition via intravitreally administered anti-VEGF agents reduces macular edema, slows progression of the neovascularization, and improves visual outcomes of patients with neovascular AMD.

See BCSC Section 12, *Retina and Vitreous,* for more discussion of AMD.

> Seddon JM, McLeod DS, Bhutto IA, et al. Histopathological insights into choroidal vascular loss in clinically documented cases of age-related macular degeneration. *JAMA Ophthalmol.* 2016;134(11):1272–1280.
>
> Shughoury A, Sevgi DD, Ciulla TA. Molecular genetic mechanisms in age-related macular degeneration. *Genes (Basel).* 2022;13(7):1233.

Polypoidal Choroidal Vasculopathy

Polypoidal choroidal vasculopathy (previously called *posterior uveal bleeding syndrome* and *multiple recurrent serosanguineous RPE detachments*) is a disorder in which dilated, thin-walled vascular channels (Fig 10-34) are interposed between the RPE and the outer aspect of Bruch membrane. Associated choroidal neovascularization is often present in these lesions, as observed in several histologic specimens. See BCSC Section 12, *Retina and Vitreous,* for more information on this condition.

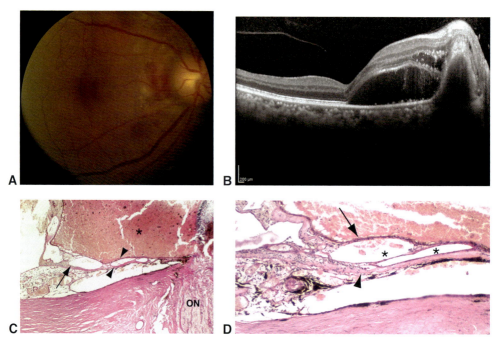

Figure 10-34 Polypoidal choroidal vasculopathy. **A,** Fundus photograph reveals elevated, red-orange, nodular subretinal lesions in the peripapillary area. **B,** OCT from the same patient shows an elevated sub-RPE lesion in the peripapillary region with associated intraretinal and subretinal fluid. **C,** Peripapillary dilated vascular channels *(arrow)* between the RPE and the outer aspect of Bruch membrane *(arrowheads)*. Note the dense subretinal hemorrhage *(asterisk)*. ON = optic nerve. **D,** Higher-magnification view of thin-walled vascular channels *(asterisks)* interposed between the RPE *(arrow)* and Bruch membrane *(arrowhead)*. *(Parts A and B courtesy of Robert M. Carroll, MD; parts C and D courtesy of Robert H. Rosa Jr, MD.)*

Dystrophies

See BCSC Section 12, *Retina and Vitreous,* for additional discussion of retinal dystrophies.

Macular Dystrophies

Fundus flavimaculatus and Stargardt disease

Fundus flavimaculatus and Stargardt disease are thought to represent opposite ends of an inherited disease spectrum characterized by yellowish flecks at the RPE level, a generalized vermilion (reddish) fundus clinically, variable late RPE atrophy, dark choroid on FA, and gradual vision loss (Fig 10-35). The inheritance pattern is generally autosomal recessive, but autosomal dominant forms have been reported. The most striking feature of Stargardt disease revealed by light and electron microscopy is the marked engorgement of RPE cells with PAS-positive lipofuscin and apical displacement of the normal RPE melanin granules (see Fig 10-35D).

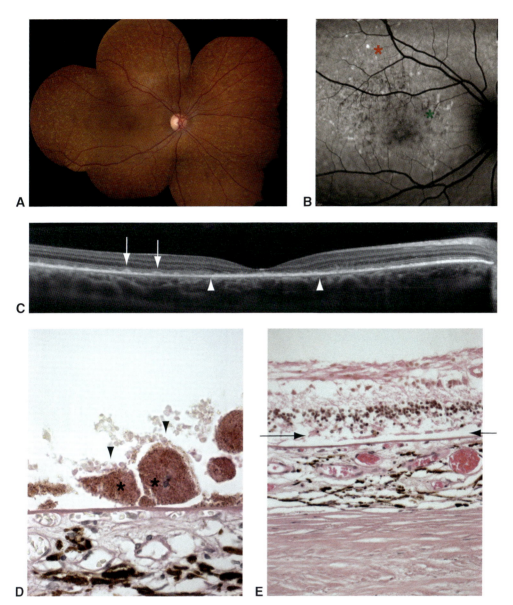

Figure 10-35 Stargardt disease. **A,** Fundus photograph shows diffuse retinal flecks. **B,** FAF imaging reveals increased autofluorescence corresponding to the retinal flecks *(red asterisk)* and decreased autofluorescence corresponding to areas of RPE atrophy *(green asterisk)*. **C,** SD-OCT image shows hyperreflectivity at the level of the RPE (corresponding histologically with enlarged RPE cells with increased lipofuscin content) *(arrows)*, markedly thinned retina in the foveal region, and focal attenuation or loss of the photoreceptor cell layer in areas corresponding to RPE atrophy *(area between arrowheads)*. **D,** Photomicrograph of a PAS-stained section demonstrates hypertrophic RPE cells *(arrowheads)* with numerous PAS-positive cytoplasmic granules containing lipofuscin *(asterisks)*. This histologic finding corresponds to the retinal flecks seen clinically. **E,** In advanced stages of Stargardt disease, geographic RPE atrophy with loss of the photoreceptor cell layer *(between arrows)* may be noted. *(Parts A–C courtesy of Tomas S. Aleman, MD; parts D and E courtesy of Sander Dubovy, MD.)*

Pattern dystrophies

The term *pattern dystrophies* refers to a heterogeneous group of inherited macular diseases characterized by varying patterns of pigment deposition in the macular RPE (Fig 10-36). The most common pathogenic variation associated with the pattern dystrophies occurs in the *PRPH2* (peripherin 2) gene. Historically, pattern dystrophies were classified by morphology. The underlying molecular genetic mechanisms are now better understood, and pattern dystrophies are classified based on genetic variation.

Spectral-domain optical coherence tomography (SD-OCT) in patients with pattern dystrophy reveals elevation of the photoreceptor layer, with localization of the dystrophic material between the photoreceptors and RPE (see Fig 10-36B). Histologic studies reveal

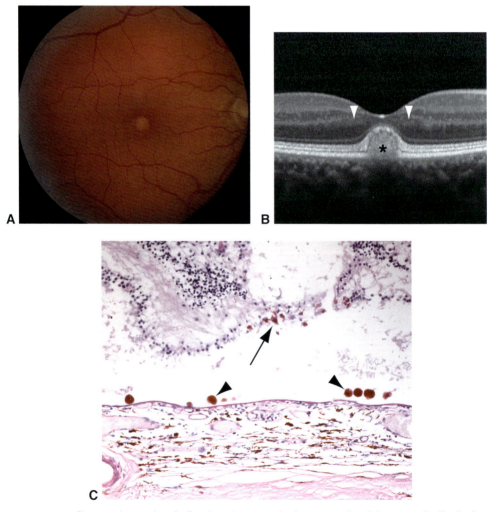

Figure 10-36 Pattern dystrophy. **A,** Fundus photograph shows a yellowish, egg yolk–like lesion with focal pigment clumping and mottling in the central macula. **B,** SD-OCT (same patient as in part A) reveals subfoveal hyperreflective material *(asterisk)*. Note the irregular RPE elevation *(between arrowheads)*. **C,** Histologic findings include pigment-containing cells in the subretinal space *(arrowheads)* and outer neurosensory retina *(arrow)*. *(Parts A and B courtesy of Tomas S. Aleman, MD; part C courtesy of Sander Dubovy, MD.)*

central loss of the RPE and photoreceptor cell layer, with a moderate number of pigment-containing histiocytes and RPE cells in the subretinal space and outer neurosensory retina (see Fig 10-36C). The adjacent RPE is distended with lipofuscin. Basal laminar and linear deposits may be present throughout the macular region. The pathologic finding of pigment-containing cells with lipofuscin and drusenlike material in the subretinal space correlates with the pattern seen clinically.

Diffuse Photoreceptor Dystrophies

Inherited dystrophies that affect the rods and cones are discussed in greater detail in BCSC Section 12, *Retina and Vitreous*. Only the most common photoreceptor dystrophy, *retinitis pigmentosa (RP)*, is discussed in this section.

RP refers to a group of inherited retinal diseases characterized by RPE and photoreceptor dysfunction and degeneration, resulting in progressive visual field loss. The inheritance patterns of RP are complex: it can be sporadic, autosomal dominant, autosomal recessive, or X-linked. Pathogenic variants in the rhodopsin gene *(RHO)* are the most common cause of autosomal dominant RP.

The term *retinitis pigmentosa* is a misnomer because clear evidence of inflammation is lacking. Ophthalmoscopic findings include pigment arranged in a bone spicule–like configuration around the retinal arterioles, arteriolar narrowing, and optic nerve head atrophy (Fig 10-37A). The disease is characterized primarily by the loss of rod photoreceptor cells via apoptosis. Cones are seldom directly affected; however, they degenerate secondary to the loss of rods. Microscopically, loss of photoreceptor cells is seen, as well as RPE migration into the neurosensory retina around retinal vessels (Fig 10-37B). The arterioles, though narrowed clinically, initially show no histologic abnormality. Later, thickening and hyalinization of the vessel walls develop (Fig 10-37C). The optic nerve may show diffuse or sectoral atrophy, with gliosis as a late-stage change.

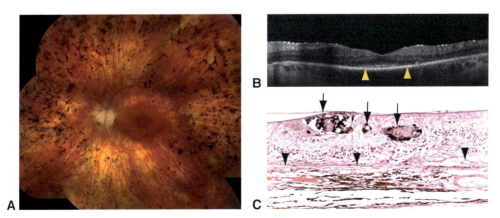

Figure 10-37 Retinitis pigmentosa. **A,** Fundus photograph shows pallor of the optic nerve, retinal arteriolar narrowing, focal depigmentation, and bone spicule–like pigmentation in the peripheral fundus. **B,** SD-OCT image shows loss of the photoreceptors outside the fovea *(outside of arrowheads)*. **C,** Histologically, marked photoreceptor cell loss *(arrowheads)* and RPE migration into the retina in a perivascular distribution *(arrows)* are apparent and correspond to the bone spicule–like pattern seen clinically. Retinal vessels are hyalinized. *(Parts A and B courtesy of Edwin M. Stone, MD, PhD; part C courtesy of Tatyana Milman, MD.)*

Neoplasia

This section discusses tumors that arise from tissue derived from the inner layer of the optic cup.

Retinoblastoma

Retinoblastoma is the most common primary intraocular malignancy in childhood, occurring in 1 in 14,000–20,000 live births. Retinoblastoma is of neuroblastic origin, arising from immature cells in the nucleated layers of the retina. Chapter 18 discusses the clinical aspects of retinoblastoma. Retinoblastoma is also discussed in BCSC Section 6, *Pediatric Ophthalmology and Strabismus*.

Histologic features

Commonly referred to as a *small blue cell tumor*, retinoblastoma consists of cells with round or oval nuclei that are approximately twice the size of a lymphocyte. On hematoxylin and eosin stain, retinoblastoma is histologically distinguished by 3 predominant colors (see Fig 10-38B), which are best appreciated at low magnification:

- blue: retinoblastoma tumor cells
- pink: areas of necrosis
- purple: areas of calcification

As the tumor expands into the vitreous or subretinal space, retinoblastoma cells surround blood vessels for sustenance, creating a characteristic pattern referred to as *pseudorosettes* (ie, viable tumor cells surrounding a blood vessel). However, they frequently outgrow their blood supply, and regions of ischemic necrosis begin 90–120 µm from the central vessel. Associated with the necrosis are foci of calcification (Fig 10-38).

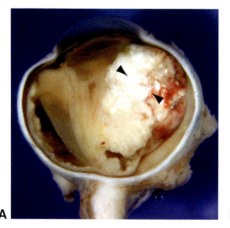 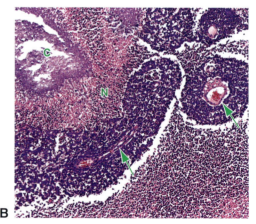

Figure 10-38 Retinoblastoma. **A,** Gross photograph of an enucleated eye with retinoblastoma. Note the bright white tumor calcifications in the anterior portion of the mass *(arrowheads)*. **B,** Histopathology demonstrates viable blue tumor surrounding a blood vessel *(arrows)* with alternating zones of pink necrosis (N) and focal purple calcification (C). *(Part A courtesy of Ralph C. Eagle Jr, MD; part B courtesy of Tatyana Milman, MD.)*

Various forms of differentiation may occur in retinoblastomas, such as

- *Homer Wright rosettes:* representing neuronal differentiation, these are circular arrangements of neoplastic nuclei with a central neurofibrillary tangle (Fig 10-39A)
- *Flexner-Wintersteiner rosettes:* representing differentiation toward the retina, these are circular arrangements of neoplastic nuclei joined by external limiting membrane–type junctions which create a central lumen (Fig 10-39B)
- *Fleurettes:* representing the greatest degree of differentiation toward the retina, fleurettes are bouquet-like arrangements of neoplastic nuclei and photoreceptor inner segments, joined by external limiting membrane (Fig 10-39C)

However, differentiation is not an important prognostic indicator. In a typical retinoblastoma, undifferentiated tumor cells greatly outnumber rosettes or fleurettes. Nuclear anaplasia (enlarged, pleomorphic nuclei with brisk mitotic activity) has been shown to be associated with unfavorable prognosis. Neovascularization of the iris, sometimes resulting in angle closure, may occur in patients with retinoblastoma, and it has been associated with high-risk histologic features (see the section "Histologic prognostic factors") (Fig 10-40).

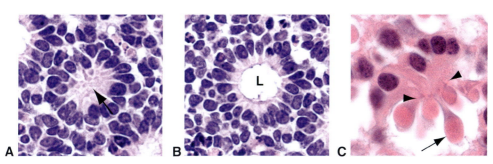

Figure 10-39 Retinoblastoma differentiation. **A,** Homer Wright rosettes have a single row of columnar cells with eosinophilic cytoplasm filled with a neurofibrillary tangle of cytoplasmic processes *(arrow)*. **B,** Flexner-Wintersteiner rosettes have a single row of columnar cells with eosinophilic cytoplasm and peripherally situated nuclei arranged radially. The cells surround a central lumen (L) lined by a refractile membranous structure that corresponds to the ELM of the retina. **C,** The fleurette resembles a bouquet of flowers composed of curvilinear rows of nuclei on 1 side of neoplastic ELM *(between arrowheads)* and bulbous eosinophilic photoreceptor inner segments on the other side *(arrow)*. *(Parts A and B courtesy of Amanda C. Maltry, MD; part C courtesy of Ralph C. Eagle, Jr. MD.)*

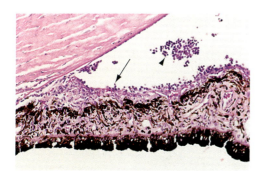

Figure 10-40 Retinoblastoma, anterior segment of the globe. Note the thick neovascular membrane *(arrow)* on the iris surface extending into the angle, resulting in angle closure. Free-floating tumor cells *(arrowhead)* are present in the anterior chamber.

> **Clinical Pearl** Homer Wright rosettes, Flexner-Wintersteiner rosettes, and fleurettes may be seen in other neuroepithelial and neuroendocrine tumors and are not pathognomonic of retinoblastoma.

Vitreous seeds Small clumps of cells shed from the tumor may remain viable in the vitreous *(vitreous seeds)* and subretinal space without a blood supply. Vitreous seeds are classified based on clinical appearance as dust, spheres, or clouds (see Chapter 18), and each has a correlating typical appearance on histopathology:

- *dust:* scattered single cells that alternate with macrophages
- *spheres:* multiple layers of viable tumor cells
- *clouds:* mostly necrotic material with some active cancer cells

Multilayered sphere seeds can shed single cells and may be more clinically aggressive, requiring higher dosage and more frequent injection of intravitreal chemotherapy compared with dust seeds. Cloud seeds, because they contain fewer viable cells, appear to respond less readily to intravitreal chemotherapy, but the low tumor burden means they may not need to be treated as intensely as sphere seeds.

Tumor seeds may eventually develop into focal tumor implants throughout the eye. It may be difficult to determine histologically whether multiple intraocular foci of the tumor represent multiple primary tumors or tumor implants due to intraocular seeding.

> Amram AL, Rico G, Kim JW, et al. Vitreous seeds in retinoblastoma: clinicopathologic classification and correlation. *Ophthalmology.* 2017;124(10):1540–1547.

Histologic prognostic factors Histologic features of retinoblastoma that are associated with higher risk of metastasis and poorer survival include

- optic nerve invasion (laminar, retrolaminar, or surgical cut end of the nerve) (Fig 10-41A)
- anterior chamber involvement (Fig 10-41B)
- direct extraocular extension (Fig 10-41C)
- massive choroidal invasion (see Fig 10-41C)

The most common route for retinoblastoma to extend out of the eye is through the optic nerve. Direct infiltration of the optic nerve can lead to extension into the brain. Cells that spread into the leptomeninges can gain access to the cerebrospinal fluid and potentially seed throughout the CNS. Therefore, invasion of the optic nerve is a poor prognostic indicator.

Massive choroidal invasion is defined as an invasive focus of a tumor with a diameter (in any dimension) of at least 3 mm and the tumor reaching at least the inner fibers of the scleral tissue. Massive choroidal invasion is a poor prognostic factor that is thought to be related to hematogenous spread of tumor via the highly vascular choroid. Choroidal involvement that is less than 3 mm in any dimension and does not reach the sclera is termed *focal choroidal invasion,* which is not associated with a worse prognosis. See Chapter 18 for further discussion of prognosis.

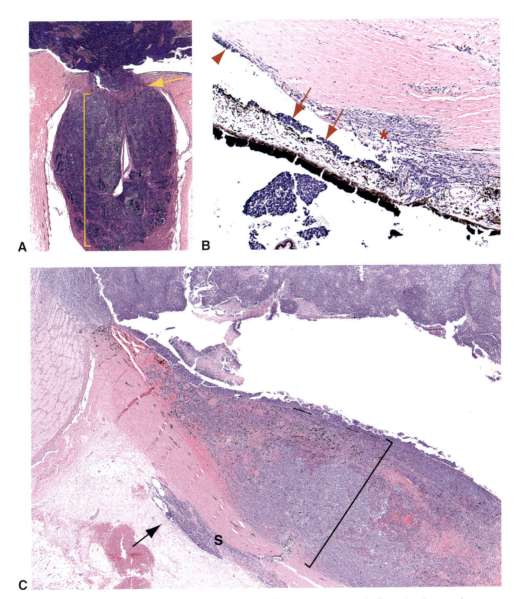

Figure 10-41 Intraocular and extraocular spread of retinoblastoma. **A,** Retrolaminar optic nerve invasion. The tumor fills the optic nerve *(bracket)* posterior to the lamina cribrosa *(arrow)*. **B,** Anterior chamber involvement. Retinoblastoma cells are seen lining the surface of the iris *(arrows)* and in the iris stroma, along Descemet membrane *(arrowhead)*, and invading the trabecular meshwork *(asterisk)*. **C,** Massive choroidal invasion and extraocular extension. Tumor thickens the choroid *(bracket)* and invades through the sclera (S) with a nodule of extraocular extension *(arrow)*. *(Parts A and C courtesy of Tatyana Milman, MD; part B courtesy of Amanda C. Maltry, MD.)*

> **Clinical Pearl** Pathologic examination findings help guide retinoblastoma management after enucleation. To prevent metastases and improve survival rates, adjuvant chemotherapy is indicated for patients with high-risk histopathologic features, including postlaminar optic nerve invasion, massive choroidal invasion, and extraocular extension.

> Sastre X, Chantada GL, Doz F, et al; International Retinoblastoma Staging Working Group. Proceedings of the consensus meetings from the International Retinoblastoma Staging Working Group on the pathology guidelines for the examination of enucleated eyes and evaluation of prognostic risk factors in retinoblastoma. *Arch Pathol Lab Med.* 2009;133(8):1199–1202.

Molecular genetics of retinoblastoma

See BCSC Section 2, *Fundamentals and Principles of Ophthalmology*, for discussion of the clinical genetics of retinoblastoma.

Initiation of molecular events Retinoblastoma develops when both copies of the retinoblastoma gene *(RB1)* become nonfunctional, either by a deletion error or by mutation. *RB1* is located on the long arm of chromosome 13 and encodes for retinoblastoma protein, pRB, which functions as a tumor suppressor.

A single normal gene copy is sufficient to suppress the development of retinoblastoma. However, when 1 abnormal gene is present, if a pathogenic variation in the remaining normal gene occurs during retinal differentiation, loss of tumor suppression occurs, and retinoblastoma is likely to develop.

In a minority (approximately 2%) of retinoblastomas that lack *RB1* gene variants, amplification of the *MYCN* oncogene underlies tumorigenesis. This type of sporadic retinoblastoma is associated with very early age (median age of 4.5 months) at diagnosis and unilateral occurrence, as well as more aggressive growth compared to retinoblastoma caused by the *RB1* pathogenic variant.

Tumors secondary to *MYCN* amplification demonstrate distinct histologic features, such as undifferentiated cells with prominent and multiple nucleoli, necrosis, apoptosis, little calcification, and absence of rosettes (Fig 10-42). Despite their aggressive growth and poor differentiation, these tumors appear unlikely to spread systemically.

Cytogenetic and molecular prognostic factors Studies suggest that, beyond biallelic inactivation of *RB1*, progression to retinoblastoma requires additional genetic aberrations.

CYTOGENETIC ALTERATIONS Chromosomal abnormalities, including gains of 1q, 2p, and 6p, and loss of 16q, likely lead to activation of oncogenes or inactivation of tumor suppressor genes at these regions. These aberrations, specifically the 6p gain, have been associated with more aggressive histopathologic features and higher likelihood of treatment failure than cases without these abnormalities. The loss of 16q is associated with diffuse vitreous seeding.

MOLECULAR GENETIC ALTERATIONS Likely pathogenic alterations have been identified beyond *RB1* in several other oncogenes and tumor suppressor genes. Pathogenic variation of the

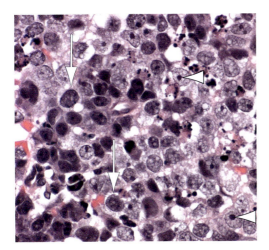

Figure 10-42 High-magnification photomicrograph of retinoblastoma cells with *MYCN* oncogene amplification. Tumor cells are very poorly differentiated and highly pleomorphic. Nuclei are often hyperchromatic and enlarged *(arrows)* or have prominent nucleoli *(arrowheads)*. *(Courtesy of Nasreen A. Syed, MD.)*

BCOR tumor suppressor gene is an example of a genetic alteration beyond *RB1* that correlates with more aggressive tumor behavior.

> Afshar AR, Pekmezci M, Bloomer MM, et al. Next-generation sequencing of retinoblastoma identifies pathogenic alterations beyond *RB1* inactivation that correlate with aggressive histopathologic features. *Ophthalmology*. 2020;127(6):804–813.
>
> Xu L, Polski A, Prabakar RK, et al. Chromosome 6p amplification in aqueous humor cell-free DNA is a prognostic biomarker for retinoblastoma ocular survival. *Mol Cancer Res*. 2020;18(8):1166–1175.

Retinocytoma

Retinocytoma is a rare, highly differentiated tumor of the neurosensory retina. Its pathogenesis is the subject of debate. Although retinocytoma harbors biallelic *RB1* mutations similar to retinoblastoma, it has greater genomic stability and lacks proliferative activity. Dedifferention may lead to malignant transformation into retinoblastoma. Retinocytoma is characterized histologically by numerous fleurettes admixed with individual cells that demonstrate varying degrees of photoreceptor differentiation (Fig 10-43). Retinocytoma differs from retinoblastoma in the following ways:

- Retinocytoma cells have more cytoplasm and more evenly dispersed nuclear chromatin.
- Mitoses are not observed in retinocytoma cells.
- Although calcification may be present in eyes with retinocytoma, necrosis is usually absent.

Medulloepithelioma

Medulloepithelioma is a neuroepithelial tumor that arises from primitive neuroepithelium (ie, the inner layer of the optic cup). This tumor usually arises from the ciliary epithelium but has been documented in the retina and optic nerve in rare instances. In the

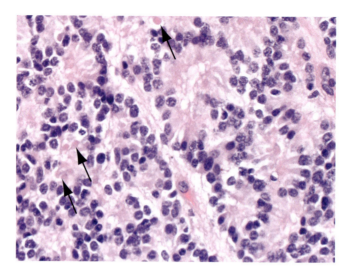

Figure 10-43 Retinocytoma consisting of curvilinear fleurettes with bulbous eosinophilic photoreceptor inner segments *(arrows)*. Note the low nucleus to cytoplasm ratios, bland nuclei without conspicuous nucleoli, lack of mitotic figures, and the absence of necrosis. *(Courtesy of Amanda C. Maltry, MD.)*

ciliary body, medulloepithelioma may appear clinically as a lightly pigmented or white multicystic mass with erosion into the anterior chamber and iris root, frequently associated with iris neovascularization (see Chapter 18, Fig 18-15). Within the tumor, undifferentiated round-to-oval cells with little cytoplasm are organized into ribbonlike structures that have a distinct cellular polarity (Fig 10-44A). Cell nuclei are stratified in 3–5 layers, and the entire structure is lined on 1 side by a thin basement membrane. One surface secretes a mucinous substance, rich in hyaluronic acid, that resembles vitreous. Stratified sheets of cells can form mucinous cysts that are clinically characteristic. Homer Wright and Flexner-Wintersteiner rosettes may also be present.

Medulloepitheliomas that contain solid masses of neuroblastic cells indistinguishable from retinoblastomas are more difficult to classify. Heteroplastic tissue, such as cartilage or muscle, may be found in medulloepitheliomas. This variant of the tumor is referred to as *teratoid medulloepithelioma* (Fig 10-44B, C). Medulloepitheliomas that have substantial numbers of undifferentiated cells with high mitotic rates and demonstrate locally aggressive behavior are considered malignant; however, patients treated with enucleation have high survival rates, and "malignant" medulloepithelioma typically follows a relatively benign course if the tumor remains confined to the eye.

In rare cases, ciliary body medulloepithelioma presents in association with pleuropulmonary blastoma as part of a familial cancer predisposition syndrome. In these cases, tumors are typically secondary to a germline pathogenic variant in the *DICER1* gene.

Schultz KA, Yang J, Doros L, et al. *DICER1*-pleuropulmonary blastoma familial tumor predisposition syndrome: a unique constellation of neoplastic conditions. *Pathol Case Rev.* 2014;19(2):90–100.

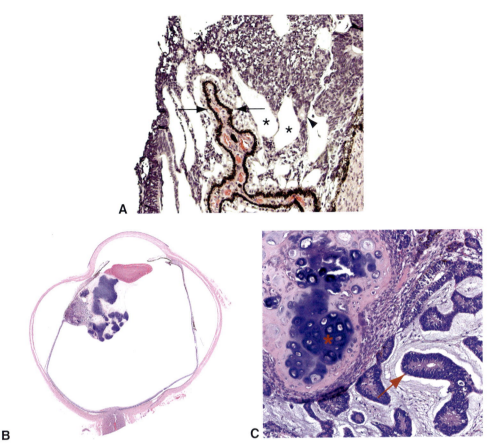

Figure 10-44 Medulloepithelioma. **A,** Photomicrograph shows ribbons, cords, and small sheets of blue tumor cells arising from the ciliary epithelium (ciliary processes of the pars plicata *between arrows*) and surrounded by pockets of vitreous *(asterisk)* and occasional Flexner-Wintersteiner rosettes *(arrowhead)*. **B,** Teratoid medulloepithelioma at low magnification. **C,** Higher magnification of part B demonstrates ribbons of polarized neuroepithelium *(arrow)* surrounded by blue pools of mucopolysaccharide and adjacent heterotopic cartilage *(asterisk)*. *(Part A courtesy of George J. Harocopos, MD; parts B and C courtesy of Tatyana Milman, MD.)*

Nodular Hyperplasia of Ciliary Body Epithelium

Nodular hyperplasia of ciliary body epithelium (formerly called Fuchs adenoma), derived from the inner layer of the optic cup, is an acquired, age-related benign tumor of the nonpigmented ciliary epithelium. This lesion usually goes undetected clinically (unless it reaches significant size) but is frequently identified upon autopsy examination of eyes of older adults. Larger lesions may be associated with sectoral cataract and may mimic other iris or ciliary body neoplasms. Histologically, this condition consists of hyperplastic nonpigmented ciliary epithelium arranged in sheets and tubules (Fig 10-45), with alternating areas of PAS-positive basement membrane material.

> Shields JA, Eagle RC Jr, Ferguson K, Shields CL. Tumors of the nonpigmented epithelium of the ciliary body: the Lorenz E. Zimmerman tribute lecture. *Retina*. 2015;35(5):957–965.

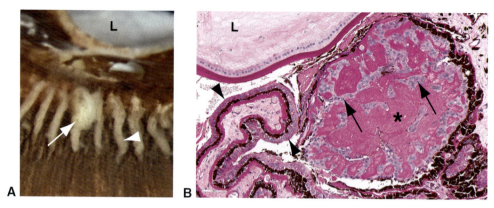

Figure 10-45 Nodular hyperplasia of ciliary body epithelium. **A,** Gross photograph of a mass *(arrow)* involving the ciliary body pars plicata. Note the adjacent ciliary processes *(arrowhead)* and the cataractous lens (L). **B,** Histology reveals a tumor arising from the ciliary body epithelium, composed of interweaving trabeculae of bland nonpigmented ciliary epithelial cells *(arrows)* associated with abundant PAS-positive basement membrane material *(asterisk)*. The neighboring ciliary process is lined by normal epithelium *(between arrowheads)*. Note the adjacent lens (L). *(Part A courtesy of Ralph C. Eagle, Jr; part B courtesy of Tatyana Milman, MD.)*

Combined Hamartoma of the Retina and RPE

A combined hamartoma of the retina and RPE is not a true neoplasm but may present as a tumorous growth in the eye. Clinically, it appears as a slightly elevated, variably pigmented mass that involves the RPE, retina, optic nerve, and overlying vitreous (see Chapter 16, Fig 16-14C). Although most common in a peripapillary location, this lesion can also be found elsewhere in the retina. Frequently, a preretinal membrane that distorts the tumor's inner surface is present. The lesion is often diagnosed in childhood, supporting a probable hamartomatous origin. Association with neurofibromatosis type 2, as well as several other syndromes, has been reported.

Histologically, the tumor is characterized by disorganized glial tissue and vascular proliferation (Fig 10-46). The RPE is hyperplastic and frequently migrates into the retina,

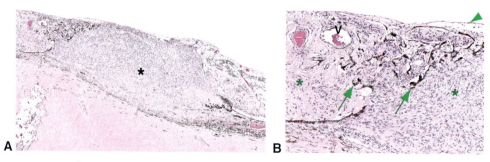

Figure 10-46 Combined hamartoma of the retina and RPE. **A,** Low-magnification photomicrograph shows masslike thickening of the peripapillary retina and RPE *(asterisk)*. **B,** Disorganized glial proliferation *(asterisks)*, associated with hyperplasia of RPE *(arrows)* and vascular proliferation (V). A glial membrane along the tumor surface is also seen at higher magnification *(arrowhead)*. *(Courtesy of Tatyana Milman, MD.)*

forming cords and tubules. Vitreous condensation and glial proliferation may be present on the surface of the tumor.

Adenomas and Adenocarcinomas of the Ciliary Body Epithelium and RPE

Neoplasia of the ciliary body epithelium and RPE is rare. Histologically, *adenomas* in this layer typically retain characteristics of ciliary body epithelial and RPE cells, including basement membranes, cell junctions, and microvilli. *Adenocarcinomas* are distinguished from adenomas by greater anaplasia, mitotic activity, and invasion of the choroid or retina. Adenoma and adenocarcinoma of the RPE may arise from CHRPE. Adenomas and adenocarcinomas may also arise from the ciliary epithelium. Metastases from adenocarcinoma of ciliary body epithelium and RPE are exceedingly rare. See also Chapter 16.

CHAPTER **11**

Uveal Tract

 Indicates that a supplemental case study is available in the Pathology Atlas *(aao.org/education/resident-course/pathology-atlas).*

Highlights

- Dalen-Fuchs nodules may be seen in some cases of sympathetic ophthalmia and are located between the retinal pigment epithelium and Bruch membrane.
- The uveal tract is the most common site of ocular involvement in sarcoidosis, a nonnecrotizing granulomatous condition.
- Tumor cell type, tumor size, extraocular extension, tumor location (including ciliary body involvement), and molecular classification are key prognostic factors in cases of posterior uveal melanoma.
- Metastatic tumors to the uvea, a highly vascularized layer, constitute the most common intraocular tumors in adults; mainly breast carcinoma in women and lung carcinoma in men.

Topography

The *iris, ciliary body,* and *choroid* constitute the uveal tract (also called *uvea*) (Fig 11-1). The constituents of the uveal tract

- have a layer of associated neuroepithelium
- are highly vascular, with blood supply from the anterior and/or posterior ciliary arteries
- have a high concentration of dendritic melanocytes

The uveal tract is embryologically derived from mesoderm and neural crest. The neuroepithelium is derived from the optic cup. See BCSC Section 2, *Fundamentals and Principles of Ophthalmology,* for more information on the uveal tract.

Clinical Pearl   Firm attachments between the uveal tract and the sclera exist at only 3 sites: the scleral spur, the emissarial canals (exit points of the vortex veins and posterior ciliary arteries/nerves), and the optic nerve. These structures delineate the extent of fluid and hemorrhage that can collect in the suprauveal space.

215

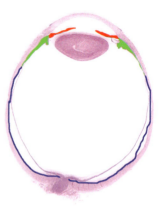

Figure 11-1 Uveal topography. The uveal tract consists of the iris *(red)*, ciliary body *(green)*, and choroid *(blue)*. *(Courtesy of Nasreen A. Syed, MD.)*

Iris

The iris sits in front of the crystalline lens. It separates the anterior segment of the eye into 2 compartments, the anterior chamber (between the cornea and iris) and the posterior chamber (between the iris and the lens/zonular fibers). The iris forms a circular aperture (pupil) that controls the amount of light transmitted into the eye. The iris comprises 4 layers (Fig 11-2):

- *anterior border layer:* a condensation of iris stroma, particularly melanocytes, that is coarsely ribbed with numerous crypts
- *stroma:* contains nerves, melanocytes, fibrocytes, histiocytes with pigment, and blood vessels. These vessels are surrounded by a thick cuff of collagen.
- *muscular layer:* 2 smooth muscles, both under autonomic control:
  - The *dilator muscle* is a flat, radially arranged muscle that extends from the peripupillary region to the iris root. This muscle is integrated with the anterior layer of pigment epithelium.
  - The *sphincter muscle* is a thicker muscle that encircles the pupil.

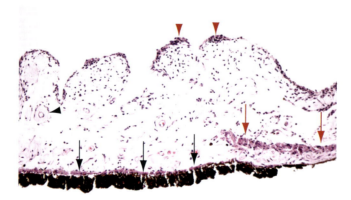

Figure 11-2 Histologic appearance of a normal iris: the anterior border layer *(red arrowheads)* is thrown into numerous crypts and folds. The sphincter muscle *(red arrows)* is present at the pupillary border, and the dilator muscle *(black arrows)* lies just anterior to the posterior pigment epithelium. Normal iris vessels are present in the stroma (not on its surface) and demonstrate a thick collagen cuff *(black arrowhead)*. *(Courtesy of Nasreen A. Syed, MD.)*

- *iris pigment epithelium:* consists of 2 layers: anterior and posterior, arranged apex to apex. The cytoplasm of these epithelial cells is packed with melanin granules.

Clinical Pearl   The number of melanin granules in the epithelium does not vary with iris color; rather, iris color is determined by the number of melanin granules and their size within the melanocytes of the anterior border layer and deep stroma.

Ciliary Body

The ciliary body is a ring-shaped structure approximately 6–7 mm wide that extends from the base of the iris and becomes continuous with the choroid at the ora serrata. The ciliary body is subdivided into 2 parts: the anterior *pars plicata* (1.5 mm wide; located 1 mm away from the limbus), which includes the ciliary processes, and the more posterior *pars plana* (3.5–4 mm wide; located 3–4 mm from the limbus) (Fig 11-3A). The zonular fibers of the lens attach to the ciliary body in the valleys of the ciliary processes and along the pars plana. The inner portion of the ciliary body is lined by a double layer of epithelial cells: the inner, nonpigmented layer and the outer, pigmented layer (Fig 11-3B).

The ciliary muscle comprises 3 layers of smooth muscle fibers: the outermost *longitudinal* layer, the middle *radial* layer, and the innermost *circular* layer. These individual muscle layers function as a unit during accommodation. Histologically, the layers are difficult to distinguish, and the muscle appears wedge-shaped in cross section.

Clinical Pearl   To access the vitreous cavity (eg, for intravitreal injection or for trocar placement for vitreoretinal surgery), the needle or trocar is inserted through the sclera at the level of the pars plana, generally 3.5–4 mm posterior to the limbus in phakic eyes and 3–3.5 mm posterior to the limbus in pseudophakic or aphakic eyes. This placement allows surgeons to avoid the lens and vascular ciliary processes anteriorly and the retina posterior to the insertion site.

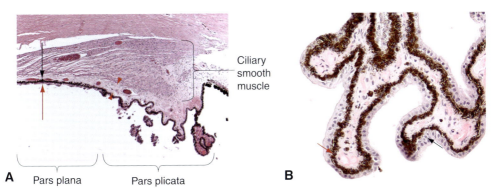

Figure 11-3 Ciliary body. **A,** Normal ciliary body. The inner face is lined with a double layer of epithelium: an inner, nonpigmented layer *(red arrow)* and an outer, pigmented layer *(black arrow).* Note the fibrovascular connective tissue interposed between the pigmented ciliary epithelium and the ciliary muscle fibers *(between arrowheads).* **B,** Higher-magnification image shows the pigmented *(red arrow)* and nonpigmented ciliary body epithelium *(black arrow)* on the surface of the pars plicata ciliary processes. *(Part A courtesy of Nasreen A. Syed, MD; part B courtesy of Nora V. Laver, MD.)*

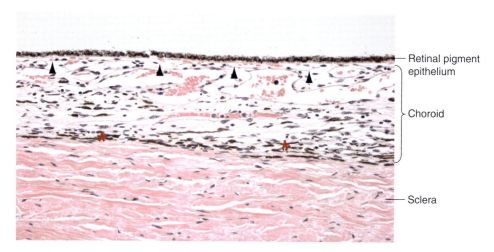

Figure 11-4 Histologic appearance of a normal choroid. The choroid is a vascular, pigmented structure located between the retinal pigment epithelium (RPE) and the sclera. The layer closest to the RPE is composed of capillaries and is known as the choriocapillaris *(arrowheads)*. The lamina fusca is also shown *(asterisks)* (hematoxylin and eosin [H&E] stain). *(Courtesy of Nasreen A. Syed, MD.)*

Choroid

The choroid is the pigmented vascular tissue situated between the retina/retinal pigment epithelium (RPE) and the sclera. It extends from the ora serrata anteriorly to the optic nerve posteriorly and consists of 3 principal layers:

- *lamina fusca:* outermost, pigmented layer with fine attachments to the sclera
- *stroma:* central layer of loose fibrovascular connective tissue with arterioles originating from posterior ciliary arteries and veins that drain primarily to the vortex veins. The outer layer of large vessels is called Sattler layer, and the middle layer of small vessels is called Haller layer.
- *choriocapillaris:* innermost layer; contains thin-walled capillaries that are contiguous with Bruch membrane

The choriocapillaris supplies blood to the RPE and the outer retinal layers (Fig 11-4). In addition to blood vessels, the choroid contains melanocytes, fibrocytes, nerves, and various inflammatory cells.

Developmental Anomalies

See BCSC Section 2, *Fundamentals and Principles of Ophthalmology,* and Section 6, *Pediatric Ophthalmology and Strabismus,* for discussion of various developmental ocular anomalies, including aniridia and coloboma.

Aniridia

True aniridia, or complete absence of the iris, is rare. Most cases of aniridia are incomplete, with a narrow peripheral rim of rudimentary iris tissue present (Fig 11-5). Aniridia is

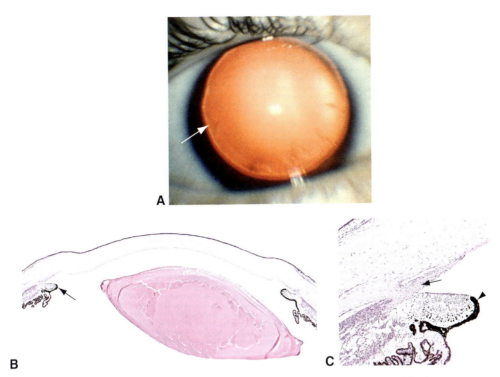

Figure 11-5 Aniridia. **A,** Retroillumination of the eye in a child with bilateral aniridia shows a zonular gap *(arrow)* between the lens and a rudimentary iris. **B,** Low-magnification view of the anterior segment of an eye (different patient than in A) with aniridia. Note the rudimentary iris *(arrow)* and cataractous lens. **C,** Higher-magnification image reveals a malformed iris *(arrowhead)*, which inserts anteriorly into the trabecular meshwork of a malformed angle *(arrow)*. *(Part A courtesy of Nora V. Laver, MD; parts B and C courtesy of Tatyana Milman, MD.)*

typically bilateral, though it may sometimes be asymmetric. Histologically, the rudimentary iris consists of underdeveloped ectodermal/mesodermal neural crest elements. The angle is often incompletely developed, and peripheral anterior synechiae that have an overgrowth of corneal endothelium are often present, most likely accounting for the high incidence of glaucoma in individuals with aniridia. Other ocular findings in aniridia include cataract, corneal limbal stem cell deficiency, and foveal hypoplasia.

Both autosomal dominant and sporadic inheritance patterns have been described. An association between sporadic aniridia and Wilms tumor has been linked to 11p13 deletions and to pathogenic variants in the *PAX6* gene, located in the same region of chromosome 11. Microcephaly, cognitive impairment, and genitourinary abnormalities have also been associated with aniridia.

> Tibrewal S, Ratna R, Gour A, et al. Clinical and molecular aspects of congenital aniridia—a review of current concepts. *Indian J Ophthalmol.* 2022;70(7):2280–2292.

Coloboma

Coloboma, a partial or complete absence of normal tissue, may affect the iris, ciliary body, or choroid or all 3 structures (Fig 11-6). Colobomas are often a result of incomplete closure

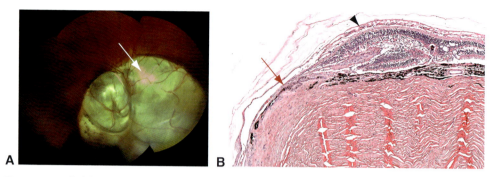

Figure 11-6 Colobomas. **A,** Choroidal coloboma. Note the RPE hyperplasia at the margin of the colobomatous defect and the fibroglial tissue within the coloboma *(arrow).* **B,** Retinochoroidal coloboma shows loss of choroid and normal retina. A glial membrane replaces the retina over the coloboma *(red arrow).* The retina is malformed at the edge of the coloboma *(black arrowhead). (Part B courtesy of Tatyana Milman, MD.)*

of the fetal fissure in the optic cup in the inferonasal meridian of the eye. Histologically, choroidal colobomas appear as an area nearly devoid of both retinal and choroidal tissues. A thin layer of glial tissue (intercalary membrane) may be the only tissue overlying the sclera.

Inflammation (Uveitis)

See BCSC Section 9, *Uveitis and Ocular Inflammation,* for in-depth discussion of the conditions described in the following sections and the immunologic processes involved. See also Chapter 9, Activity 9-1, on common patterns of ocular inflammation.

Infectious Uveitis

Infectious processes in the uveal tract may be restricted to that layer of the eye or may be part of a generalized inflammatory process that affects multiple or all layers of the eye. If the eye is the primary source of the infection (eg, as in posttraumatic bacterial infection), that infection is termed *exogenous*. If, however, the infection originates elsewhere in the body (eg, a ruptured diverticulum) and subsequently spreads hematogenously to involve the uveal tract, the infection is referred to as *endogenous*. A wide variety of organisms can cause infections of the uveal tract, including bacteria, fungi, viruses, and protozoa.

Histologic examination often shows a mix of acute and chronic inflammatory cells within the choroid, ciliary body, or iris stroma. In cases of infection with viral, fungal, or protozoal (eg, toxoplasmosis) agents, epithelioid histiocytes are typically present (granulomatous inflammation). If infection is suspected, special stains for microorganisms may be helpful. See Chapter 2, Table 2-2, as well as Figure 2-6F–H for examples of histochemical stains for infectious organisms commonly used in ophthalmic pathology.

Noninfectious Uveitis

Noninfectious uveitis can be divided into nonspecific and specific forms. Most uveitides are nonspecific with no etiologic causes found and likely represent localized autoimmune disease. Several types of specific uveitis are discussed in the following sections.

Sympathetic ophthalmia

Sympathetic ophthalmia is a rare bilateral granulomatous panuveitis that occurs after accidental or surgical injury to one eye (the *exciting,* or *inciting, eye*), followed by a latent period of weeks to years before development of uveitis in the uninjured globe (the *sympathizing eye*).

> Sympathetic ophthalmia is a clinical diagnosis. The histologic findings are not pathognomonic.

Immunomodulatory therapy may modify the histologic findings in sympathetic ophthalmia. Histologically, a diffuse granulomatous inflammatory reaction occurs within the uveal tract and is composed of lymphocytes and epithelioid histiocytes containing phagocytosed melanin (Figs 11-7, 11-8). Plasma cells are usually scant, suggesting a cell-mediated response. Classically, in the early stages of the disease, the choriocapillaris is spared, a finding that may help distinguish sympathetic ophthalmia from Vogt-Koyanagi-Harada (VKH) syndrome. Varying degrees of inflammation may be present in the anterior chamber, such as clusters of histiocytes deposited on the corneal endothelium *(mutton-fat keratic precipitates)*. *Dalen-Fuchs nodules,* which are accumulations of epithelioid histiocytes and lymphocytes between the RPE and Bruch membrane, may be seen in some cases (see Fig 11-8). These nodules may also be present in other diseases (eg, VKH syndrome and sarcoidosis) and thus are not pathognomonic of sympathetic ophthalmia.

See BCSC Section 7, *Oculofacial Plastic and Orbital Surgery,* for additional discussion.

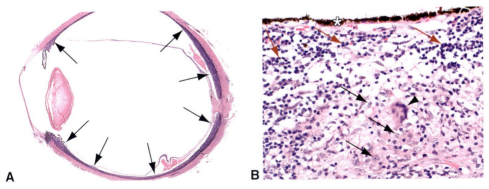

Figure 11-7 Sympathetic ophthalmia. **A,** Diffuse infiltration of the uveal tract by chronic inflammatory cells, seen as a purple layer beneath the retina *(arrows)*. **B,** Higher magnification of the RPE *(asterisk)* and choroid shows a multinucleated giant cell *(arrowhead)*, epithelioid histiocytes *(black arrows)*, and lymphocytes *(red arrows)*. Note the relative sparing of the choriocapillaris beneath the RPE. *(Part A courtesy of Hans E. Grossniklaus, MD; part B courtesy of Michele M. Bloomer, MD.)*

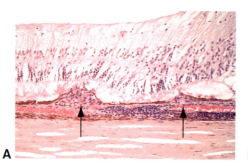 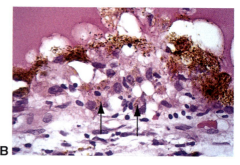

Figure 11-8 Dalen-Fuchs nodules in sympathetic ophthalmia. **A,** Focal aggregates of inflammatory cells are present between the RPE and Bruch membrane *(arrows).* **B,** Higher magnification demonstrates epithelioid histiocytes containing cytoplasmic pigment *(arrows)* within the nodules (H&E stain). *(Courtesy of Hans E. Grossniklaus, MD.)*

Sarcoidosis

Sarcoidosis is an inflammatory disorder (or group of disorders) that can affect nearly all systems of the body. The disease is characterized by granulomatous inflammation, specifically, the formation of granulomas, in various organs and tissues. The uveal tract is the most common site of ocular involvement. Anteriorly, granulomas of the iris may develop, either at the pupillary margin *(Koeppe nodules)* or elsewhere in the iris stroma *(Busacca nodules).* In the posterior segment, chorioretinitis (Fig 11-9A, B), periphlebitis, and chorioretinal nodules may be present. Periphlebitis may appear clinically as inflammatory lesions, referred to as *candlewax drippings* (perivenous exudates). Inflammatory cell infiltration may cause the optic nerve head to become swollen.

Histologically, the classic sarcoid nodule is a nonnecrotizing granuloma. These granulomas are collections of epithelioid histiocytes, sometimes accompanied by multinucleated giant cells, surrounded by a narrow cuff of lymphocytes (Fig 11-9C). In the uveal tract, the inflammatory infiltrate may show a more diffuse distribution of lymphocytes and epithelioid histiocytes (granulomatous inflammation). Multinucleated giant cells may contain *asteroid bodies* (star-shaped, acidophilic inclusion bodies) (Fig 11-9D) and/or *Schaumann bodies* (spherical, basophilic, calcified inclusion bodies) in their cytoplasm. Neither asteroid nor Schaumann bodies are pathognomonic for sarcoidosis.

Juvenile xanthogranuloma

Juvenile xanthogranuloma is an uncommon inflammatory condition that occurs in children. The skin and uvea are commonly affected. In the uveal tract, lesions may present as a solid mass, mimicking a neoplastic process. The lesions are often vascularized, and the blood vessels tend to be fragile, resulting in intralesional hemorrhage. Iris lesions in juvenile xanthogranuloma may cause a spontaneous hyphema (Fig 11-10A). The characteristic histologic features of the lesions include lipid-laden histiocytes, Touton giant cells, lymphocytes, and occasional eosinophils (Fig 11-10B).

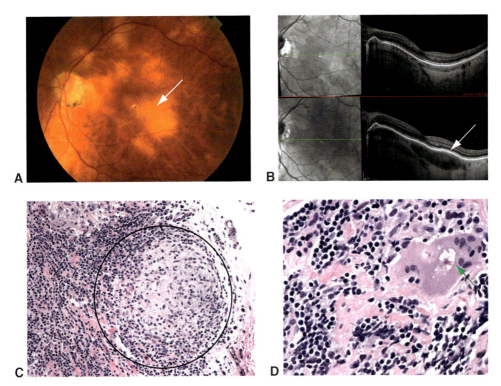

Figure 11-9 Sarcoidosis. **A,** Creamy choroidal infiltrates with irregular borders *(arrow).* **B,** Optical coherence tomography (OCT) images of the unaffected eye *(top)* and the eye with chorioretinitis *(bottom)* demonstrate thickening of the choroid with obscuration of choroidal vasculature *(arrow)* in the involved eye. **C,** Biopsy of a sarcoid nodule showing epithelioid histiocytes and lymphocytes (granulomatous inflammation) arranged as a nonnecrotizing granuloma *(circle).* **D,** High-magnification photomicrograph of a sarcoid nodule demonstrates a star-shaped pink, proteinaceous inclusion, an asteroid body *(arrow),* within a multinucleated giant cell. *(Parts A and B courtesy of H. Josefine Fuchs, MD; parts C and D courtesy of Nasreen A. Syed, MD.)*

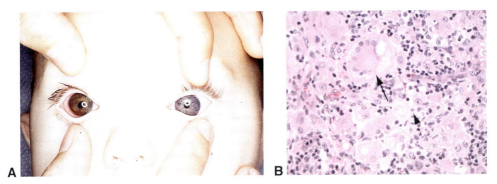

Figure 11-10 Juvenile xanthogranuloma. **A,** 20-month-old child with right unilateral spontaneous hyphema due to xanthogranulomatous inflammation involving the iris in juvenile xanthogranuloma. **B,** Touton giant cells *(arrow)* with a ring of nuclei, inner eosinophilic cytoplasm, and outer vacuolated or foamy cytoplasm; foamy histiocytes *(arrowhead);* and lymphocytes are admixed. *(Part A courtesy of Nora V. Laver, MD; part B courtesy of Nasreen A. Syed, MD.)*

Degenerations

Neovascularization of the Iris (Rubeosis Iridis)

Neovascularization of the iris (NVI) is commonly found in surgically enucleated blind eyes. NVI occurs often due to severe inflammation or ischemia, leading to production of vascular endothelial growth factor in the eye. See BCSC Section 10, *Glaucoma*, for other conditions associated with NVI.

Histologically, the new vessels tend to lack supporting tissue and do not possess the thick collagenous cuff that encircles normal iris vessels. The new vessels grow on the anterior surface of the iris, eventually forming a fibrovascular membrane, which often flattens the anterior surface of the iris and may extend into the anterior chamber angle. The neovascular membrane has a myofibroblastic component, which contracts and eventually leads to angle closure due to formation of peripheral anterior synechiae. Neovascularization of the angle often results in *neovascular glaucoma,* a secondary form of angle-closure glaucoma (see Chapter 10, Fig 10-25). Membrane contraction may drag the posterior iris pigment epithelial layer onto the anterior iris surface at the pupillary border, resulting in an *ectropion uveae* (Fig 11-11). In advanced cases, atrophy of the dilator muscle, attenuation of the pigment epithelium, and stromal fibrosis may occur.

Hyalinization of the Ciliary Body

With age, the ciliary processes become hyalinized and fibrosed, losing stromal cellularity; occasionally, dystrophic calcification develops. The thin, delicate processes become blunted and attenuated, and the stroma becomes more eosinophilic (Fig 11-12). This process is a normal age-related change to the ciliary body and is not considered pathologic, although it does contribute functionally to the development of presbyopia.

Choroidal Neovascularization

Choroidal neovascularization is discussed in Chapter 10 and in BCSC Section 12, *Retina and Vitreous*.

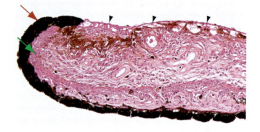

Figure 11-11 Iris neovascularization (rubeosis iridis). Tiny blood vessels sprout from existing iris vasculature, typically on the anterior surface of the iris *(black arrowheads)*, flattening the anterior surface of the iris. The contractile component of the neovascular membrane may result in dragging of the posterior iris pigment epithelium *(red arrow)* and sphincter muscle *(green arrow)* anteriorly at the pupillary margin, resulting in ectropion uveae. *(Courtesy of Tatyana Milman, MD.)*

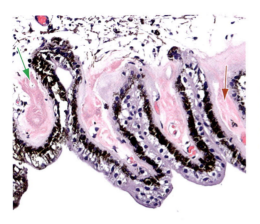

Figure 11-12 Age-related changes in the ciliary body. Blunting of ciliary processes with sclerotic vessels *(green arrow)* and hyalinization *(red arrow)* develop with increasing age. *(Courtesy of Nora V. Laver, MD.)*

Neoplasia

Uveal neoplasms are also discussed in detail in Chapters 16, 17, and 19. This chapter's discussion of uveal neoplasms focuses primarily on histology.

Iris

Nevus

An *iris nevus* is a localized proliferation of melanocytic cells that generally appears as a darkly pigmented lesion of the iris stroma with minimal distortion of the iris architecture (see Chapter 16, Fig 16-1).

An iris nevus appears histologically as a combination of, or an accumulation of, any of the following:

- branching dendritic nevus cells
- spindle nevus cells
- epithelioid nevus cells (least common)

All of these cell types usually contain melanin granules in the cytoplasm. A nevus cell nucleus is typically oblong or ovoid with a bland appearance and indistinct nucleoli. Less commonly, epithelioid nevus cells may be present. A variety of growth patterns and cytologic appearances are possible, but cellular atypia and significant mitotic activity are not present. The nevus cells aggregate within the stroma and sometimes also appear as a plaque on the surface of the iris (Fig 11-13). Occasionally, nevus cells may extend into the adjacent anterior chamber angle structures.

Melanoma

Melanomas that arise in the iris typically follow a relatively nonaggressive clinical course, in contrast to posterior (ciliochoroidal) melanomas. Most iris melanomas develop in the inferior sectors of the iris (see Chapter 16, Fig 16-2). The lesions can be quite vascularized and may occasionally cause spontaneous hyphema.

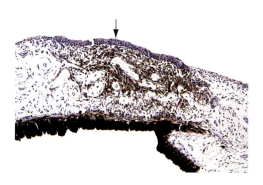

Figure 11-13 Iris nevus. Circumscribed lesion composed of darkly pigmented spindle melanocytes in the iris stroma with an overlying placoid proliferation of amelanotic melanocytes *(arrow)*. *(Courtesy of Tatyana Milman, MD.)*

Iris melanomas can be composed of spindle melanoma cells, epithelioid melanoma cells, or a combination of both. Histologically, spindle cells possess plump, spindle-shaped nuclei that have a coarse, granular appearance and prominent nucleoli. These cells are the equivalent of the spindle-B cells in posterior uveal melanoma (see the "Melanoma" subsection under Choroid and Ciliary Body). Epithelioid cells are polyhedral, with large, round nuclei that have a clumped chromatin pattern and prominent eosinophilic nucleoli. Both spindle and epithelioid cells tend to have a high nuclear-to-cytoplasmic ratio. The cytoplasm of melanoma cells can range from amelanotic to heavily pigmented.

Typically, iris melanomas grow as a solid mass in the stroma, sometimes covered by a surface plaque. Occasionally, the tumor demonstrates satellite lesions or a diffuse growth pattern and replaces normal iris stroma (Fig 11-14). In some cases, iris melanoma may be seen arising from a nevus on histologic examination. The modified Callender classification for posterior melanomas (see the "Melanoma" subsection under Choroid and Ciliary Body) is not applicable to iris melanomas in terms of prognostic significance. Iris melanomas are classified by a separate staging system that is based on infiltration of adjacent structures and the presence or absence of coexisting glaucoma. Distinguishing between iris nevus and melanoma based on histology may sometimes be challenging, requiring the expertise of an experienced ophthalmic pathologist.

Although iris melanomas may grow in a locally aggressive fashion, they rarely metastasize. One exception occurs when melanomas grow to diffusely involve the entire iris stroma (ring melanoma); patients present with unilateral hyperchromic heterochromia and glaucoma. This diffuse form of melanoma may invade the anterior chamber angle and extend posteriorly to involve the ciliary body.

Kivelä T, Simpson ER, Grossniklaus HE, et al. Uveal melanoma. In: Amin MB, Edge SB, Greene FL, eds. *AJCC Cancer Staging Manual*. 8th ed. Springer; 2017:805–817.

Choroid and Ciliary Body

Nevus

Most uveal nevi (>90%) develop in the choroid (see Chapter 16, Fig 16-4). Choroidal nevi may be composed of 4 types of nevus cells:

- *plump polyhedral nevus cells:* abundant cytoplasm is filled with pigment; has a small round to oval nucleus with a bland appearance

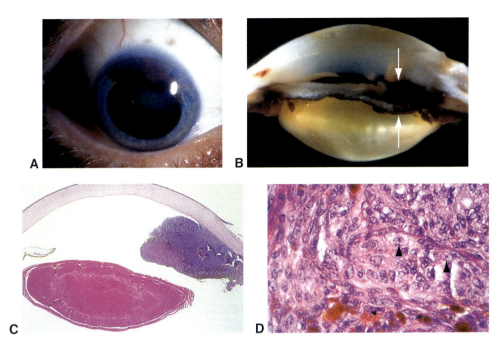

Figure 11-14 Iris melanoma. **A,** Clinical photograph. The pigmented tumor is visible between the 10:30 and 2:00 clock-hours. **B,** Gross appearance of a pigmented iris mass *(between arrows)*. **C,** Low magnification shows that the melanoma has completely replaced the normal iris stroma, extending into the anterior chamber, touching the posterior cornea, and occluding the angle. **D,** Histologic examination shows numerous plump epithelioid melanoma cells containing prominent nucleoli *(arrowheads)*. *(Courtesy of Hans E. Grossniklaus, MD.)*

- *slender spindle nevus cells* (Fig 11-15): the cytoplasm contains scant pigment; has a small, dark, elongated nucleus
- *plump fusiform dendritic nevus cells:* morphology is intermediate, between that of plump polyhedral and slender spindle cells
- *balloon cells:* abundant, foamy cytoplasm lacks pigment; has a bland nucleus

Depending on the size and location of the nevus, it may exert nonspecific effects on adjacent ocular tissues. The associated choriocapillaris may become compressed or obliterated, and drusen may form along Bruch membrane overlying the nevus. In rare cases, a choroidal nevus may be associated with localized serous detachments of the overlying RPE or neurosensory retina; secondary choroidal neovascularization may also occur.

Most choroidal nevi remain stationary over long periods of observation. However, the presence of nevus cells contiguous with a choroidal melanoma on histologic examination supports the theory that melanomas arise from choroidal nevi.

Melanocytoma

Uveal melanocytoma (magnocellular nevus) is a specific type of uveal nevus that warrants separate consideration. These benign dark-brown to jet-black lesions can occur anywhere in the uveal tract but appear most commonly in the peripapillary region (see Chapter 14, Fig 14-12A, B).

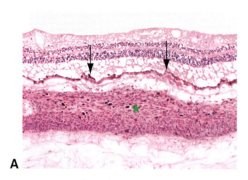 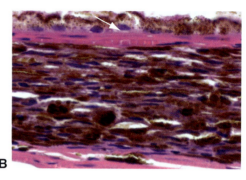

Figure 11-15 Choroidal nevi. **A,** Low-magnification image of a spindle-cell choroidal nevus *(asterisk)*. Drusen, typically associated with nevi, are present *(arrows)*. **B,** Higher-magnification image of a choroidal nevus composed of slender spindle cells with elongated thin nuclei and melanin pigment. Note the overlying RPE *(arrow)*. *(Part A courtesy of Nasreen A. Syed, MD; part B courtesy of Nora V. Laver, MD.)*

Histologically, a melanocytoma is composed of large polyhedral cells with small round to oval nuclei, finely dispersed chromatin, small nucleoli, and abundant cytoplasm. Mitotic figures are usually absent. Because the nevus cells are so heavily pigmented, it is usually necessary to apply melanin bleaching techniques to sections to accurately study the cytologic features (see Chapter 14, Fig 14-12C, D). Areas of cystic degeneration or necrosis may be observed in these nevi. In rare cases, melanocytoma can give rise to melanoma.

Melanoma

The most common primary intraocular malignancy in adults is melanoma that arises from the ciliary body and/or choroid. When this type of tumor grows to a significant size, it may extend beyond its site of origin (ie, from the choroid to the ciliary body and vice versa). Ciliary body and choroidal melanomas exhibit overlapping clinical features with similar prognostic implications and may be referred to collectively as *posterior uveal melanomas*.

Histologically, posterior uveal melanomas are composed of spindle cells and/or epithelioid melanoma cells (Table 11-1). Less commonly, balloon cells similar to those seen in choroidal nevi may be present. *Spindle cell melanoma* consists primarily of spindle-B melanoma cells. It may also contain spindle-A cells (however, a tumor that consists entirely of spindle-A cells is considered a nevus).

The cytoplasmic melanin content in melanoma cells can vary considerably. The mitotic rate in posterior uveal melanomas tends to be quite low (1–2 mitoses per 10 high-power fields [HPFs]), and mitotic counts by the pathologist typically require 40 HPFs. These tumors may exhibit variable amounts of necrosis.

Choroidal melanomas typically start as dome-shaped lesions and, as they grow and break through Bruch membrane, they acquire a mushroom or collar-button shape (Fig 11-16A, B). In some cases, tumors may involve both the choroid and the ciliary body (ciliochoroidal melanoma), and it may be difficult to determine where the lesion originated. Less commonly, choroidal lesions grow in a diffuse pattern, replacing normal choroid without achieving

Table 11-1 Posterior Uveal Melanoma Cell Types

Type	Description	Histopathology Image
Spindle A	• Has slender, elongated nuclei with finely dispersed chromatin and small nucleoli • A central stripe may be present along the long axis of the nucleus • Grows in a syncytial arrangement without clearly delineated borders	
Spindle B	• Has coarse, granular chromatin and plump ovoid nuclei • Has prominent nucleoli • Grows in a syncytial arrangement without clearly delineated borders	
Epithelioid	• Resembles epithelium because of the abundant eosinophilic cytoplasm and enlarged round to oval nuclei with coarse chromatin and large purple nucleoli • Border of the nucleus appears purple because chromatin marginates there • Is discohesive, with marked pleomorphism	

Illustrations courtesy of Mark Miller; histopathology images courtesy of Nora V. Laver, MD, except for the spindle-B histopathology image, which is courtesy of Nasreen A. Syed, MD.

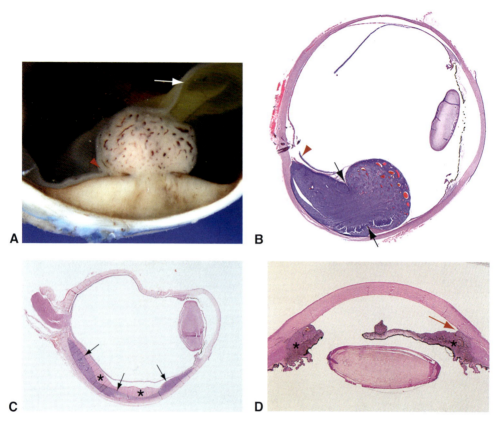

Figure 11-16 Growth patterns of posterior uveal melanoma. **A,** Gross photograph of choroidal melanoma that appears as a mushroom-shaped, predominantly amelanotic mass associated with retinal detachment *(arrow)*. The shape is a direct result of rupture through Bruch membrane *(arrowhead)*. **B,** Low-magnification microscopic appearance of a choroidal melanoma with rupture through Bruch membrane *(arrows)* and overlying retinal detachment *(arrowhead)*. **C,** A diffuse choroidal melanoma grows in a placoid fashion without achieving significant height *(arrows)*. Eosinophilic proteinaceous fluid *(asterisks)* is interposed between the retina and the tumor, corresponding to the exudative retinal detachment overlying the tumor. **D,** Ciliary body ring melanoma. By definition, a ring melanoma *(asterisks)* follows the major arterial circle of the iris at the iris root circumferentially around the eye. The melanoma has invaded the anterior chamber angle *(arrow)*, which can result in glaucoma. *(Part A courtesy of Ralph C. Eagle Jr, MD; part B courtesy of Tatyana Milman, MD.)*

significant height (Fig 11-16C). In the ciliary body, tumors usually grow in a fashion like that of their choroidal counterparts. Likewise, there is a ciliary equivalent of the diffuse pattern seen in the choroid, known as a *ring melanoma,* in which the tumor extends over the entire circumference of the ciliary body (Fig 11-16D).

Choroidal melanomas may cause serous detachments of the overlying and adjacent retina, with subsequent degenerative changes in the outer segments of the photoreceptors (see Fig 11-16). Melanoma may extend through the scleral emissary canals to gain access to the episcleral surface and the orbit (extrascleral tumor extension) (Fig 11-17). Less commonly, melanoma may directly invade the underlying sclera or overlying retina (Fig 11-18). Direct invasion of the anterior chamber or mechanical blockage of the chamber due to anterior iris displacement

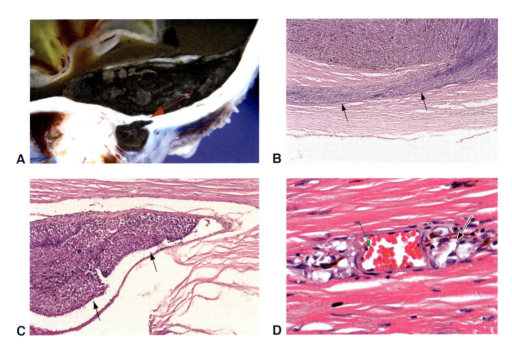

Figure 11-17 Invasion of scleral emissary canals by posterior melanoma. **A,** Macroscopic examination of a pigmented uveal melanoma with tumor extension into an emissary canal *(arrow)* and orbital tumor seeding. **B,** Melanoma cells track along an emissary canal within the sclera *(arrows)*. **C,** Melanoma is found within the vortex vein *(arrows)*. **D,** Melanoma cells focally pigmented with foamy cytoplasm *(black arrow)* spread by tracking along the outer sheaths of posterior ciliary vessels *(green arrow)*. *(Part A courtesy of Ralph C. Eagle Jr, MD; part D courtesy of Nora V. Laver, MD.)*

may lead to secondary glaucoma (see Chapter 6, Fig 6-16). In addition, tumor necrosis may lead to the dispersion of melanin in the anterior chamber and angle. The trabecular meshwork then becomes obstructed by histiocytes that have ingested this pigment, causing a type of secondary glaucoma called *melanomalytic glaucoma* (see Chapter 6, Fig 6-15).

Histologic prognostic factors Statistically, the most important histologic variables associated with survival in patients with posterior uveal melanomas are

- tumor cell type (modified Callender classification; see Table 11-1)
- size of tumor in contact with the sclera (greatest basal dimension of tumor)
- direct extraocular extension
- tumor location
- complexity of extravascular matrix patterns and high microvascular density

TUMOR CELL TYPE As defined by the modified Callender classification, tumor cell type is the most important histologic parameter in uveal melanoma risk stratification:

- *spindle cell melanoma:* more than 90% spindle cells; has the best prognosis
- *epithelioid melanoma:* more than 90% epithelioid cells; has the worst prognosis
- *mixed-cell type:* mixture of spindle and epithelioid cells; has an intermediate prognosis

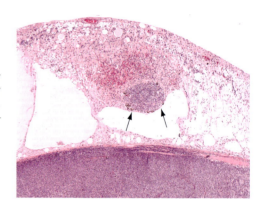

Figure 11-18 Invasion of the neurosensory retina by melanoma *(arrows)*. Note the atrophy of the overlying outer retina, cystoid edema, and intraretinal hemorrhage. *(Courtesy of Nasreen A. Syed, MD.)*

In rare cases, a melanoma undergoes extensive necrosis and is unable to be classified according to the Callender classification system. The prognosis for completely necrotic melanomas is the same as that for mixed-cell melanomas.

TUMOR SIZE Most studies have demonstrated that tumor size is an independent risk factor for patient survival; the larger the tumor, the worse the survival rate. Methodical measurements of tumor size are obtained on clinical and pathologic examination of tumors in eyes that have been treated with enucleation. Many studies use greatest basal dimension (arc of contact with the sclera) and greatest tumor thickness (apical height) to classify tumors based on size. The American Joint Committee on Cancer (AJCC) staging system stratifies uveal melanoma by size into 4 categories; these categories are described in Chapter 16.

EXTRAOCULAR EXTENSION Extension of posterior uveal melanomas may be classified as macroscopic (extension that can be detected clinically or by ultrasonography or, for enucleated eyes, seen on gross examination) or microscopic (extension seen only under the microscope in enucleated specimens). The AJCC staging system categorizes extrascleral extension as *present* or *not present*; if it is present, the largest diameter of the extrascleral component is categorized according to size: (1) 5 mm or less, or (2) greater than 5 mm. In general, extrascleral extension, particularly macroscopic extension, is associated with a less favorable outcome.

LOCATION Posterior uveal melanomas with any ciliary body involvement are also associated with a worse prognosis. Tumors with a scleral base located 1 mm or less from the optic disc (juxtapapillary) have a less favorable prognosis due to their less favorable location for treatment.

EXTRAVASCULAR MATRIX PATTERNS Intrinsic tumor extravascular matrix patterns are difficult to assess without histologic evaluation. Tumors demonstrating complex extravascular matrix patterns, such as closed loops or networks (3 or more back-to-back loops), are associated with a higher rate of subsequent metastases (Fig 11-19).

OTHER FACTORS Other histologic factors have some association with rates of survival and/or metastasis. The presence of many tumor-infiltrating lymphocytes and/or histiocytes

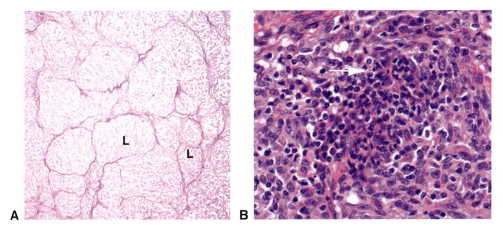

Figure 11-19 Unfavorable histologic prognostic factors in uveal melanoma. **A,** Complex extravascular matrix patterns in uveal melanoma (periodic acid–Schiff [PAS] stain) with closed loop (L) and networks (3 or more back-to-back loops). **B,** Melanoma with brisk tumor-infiltrating lymphocytes *(arrow)*. *(Part A courtesy of Nasreen A. Syed, MD; part B courtesy of Nora V. Laver, MD.)*

is associated with a higher metastatic rate. It is important to note that invasion through Bruch membrane is *not* associated with a decrease in survival rates.

Some types of posterior uveal melanomas exhibit biological behavior that cannot be predicted according to the criteria previously discussed. Survival rates of patients with diffuse ciliary body melanomas (ring melanoma) are particularly poor. These relatively flat tumors, which are almost always of mixed-cell type, may grow circumferentially without becoming significantly elevated. Diffuse choroidal melanomas have a similarly poor prognosis. Recent studies demonstrated that these tumors have an unfavorable molecular genetic profile.

Molecular genetics of uveal melanoma Molecular genetic studies of posterior uveal melanoma have shown that mutually exclusive pathogenic variants in *GNAQ* and *GNA11* are an initiating event in the development of uveal melanomas and nevi from melanocytes. However, these genetic variants are not prognostically relevant. Molecular profiling of uveal melanoma has emerged as the most powerful predictor of survival (Table 11-2).

CYTOGENIC ALTERATIONS In approximately half of all cases of uveal melanomas, monosomy of chromosome 3 is present; in a smaller proportion of cases, there is a gain or loss of a chromosome in chromosomes 1, 6, or 8. Tumors in individuals with monosomy 3, especially those with gains in 8q, are associated with increased mortality. The Cancer Genome Atlas (TCGA) classification for uveal melanoma groups tumors into 4 groups (A, B, C, and D) based on chromosome 3, 6, and 8 status (see Table 11-2).

GENE EXPRESSION PROFILING Molecular analysis of posterior uveal melanomas by gene expression profiling (GEP) classifies uveal melanoma prognoses as follows:

- *class 1A:* low metastatic potential
- *class 1B:* intermediate metastatic potential
- *class 2:* high metastatic potential

Table 11-2 TCGA Prognostic Classification of Uveal Melanoma

	TCGA Group A	TCGA Group B	TCGA Group C	TCGA Group D
Chromosome 3	Disomy 3	Disomy 3	Monosomy 3	Monosomy 3
Chromosome 6	Extra 6p	Extra 6p	—	—
Chromosome 8	Normal 8q	Partial extra 8q	Extra 8q	Extra 8q (multiple)
mRNA GEP	Class 1A	Class 1B	Class 2	Class 2
Frequent genetic alterations	E1F1AX	SF3B1	BAP1	BAP1
Prognosis	Favorable	Late metastasis	Unfavorable	Unfavorable

GEP = gene expression profiling; TCGA = The Cancer Genome Atlas.

Adapted from Jager MJ, Brouwer NJ, Esmaeli B. The Cancer Genome Atlas Project: an integrated molecular view of uveal melanoma. *Ophthalmology.* 2018;125(8):1139–1142.

In addition to GEP, *PRAME* gene mRNA expression in tumors is associated with increased metastatic risk in patients with class 1 or disomy 3 tumors as an independent prognostic factor. Resent research suggests that *PRAME* may also be a useful treatment target for patients with high-risk uveal melanomas.

MOLECULAR GENETIC ALTERATIONS Pathogenic variants in *BAP1* (BRCA1-associated protein-1) that lead to inactivation of *BAP1* within the tumor are associated with monosomy 3 (TCGA groups C and D), class 2 GEP, and a higher rate of metastasis. Pathogenic variants in *SF3B1* are associated with TCGA group B, class 1B GEP, and late metastasis.

 See Chapter 16 for further discussion of posterior uveal melanomas. Also see the Posterior Uveal Lesion Interactive Case Study in the online *Pathology Atlas*.

> Metastases almost invariably result from the hematogenous spread of melanoma to the liver; in more than 95% of tumor-related deaths, there is liver involvement. In as many as one-third of tumor-related deaths, the liver is the sole site of metastasis.

Field MG, Decatur CL, Kurtenbach S, et al. PRAME as an independent biomarker for metastasis in uveal melanoma. *Clin Cancer Res.* 2016;22(5):1234–1242.

Field MG, Durante MA, Anbunathan H, et al. Punctuated evolution of canonical genomic aberrations in uveal melanoma. *Nat Commun.* 2018;9(1):116.

Jager MJ, Brouwer NJ, Esmaeli B. The Cancer Genome Atlas Project: an integrated molecular view of uveal melanoma. *Ophthalmology.* 2018;125(8):1139–1142.

Metastatic Tumors

Tumors that have metastasized to the uveal tract are the most common intraocular tumors in adults. When these lesions are identified clinically, they most often involve the posterior choroid, with its rich vascular supply, but metastatic disease can affect any part of the uvea. Unlike primary uveal melanoma, metastases to the uvea are often multiple and may be bilateral. Most metastases are nonpigmented and flat; rare cases of mushroom-shaped metastases have been reported. The most common primary tumors that metastasize to the eye are breast carcinoma in women and lung carcinoma in men (Fig 11-20), although metastases from many different primary sites have been reported. Histologically, metastatic tumors may recapitulate the appearance of the primary lesion, or they may appear less differentiated. Special histochemical stains and a panel of immunohistochemical stains can be helpful in diagnosing metastatic lesions, determining the origin of the primary tumor, and, in some cases, guiding therapy for that tumor. See Chapter 19 for further discussion.

Clinical Pearl The importance of a careful clinical history in patients presenting with uveal melanoma cannot be overemphasized.

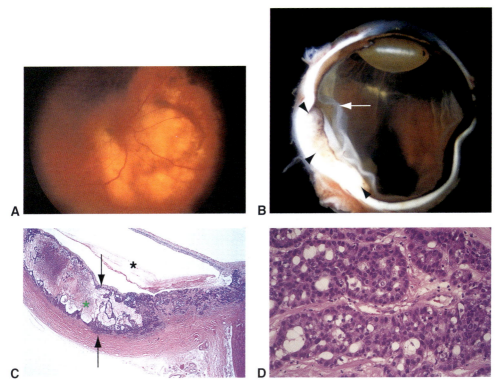

Figure 11-20 Choroidal metastases. **A,** Clinical appearance of a metastatic lesion from a primary lung tumor. **B,** Gross appearance of the same lesion shown in A *(between arrowheads),* associated with serous retinal detachment *(arrow).* **C,** Choroidal metastasis from lung adenocarcinoma; histology shows adenocarcinoma *(between arrows)* with mucin production *(green asterisk).* Note the overlying exudative retinal detachment *(asterisk).* **D,** Higher-magnification image depicts a well-differentiated adenocarcinoma with a distinct glandular morphology. *(Courtesy of Hans E. Grossniklaus, MD.)*

Other Uveal Tumors

Hemangioma

Hemangiomas of the choroid occur in 2 specific forms: circumscribed (ie, localized) and diffuse. *Circumscribed* choroidal hemangioma typically occurs in patients without systemic disorders. *Diffuse* choroidal hemangioma is generally seen in patients with encephalofacial angiomatosis (Sturge-Weber syndrome).

Histologically, in both forms of choroidal hemangioma, collections of variably sized vessels are present within the choroid (Fig 11-21). The lesions may appear as predominantly capillary hemangiomas, cavernous hemangiomas, or a mix of the two. There may be compressed melanocytes, hyperplastic RPE, and fibrous tissue proliferation in the adjacent and overlying choroid. See Chapters 16 and 17 (Figs 17-1, 17-2) in this volume for further discussion of choroidal hemangiomas. See also BCSC Section 12, *Retina and Vitreous*.

Choroidal osteoma

Choroidal osteomas are benign bony tumors that typically arise from the juxtapapillary choroid of young adults, most commonly young women. Histologically, choroidal osteomas are composed of compact mature lamellar bone in choroidal stroma (Fig 11-22A). The intratrabecular spaces are filled with loose connective tissue that contains large and small blood vessels, vacuolated mesenchymal cells, and scattered mast cells. The bony trabeculae contain osteocytes, mineralization lines, and occasional osteoclasts (Fig 11-22B). See Chapter 16 (Fig 16-12D) in this volume for detailed discussion of choroidal osteoma.

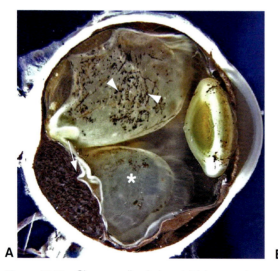 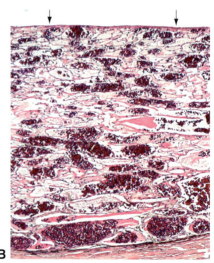

Figure 11-21 Circumscribed choroidal hemangioma. **A,** Macroscopic examination of an enucleated eye shows a circumscribed vascular mass *(arrow)* associated with a chronic bullous serous retinal detachment *(asterisk)*. Note the RPE hyperplasia in the detached retina *(arrowheads)*, which are indicative of chronicity of detachment. **B,** Histology demonstrates numerous thin-walled choroidal blood vessels; *arrows* designate Bruch membrane. *(Part A courtesy of Tatyana Milman, MD; part B courtesy of Steffen Heegaard, MD.)*

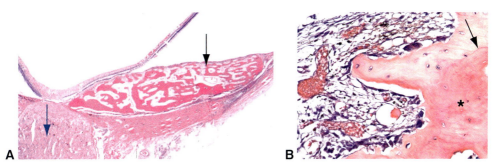

Figure 11-22 Choroidal osteoma. **A,** Circumscribed mass in choroidal stroma *(black arrow),* adjacent to the optic nerve *(blue arrow).* **B,** Higher-magnification image shows that the lesion is composed of compact, mature lamellar bone *(asterisk)* with mineralization lines *(arrow)* and intratrabecular connective tissue. *(Part A courtesy of Nora V. Laver, MD; part B courtesy of Steffen Heegaard, MD.)*

Clinical Pearl   Both choroidal osteoma and osseous metaplasia of the RPE in a phthisical eye are composed of a mature lamellar bone. The key difference between these lesions is in location: choroidal osteoma involves choroidal stroma, while osseous metaplasia of the RPE is situated internal to Bruch membrane, in subretinal space.

Lymphoid proliferation

The choroid may be the site of lymphoid proliferation, either as a primary ocular process or in association with systemic lymphoproliferative disease.

Primary choroidal lymphomas (previously known as *uveal lymphoid hyperplasia* or *uveal lymphoid infiltration*) are typically low-grade, extranodal marginal zone B-cell lymphomas similar to those that occur in the ocular adnexa and elsewhere in the body. High-grade choroidal lymphomas (Fig 11-23) are usually secondary to systemic disease. See Chapter 13 for discussion of the classification of lymphoproliferative lesions and Chapter 19 for additional information on uveal lymphoma.

Sagoo MS, Mehta H, Swampillai AJ, et al. Primary intraocular lymphoma. *Surv Ophthalmol.* 2014;59(5):503–516.

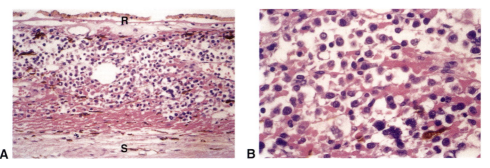

Figure 11-23 Choroidal lymphoma. **A,** Diffuse infiltration of the choroid by lymphoma *(blue cells).* R = RPE; S = sclera. **B,** Higher-magnification image demonstrates atypical pleomorphic lymphocytes. *(Courtesy of Hans E. Grossniklaus, MD.)*

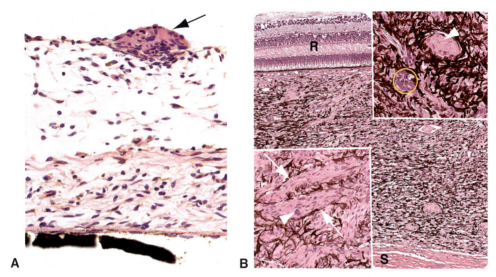

Figure 11-24 Neurofibromatosis 1. **A,** Lisch nodule on the anterior surface of the iris *(arrow)* is a hamartomatous proliferation of melanocytes and neural elements. **B,** Choroidal neurofibroma appears as a disorganized proliferation of neural elements and pigmented melanocytes diffusely involving choroidal stroma. S = underlying sclera; R = overlying retina. *Lower left inset:* Enlarged choroidal nerves *(arrows)* and ganglion cell *(arrowhead)*. *Upper right inset:* Proliferation of Schwann cells with concentric processes, known as an ovoid body *(arrowhead)* and a cluster of ganglion cells *(circle)*. *(Courtesy of Tatyana Milman, MD.)*

Neural sheath tumors

Schwannomas (neurilemomas) and neurofibromas are rare in the uveal tract. Multiple neurofibromas may occur in the ciliary body, iris, and choroid in patients with neurofibromatosis 1 (Fig 11-24; see Chapter 16, Fig 16-3B for an image of Lisch nodules [melanocytic hamartomas]). For more information on neural sheath tumors, see Chapter 13.

Leiomyoma

Uveal leiomyoma is a rare neoplasm that most commonly arises from the smooth muscle of the ciliary body in young adult women. Clinically, leiomyoma may be confused with amelanotic melanoma or neurofibroma. However, unlike melanoma, leiomyoma tends to transmit light with transillumination. Histologically, leiomyoma is identical to leiomyoma of the uterus (uterine fibroid) and consists of a proliferation of tightly packed, slender amelanotic spindle cells that express smooth muscle markers, such as SMA (smooth muscle actin) and desmin (see Chapter 2). Under light microscopy and transmission electron microscopy, leiomyoma sometimes exhibits both myogenic and neurogenic differentiation. In such cases, the tumor is called *mesectodermal leiomyoma*.

CHAPTER **12**

Eyelids

 This chapter includes a related video. Go to aao.org/bcscvideo_section04 or scan the QR code in the text to access this content.

Highlights

- The eyelid contains distinct structures including meibomian glands, sweat glands, and hair follicles, all of which can give rise to various pathologic conditions.
- Benign neoplasms of the eyelid are common in both children and adults.
- Malignant eyelid neoplasms increase in incidence with age. In North America and Europe, basal cell carcinoma is most common, followed by squamous cell carcinoma and sebaceous carcinoma. In Asian countries, sebaceous carcinoma is most common.
- Sebaceous carcinoma frequently propagates along the eyelids and ocular surface via intraepidermal and intraepithelial pagetoid spread.
- Eyelid nevi are common, and they evolve and proliferate with age.

Topography

The eyelids, which extend from the eyebrow superiorly to the cheek inferiorly, can be divided into orbital and tarsal components. At the level of the tarsus, the eyelid consists of 4 main histologic layers, from anterior to posterior (Video 12-1; Fig 12-1):

- skin
- orbicularis oculi muscle
- tarsus
- palpebral conjunctiva

VIDEO 12-1 Eyelid histology.
From Resident Lectures, Eyelid Histology. © American Academy of Ophthalmology 2023. Courtesy of Nora V. Laver, MD.
Available at aao.org/bcscvideo_section04

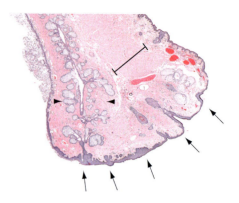

Figure 12-1 Cross section of an eyelid. Proceeding from left (posterior) to right (anterior) are the palpebral conjunctiva; the tarsus, containing the meibomian glands *(between arrowheads)*; the orbicularis oculi muscle *(bracket)*; and the dermis, underlying the epidermis. *Arrows* indicate the eyelid margin. *(Courtesy of Heather Potter, MD.)*

Clinical Pearl A surgical plane of dissection into the eyelid that functionally separates the eyelid into anterior and posterior lamellae can be accessed through an incision starting at the gray line, an isolated slip of orbicularis muscle known as the *Riolan muscle*.

The skin of the eyelids is thinner than that of most other body sites. The surface epidermis consists of keratinized stratified squamous epithelium, which contains melanocytes and antigen-presenting Langerhans cells. Deep to the epidermis is the dermis (stromal tissue), which is composed of loose collagenous connective tissue and contains the following:

- cilia (eyelashes) and associated sebaceous glands (glands of Zeis; specialized pilosebaceous units)
- apocrine sweat glands (glands of Moll)
- eccrine sweat glands
- pilosebaceous units (vellus hairs)

The eyelid has no subcutis; the dermis of the eyelid rests directly on the skeletal muscle, the orbicularis oculi. This characteristic helps in tissue site identification. The *tarsal plate*—a thick plaque of dense, collagenous connective tissue—contains the meibomian glands (specialized sebaceous glands). Also present near the upper border of the superior tarsal plate (and less so along the lower border of the inferior tarsal plate) are the accessory lacrimal glands of Wolfring; the accessory lacrimal glands of Krause are located in the conjunctival fornices. The *palpebral conjunctiva* adheres tightly to the posterior surface of the tarsus.

Eyelid glands secrete their products in various ways. Sebaceous glands are holocrine glands, meaning that their secretion contains entire secreting cells. The secretion from apocrine sweat glands contains the apical part of the secreting cells (decapitation secretion). Eccrine sweat glands and lacrimal glands secrete sweat and tears, respectively, without loss of any part of the secreting cells.

For detailed information on the topography and anatomy of the eyelids, see also BCSC Section 7, *Oculofacial Plastic and Orbital Surgery*.

The following are some common dermatopathologic terms that are also applicable to eyelid pathology:

- *acanthosis:* increased thickness (hyperplasia) of the stratum Malpighii (cellular layers of the epidermis)
- *hyperkeratosis:* increased thickness of the stratum corneum (keratin layer)
- *parakeratosis:* retention of nuclei within the stratum corneum
- *papillomatosis:* formation of fingerlike upward projections of epidermis surrounding fibrovascular cores
- *dyskeratosis:* premature keratinization of individual squamous cells
- *acantholysis:* loss of cohesion (dissolution of intercellular bridges) between adjacent squamous epithelial cells

Developmental Anomalies

For additional discussion of the developmental anomalies covered in this chapter, see BCSC Section 7, *Oculofacial Plastic and Orbital Surgery*.

Distichiasis

Distichiasis is the aberrant formation of cilia within the tarsus, which causes them to exit the eyelid margin through the orifices of the meibomian glands, resulting in an extra (partial or complete) row of eyelashes. The pathogenesis of distichiasis is thought to be an anomalous formation within the tarsus of a complete pilosebaceous unit rather than just the normal sebaceous (meibomian) gland. Histologically, hair follicles can be seen within the tarsal plate. The tarsus may be rudimentary, and the glands of Moll are often hypertrophic. See BCSC Section 6, *Pediatric Ophthalmology and Strabismus,* and Section 8, *External Disease and Cornea,* for additional discussion.

Phakomatous Choristoma

A rare developmental tumor, phakomatous choristoma (Zimmerman tumor) results from the aberrant retention of parts of the lens placode in the lower eyelid during embryologic development. As a result, lens epithelium proliferates within the inferonasal portion of the lower eyelid. The epithelial cells may undergo cytoplasmic enlargement, identical to the enlargement of "bladder" cells associated with posterior subcapsular cataract (Fig 12-2). Basement membrane material is produced, recapitulating the lens capsule; this material stains positively with periodic acid–Schiff (PAS) stain. The eyelid mass formed is usually present at birth and enlarges slowly. Complete excision is curative.

Dermoid Cyst

Dermoid cysts are not uncommon in the lateral portion of the upper eyelid and eyebrow in young children. However, they are more traditionally regarded as orbital lesions and are therefore discussed in Chapter 13 of this volume.

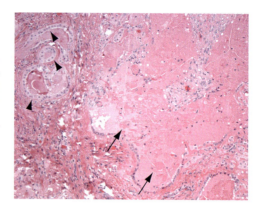

Figure 12-2 Phakomatous choristoma of the eyelid. The dermis displays a disorganized proliferation of lens epithelium *(arrowheads)* and occasional "bladder" cells *(arrows)* similar to those seen in posterior subcapsular cataract. Note the large amount of eosinophilic material, which represents lens crystalline proteins. *(Courtesy of Nasreen A. Syed, MD.)*

Inflammation

Infectious Inflammatory Disorders

Infectious organisms can cause disease that is localized (eg, hordeolum), multicentric (eg, papillomas), or diffuse (eg, cellulitis), depending on the causative agent. Common routes of infection include primary inoculation through a bite or wound and direct spread from a contiguous site, such as an infected paranasal sinus. Infectious agents may be

- bacterial, such as *Staphylococcus aureus* in hordeolum and infectious blepharitis
- fungal, such as *Trichophyton rubrum* in tinea faciei
- viral, such as poxvirus in molluscum contagiosum
- parasitic, such as *Demodex folliculorum*

Bacterial infections

Hordeolum A hordeolum (also called a *stye*) is an acute, generally self-limited primary infectious process typically involving the glands of Zeis (external hordeolum) or, less often, the meibomian glands (internal hordeolum). A small abscess, or focal collection of neutrophils and necrotic debris (ie, pus), forms at the site of infection, which is usually caused by *S aureus*. Lesions may drain spontaneously or require surgical management.

Cellulitis The diffuse spread of acute inflammatory cells through tissue planes is known as *cellulitis*. *Preseptal* cellulitis involves the tissues of the eyelid anterior to the orbital septum, which is the collagenous membrane that connects the nonmarginal borders of the tarsal plates to the bony orbital rim. Cellulitis is most often secondary to bacterial infection of the paranasal sinuses. Histologic examination reveals neutrophilic infiltration of the soft tissues, accompanied by interstitial edema and, occasionally, necrosis (Fig 12-3). See BCSC Section 7, *Oculofacial Plastic and Orbital Surgery*, for additional discussion.

Viral infections

Human papillomavirus may infect the skin of the eyelids, typically manifesting as *verruca vulgaris*, or *wart*. Clinically, verruca vulgaris is usually an elevated lesion with fine papillary projections. Histologically, the lesions exhibit a papillary growth pattern with fingerlike projections, acanthosis, compact hyperkeratosis, and apical parakeratosis (Fig 12-4A).

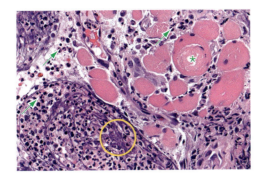

Figure 12-3 Preseptal cellulitis of the eyelid. Neutrophils *(arrows)* in the background of basophilic smudgy necrosis *(circle)* infiltrate between the skeletal muscle fibers *(asterisk)* of the orbicularis oculi muscle. *(Courtesy of Tatyana Milman, MD.)*

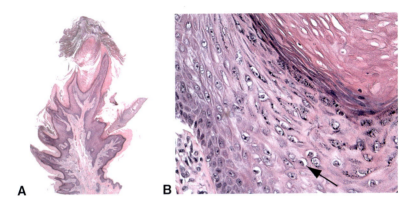

Figure 12-4 Verruca vulgaris. **A,** Verruca vulgaris is a form of human papillomavirus (HPV) infection of the eyelid epidermis. The resulting "wart" has a papillary growth pattern with fingerlike projections. **B,** Occasional koilocytes with nuclear contraction and cytoplasmic clearing are present *(arrow).* *(Courtesy of Nasreen A. Syed, MD.)*

Infected epidermal cells may demonstrate cytoplasmic clearing (koilocytosis) (Fig 12-4B). A mixed inflammatory cell infiltrate is typically present in the superficial dermis.

Molluscum contagiosum, which is caused by a member of the poxvirus family, is characterized by the formation of small, waxy, dome-shaped epidermal nodules with central umbilication. When these nodules are present on the eyelid margin, an associated follicular conjunctivitis may develop because of shedding of virus onto the conjunctival surface (Fig 12-5). The lesions have a distinctive histologic appearance; prominent molluscum (Henderson-Patterson) bodies, which are intracytoplasmic eosinophilic inclusions that contain virus particles, are present (Fig 12-6).

Parasitic infections
Infection of the eyelid with the mite *Demodex folliculorum* is a common cause of chronic eyelid and conjunctival inflammation. The conditions caused by this parasite are discussed in BCSC Section 8, *External Disease and Cornea.*

Fungal infections
Periocular fungal infection is rare and is often misdiagnosed. Tinea faciei in the periocular area can occur due to infection from a dermatophyte fungus such as *Trichophyton rubrum.*

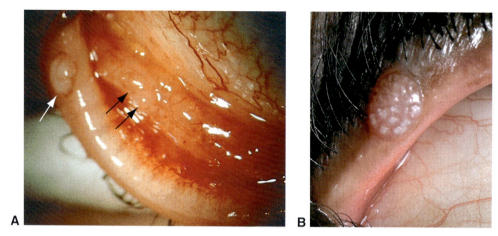

Figure 12-5 Clinical photos of molluscum contagiosum. **A,** Molluscum contagiosum involving the eyelid margin *(white arrow)* with associated follicular conjunctivitis *(black arrows)*. **B,** Solitary molluscum contagiosum involving the eyelid margin. *(Part B courtesy of Swathi Kaliki, MD.)*

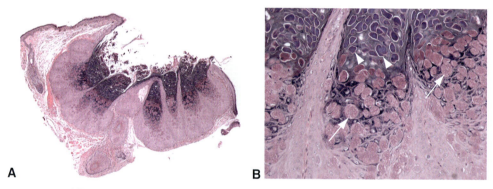

Figure 12-6 Histologic appearance of molluscum contagiosum. **A,** Note the cup-shaped, thickened epidermis with a central crater. **B,** In the more central portion of the epidermis, cell nuclei are displaced peripherally by large eosinophilic viral inclusions known as molluscum bodies *(arrows)*. The molluscum bodies become more basophilic near the surface of the epithelium *(arrowheads)*. *(Courtesy of Nasreen A. Syed, MD.)*

Tinea faciei appears as red scaly patches in the eyelids often aggravated by sunlight exposure. Diagnosis is made by microscopic identification of fungus in skin scrapings.

Noninfectious Inflammatory Disorders

Chalazia

A chalazion is a noninfectious inflammatory lesion that presents as a chronic, often painless nodule of the eyelid that develops when the lipid secretions of the meibomian glands or, less often, the glands of Zeis are discharged into the surrounding tissues, inciting a lipogranulomatous reaction (Fig 12-7). Chalazia may occur due to residual tissue lipid after the acute inflammation of a hordeolum subsides.

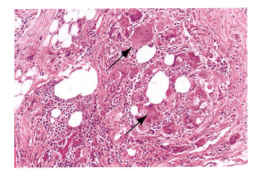

Figure 12-7 Chalazion. Granulomatous inflammation consists of epithelioid histiocytes and multinucleated foreign body–type giant cells *(arrows)* surrounding clear spaces (lipogranuloma). Because the lipid is dissolved by solvents during routine tissue processing, optically clear ("lipid dropout") spaces remain. Lymphocytes, plasma cells, and neutrophils are also often present.

Degenerations and Deposits

Xanthelasma

A type of xanthoma, xanthelasma consists of single or multiple soft, yellow plaques that occur in the medial canthal region of the eyelids (Fig 12-8A). Associated hyperlipoproteinemic states, particularly hyperlipoproteinemia types II and III, are present in 30%–40% of patients with xanthelasma. Associated inflammatory signs are minimal. Histologically, xanthelasma consists of aggregates of histiocytes with foamy, lipid-laden cytoplasm distributed diffusely and often around blood vessels within the dermis (Fig 12-8B). The histiocytes are postulated to phagocytose lipid that leaks from the blood vessels in the eyelid, although why the eyelid is often affected remains unclear.

Clinical Pearl   The differential diagnosis of extensive or atypical eyelid xanthelasma associated with orbital fullness includes:

- adult-onset xanthogranuloma
- adult-onset asthma and periocular xanthogranuloma
- necrobiotic xanthogranuloma
- Erdheim-Chester disease

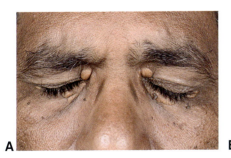
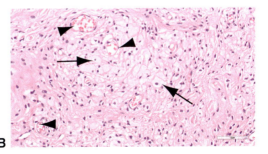

A **B**

Figure 12-8 Xanthelasma. **A,** Patient with prominent xanthelasma. Note the yellow plaques on the medial upper eyelid and lower eyelids. **B,** Aggregates of foamy lipid-laden histiocytes *(arrows)* are present in the dermis, focally surrounding blood vessels *(arrowheads)*. *(Part A courtesy of Swathi Kaliki, MD; part B courtesy of Saumya Jakati, MD.)*

The histopathology of xanthogranuloma is similar to that of xanthelasma, with foamy xanthoma cells, but the cells present in cases of xanthogranuloma are more deeply infiltrative, involving tissue deep to the orbicularis muscle. Touton giant cells (see Chapter 1, Fig 1-10B and Chapter 11, Fig 11-10B) and a prominent inflammatory infiltrate are also present. These entities may be associated with immunoglobulin G4–related disease.

Amyloidosis

The term *amyloid* refers to a heterogeneous group of extracellular proteins that have a β-pleated sheet configuration and exhibit birefringence and dichroism under polarized light when stained with Congo red (see Chapter 4, Fig 4-11D). Amyloid deposition in the skin is usually bilateral and symmetric and presents as multiple waxy yellow-white papules (Fig 12-9). The deposition of amyloid within blood vessel walls in the skin causes increased vascular fragility and often results in intradermal hemorrhages, accounting for the purpura seen clinically. On routine histologic sections, amyloid appears as an amorphous, eosinophilic extracellular deposit (see Fig 4-11B).

The amyloidoses are a group of diseases characterized by the deposition of specific amyloid proteins in various tissues and organs, often causing dysfunction of the affected tissues and organs. Common sources of amyloid proteins include

- immunoglobulin amyloid light (AL) chain fragments, in plasma cell and B-cell dyscrasias
- transthyretin, pathogenic variants in familial amyloid polyneuropathy types I and II
- gelsolin, pathogenic variants in familial amyloidosis, Finnish type (also known as *gelsolin amyloidosis* or *Meretoja syndrome*)

Amyloid deposits within the eyelid skin are highly indicative of a systemic disease process, either primary or secondary, whereas deposits elsewhere in the ocular adnexa are more likely to represent a localized disease process. Other systemic diseases with eyelid manifestations are listed in Table 12-1. See Chapter 4 for additional discussion on amyloidosis. Also see BCSC Section 8, *External Disease and Cornea,* which discusses the classification of amyloidosis.

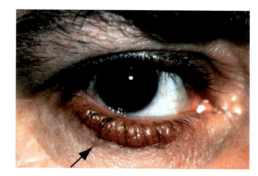

Figure 12-9 Cutaneous amyloidosis of the eyelid in a patient with plasma cell myeloma. Note the waxy elevation and the associated purpura of the lower eyelid, under the lesion *(arrow). (Courtesy of John B. Holds, MD.)*

Table 12-1 Eyelid Manifestations of Systemic Diseases

Systemic Condition	Eyelid Manifestations
Amyloidosis	Waxy papules/nodules, ptosis, purpura
Carney complex	Myxoma
Fraser syndrome	Cryptophthalmos
Dermatomyositis	Edema, erythema
Erdheim-Chester disease	Xanthogranuloma
Granulomatosis with polyangiitis (formerly Wegener granulomatosis)	Edema, ptosis, lower eyelid retraction
Hyperlipoproteinemia	Xanthelasma
Mandibulofacial dysostosis (Treacher Collins syndrome)	Lower eyelid pseudocoloboma
Neurofibromatosis 1	Cutaneous neurofibromas, plexiform neurofibroma of upper eyelid
Polyarteritis nodosa	Focal infarction
Relapsing polychondritis	Inflammatory papules, unilateral or bilateral edema, ptosis or eyelid retraction
Sarcoidosis	Inflammatory papules
Scleroderma	Reduced mobility, taut skin, telangiectasias
Systemic lupus erythematosus	Telangiectasias, edema, discoid cutaneous lesions
Thyroid eye disease	Swelling, eyelid retraction

Modified from Wiggs JL, Jakobiec FA. Eyelid manifestations of systemic disease. In: Albert DM, Jakobiec FA, eds. *Principles and Practice of Ophthalmology*. Saunders; 1994:1859.

Cysts

See BCSC Section 7, *Oculofacial Plastic and Orbital Surgery*, for further information on the entities discussed in the following subsections.

Epidermoid Cysts

Epidermoid cysts, also called *epidermal inclusion cysts*, are common in the eyelids. They may arise spontaneously, frequently from the blockage of hair follicle infundibulum, or as a result of the entrapment of epidermis beneath the skin's surface following surgery or trauma. Epidermoid cysts are lined with keratinized stratified squamous epithelium and contain keratin (Fig 12-10).

Ductal Cysts

The eyelid contains the ducts of numerous structures, including the lacrimal gland and the apocrine and eccrine sweat glands. Cysts may develop in any of these ducts. A cyst arising from the duct of the lacrimal gland is called *dacryops*. Cysts arising from sweat ducts are referred to as either *apocrine* or *eccrine hidrocystomas* (Fig 12-11). Histologically, ductal cysts typically are lined with a double layer of cuboidal epithelium, as are the ducts from which they arise. The lumen of the cyst typically appears empty.

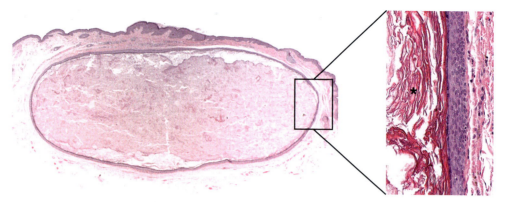

Figure 12-10 Epidermoid (epidermal inclusion) cyst in the dermis. *Detail:* The cyst lining resembles epidermis but does not contain skin appendages. The lumen contains keratin *(asterisk)*. *(Courtesy of Nasreen A. Syed, MD; detail image courtesy of Tatyana Milman, MD.)*

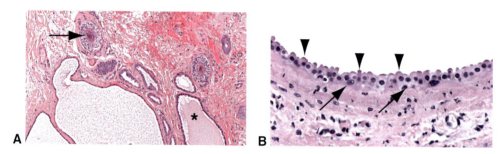

Figure 12-11 Apocrine hidrocystoma. **A,** Multiloculated cyst associated with the hair follicle *(arrow)* and filled with proteinaceous secretion *(asterisk).* **B,** The cyst is lined by a double layer of epithelium: an inner, cuboidal layer with apical projections (snouts; *arrowheads*), indicative of apocrine secretion, and an outer, flattened myoepithelial layer *(arrows)*. *(Part A courtesy of Tatyana Milman, MD; part B courtesy of Nasreen A Syed, MD.)*

Neoplasia

See BCSC Section 7, *Oculofacial Plastic and Orbital Surgery,* for further information on the entities discussed in the following subsections.

Epidermal Neoplasms

Seborrheic keratosis

Seborrheic keratosis is a common benign epidermal proliferation typically occurring in middle age. Clinically, it is a well-circumscribed round to oval, dome-shaped verrucoid "stuck-on" papule, appearing tan-pink to dark brown. Histologically, several architectural patterns are possible, but all lesions demonstrate hyperkeratosis, acanthosis, and some degree of papillomatosis. The acanthosis is a result of the proliferation of either polygonal or basaloid squamous cells without dysplasia. In more pigmented lesions, the basal epidermal layer contains an increased amount of melanin. *Pseudohorn cysts,* concentrically laminated collections of surface keratin within an epidermal crypt, are a characteristic histologic finding in most types of seborrheic keratosis (Fig 12-12).

In cases of *irritated seborrheic keratosis,* also termed *inverted follicular keratosis,* nonkeratinized squamous epithelial whorling, or squamous "eddies," and acantholysis are present within the proliferating epidermis (Fig 12-13). Sudden onset of multiple seborrheic keratoses

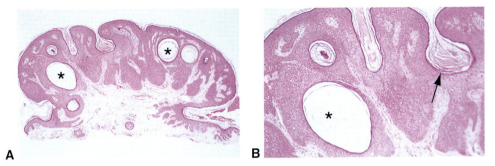

Figure 12-12 Seborrheic keratosis. **A,** The epidermis is acanthotic with a papillary configuration. Note the keratin-filled pseudohorn cysts *(asterisks).* **B,** When serial histologic sections are studied, pseudohorn cysts *(asterisk)* within the epidermis are found to represent crevices or infoldings of epidermis *(arrow)* rather than true cysts. *(Courtesy of Hans E. Grossniklaus, MD.)*

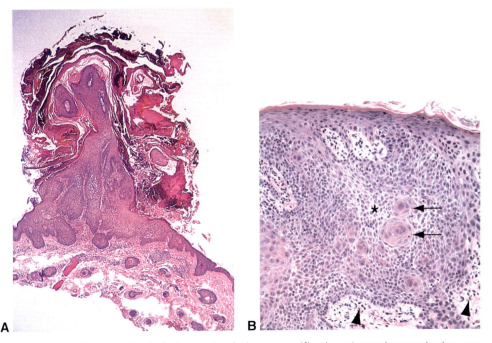

Figure 12-13 Irritated seborrheic keratosis. **A,** Low-magnification photomicrograph shows a papillary epidermal proliferation with hyperkeratosis on the surface. Clinically, this lesion appeared as a cutaneous horn. **B,** High-magnification photomicrograph of a different lesion. The epidermis often shows whorls of cells, known as squamous "eddies" *(arrows),* separation between squamous cells, or *acantholysis (asterisk),* and mild disorganization. Increased inflammatory infiltrate *(arrowheads)* is present in the underlying dermis. *(Part B courtesy of Nasreen A. Syed, MD.)*

Table 12-2 Eyelid Neoplasms Associated With Systemic Neoplastic Syndromes

Syndrome	Eyelid Manifestations
Basal cell nevus syndrome/Gorlin syndrome (medulloblastoma, fibrosarcoma)	Multiple basal cell carcinomas
Cowden disease (breast carcinoma; fibrous hamartomas of breast, thyroid, gastrointestinal tract)	Multiple trichilemmomas
Muir-Torre syndrome (visceral carcinoma, usually colorectal)	Multiple sebaceous neoplasms (adenoma, carcinoma), keratoacanthoma

Modified from Wiggs JL, Jakobiec FA. Eyelid manifestations of systemic disease. In: Albert DM, Jakobiec FA, eds. *Principles and Practice of Ophthalmology*. Saunders; 1994:1859.

is known as the *Leser-Trélat sign* and is associated with visceral malignancy, usually a gastrointestinal adenocarcinoma; these keratoses may in fact represent evolving acanthosis nigricans, which manifests as dark, thickened, and velvety skin. Table 12-2 lists other systemic neoplastic syndromes with possible eyelid manifestations.

Actinic keratosis

Actinic keratoses are precancerous squamous lesions that typically occur starting in middle age. They appear clinically as erythematous, scaly macules or papules on sun-exposed skin, particularly the face and the dorsal surfaces of the hands. Actinic keratoses range from a few millimeters to 1 centimeter in diameter. Hyperkeratotic types of these lesions may form a cutaneous horn, and hyperpigmented types may clinically simulate melanocytic lesions. Squamous cell carcinoma may develop from preexisting actinic keratosis, although most studies indicate that the risk is 0.24% per year for an individual actinic keratosis and 12%–20% for multiple actinic keratoses. When squamous cell carcinoma arises in individuals with actinic keratosis, the risk of subsequent metastatic dissemination is very low (0.5%–3.0%).

Histologically, actinic keratosis has several variants. All types demonstrate changes in the epidermis with hyperkeratosis and parakeratosis. Cellular atypia (nuclear hyperchromatism and/or pleomorphism and an increased nuclear-to-cytoplasmic ratio) is present and ranges from mild (involving only the basal epithelial layers) to frank carcinoma in situ (full-thickness involvement of the epidermis). Loss of the granular cell layer, dyskeratosis (premature keratinization of individual cells), and mitotic figures above the basal epithelial layer are often present (Fig 12-14A, B). The underlying dermis often shows solar elastosis (Fig 12-14C; also see Chapter 4, Fig 4-10B), which manifests as fragmentation, clumping, and basophilic discoloration of the dermal elastin and collagen. A chronic inflammatory cell infiltrate is usually observed at the base of the lesion in the superficial dermis. Histologic examination of the base of the lesion is necessary to determine whether invasion through the epidermal basement membrane, indicative of squamous cell carcinoma, is present.

Epidermal malignancies

Basal cell carcinoma Basal cell carcinoma (BCC), the most common malignant neoplasm of the eyelids, accounts for more than 90% of all malignant eyelid tumors. Although exposure to sunlight is the main risk factor, genetic factors can play a role in individuals with familial syndromes. The hedgehog signaling pathway is involved in the pathogenesis of BCC.

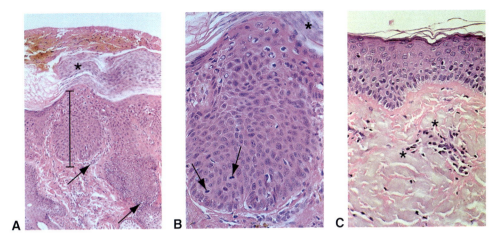

Figure 12-14 Actinic keratosis and actinic (solar) elastosis. **A,** Actinic keratosis. Note the epidermal acanthosis *(bracket)*, disorganization within the epidermis (dysplasia), parakeratosis *(asterisk)*, and inflammation within the dermis *(arrows)*. **B,** Higher magnification of part A; note the epidermal dysplasia and mitotic figures *(arrows)* and parakeratosis *(asterisk)*, with loss of granular cell layer. **C,** Actinic elastosis of the dermis. The dermal stroma appears bluish *(asterisks)* instead of pink in this hematoxylin and eosin (H&E)–stained section. This is a histologic indicator of ultraviolet light–induced tissue damage.

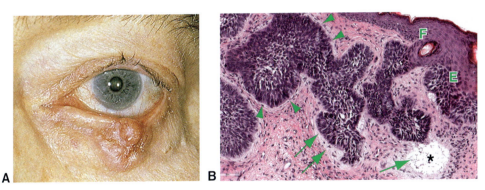

Figure 12-15 Basal cell carcinoma (BCC), nodular type. **A,** Pearly to pink centrally ulcerated nodule with elevated, rolled edges. Note the loss of eyelashes lashes in the area of the tumor. **B,** Histologic appearance. Nests of basaloid cells with peripheral palisading *(arrowheads)* and retraction artifact *(asterisk)* from desmoplastic stroma (fibrotic stroma with myxoid change; *arrows*). The tumor arises from the basal layer of the surface epidermis (E) and the hair follicle (F) infundibulum. *(Part B courtesy of Tatyana Milman, MD.)*

The lower eyelid and medial canthus are the most common sites of involvement. Tumors in the medial canthal area are more likely to be deeply invasive and to involve the orbit.

Nodular BCC (the most common subtype) is a slow-growing, slightly elevated lesion, often with ulceration and pearly, raised, rolled edges (Fig 12-15A). The *morpheaform,* or sclerosing, variant of BCC is a flat or slightly elevated pale-yellow indurated plaque; this type is often infiltrative, and its extent is difficult to determine clinically. A small percentage of BCCs are pigmented or multicentric.

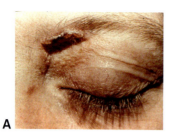 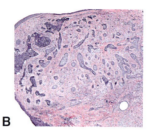 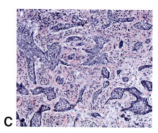

Figure 12-16 BCC, morpheaform (sclerosing) type. **A,** Note the lesion in the brow region resembles a thick scar without distinct margins. **B,** Histopathology shows thin cords and strands of basophilic (blue) tumor cells. **C,** Tumor cells infiltrate the dermis and are surrounded by fibrotic (desmoplastic) dermal tissue. *(Courtesy of Nora V. Laver, MD.)*

As the name implies, BCCs originate from the basal layer of the epidermis and the outer root sheath of the hair follicle and occur almost exclusively in hair-bearing tissue. Tumor cells are characterized by relatively bland oval nuclei and a high nuclear-to-cytoplasmic ratio. BCC forms cohesive islands with palisading of the peripheral cell layer, mimicking the hair follicle infundibulum (Fig 12-15B). In the morpheaform BCC, thin cords and strands of tumor cells are set in a fibrotic (desmoplastic) stroma (Fig 12-16).

To treat this tumor adequately, margin control is required via either frozen section (conventional or Mohs technique) or permanent section (see Chapter 2). Nonsurgical treatment options for localized BCCs include 5-fluorouracil, imiquimod, and photodynamic therapy. Radiotherapy may be an option in some cases. The Food and Drug Administration (FDA) has approved hedgehog pathway inhibitors (eg, vismodegib) and PD-1 inhibitors (eg, cemiplimab) for use in cases of unresectable and metastatic BCCs. Morbidity in BCCs is almost always the result of local spread; metastasis is extremely unusual.

Squamous cell carcinoma *Squamous cell carcinoma (SCC)* is far less common than BCC in eyelid skin. Like BCCs, most SCCs arise in solar-damaged skin and have a predilection for the lower eyelid. The clinical appearance of SCC is diverse, ranging from ulcers to plaques to fungiform or nodular growths. Accordingly, the clinical differential diagnosis is extensive; an accurate diagnosis requires pathologic examination of tissue.

Histologic examination shows atypical squamous cells that extend beyond the epidermal basement membrane into the dermis, forming nests and strands, and incite a desmoplastic tissue reaction (Fig 12-17). Tumor cells may be well differentiated (forming keratin, with intercellular bridges, and easily recognizable as squamous), moderately differentiated, or poorly differentiated (requiring ancillary studies to confirm the nature of the neoplasm). Metastases via perineural and lymphatic invasion may be present and are important to include in the pathology report when identified microscopically, as this finding may be associated with a less favorable prognosis. To treat this tumor adequately, frozen section (conventional or Mohs technique) or permanent section margin control is required. Regional lymph node metastasis may occur in patients with SCC of the eyelid.

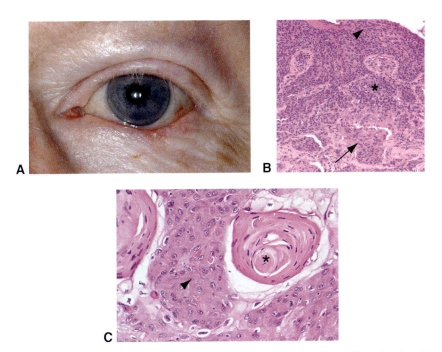

Figure 12-17 Squamous cell carcinoma (SCC). **A,** Clinical appearance. Note the focal loss of eyelashes (madarosis) and scaly appearance of the lower eyelid. **B,** Photomicrograph shows tumor cells invading the dermis *(arrow)* from the overlying epidermis, which is involved by the carcinoma in situ *(arrowhead)*. Inflammatory cell infiltrate *(asterisk)* is present at the base of the lesion. **C,** Well-differentiated SCC with invasive tumor nest *(arrowhead)* that is morphologically similar to the epidermis and a keratin pearl *(asterisk)*, an aggregate of dyskeratotic malignant cells in the dermis. *(Part A courtesy of Keith D. Carter, MD; part B courtesy of Saumya Jakati, MD.)*

KERATOACANTHOMA Keratoacanthoma is a rapidly growing epithelial proliferation with the potential for spontaneous involution. Strong evidence supports the idea that keratoacanthomas are a variant of a well-differentiated SCC. These dome-shaped nodules, which have keratin-filled central craters, may attain considerable size, up to 2.5 cm in diameter, within a matter of weeks to a few months (Fig 12-18). The natural history is typically spontaneous involution over several months, resulting in a slightly depressed scar. The incidence of keratoacanthoma is higher in immunosuppressed individuals.

Histologically, keratoacanthomas show a cup-shaped invagination of well-differentiated squamous cells into the markedly inflamed dermis, forming a so-called "pushing," or noninfiltrative, margin. Mitotic activity, dyskeratosis, and nuclear atypia may occur, similar to those seen in cases of typical SCC. Many dermatopathologists and ophthalmic pathologists prefer to call this lesion *well-differentiated squamous cell carcinoma with keratoacanthoma-like differentiation* because of the possibility of perineural invasion and metastasis. Complete excision is generally recommended.

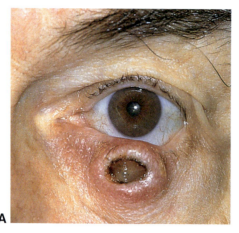
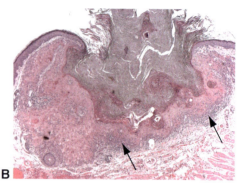

Figure 12-18 Keratoacanthoma. **A,** Clinical photograph. Note the elevated lesion with a central ulcerated crater and focal loss of eyelashes. In this case, the central crater was originally filled with keratin. **B,** Low-magnification histologic section illustrates a cup-shaped lesion with the central keratin-filled crater and an intense inflammatory infiltrate in the surrounding dermis *(arrows).* *(Part B courtesy of Nasreen A. Syed, MD.)*

Dermal Neoplasms

Infantile (capillary) hemangiomas are common in the eyelids of children. These benign neoplasms usually appear shortly after birth as a bright red lesion, grow over weeks to months, and typically involute by the time the child has reached school age.

The histologic appearance of the lesion depends on the stage of evolution of the hemangioma. Early lesions may be very cellular, with solid nests of plump endothelial cells and correspondingly little vascular lumen formation. Established lesions typically demonstrate well-developed capillary channels lined with plump endothelial cells in a lobular configuration (Fig 12-19). Involuting lesions demonstrate increased fibrosis and hyalinization of capillary walls with luminal occlusion.

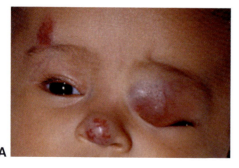
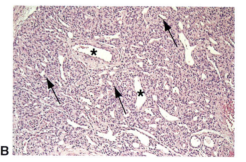

Figure 12-19 Infantile (capillary) hemangioma. **A,** Infant with multiple facial infantile hemangiomas, including a large lesion of the left upper eyelid. **B,** Histology shows small capillary-sized vessels *(arrows)* lining the numerous plump endothelial cells, surrounding larger vascular channels *(asterisks).* *(Part A courtesy of Sander Dubovy, MD.)*

Intervention is reserved for lesions that affect vision because of ptosis or astigmatism, leading to amblyopia. For infantile hemangiomas that require therapy, β-blockers are often used as first-line treatment and usually result in a significant reduction in size.

Neoplasms and Proliferations of the Dermal Appendages

Dermal appendages of the eyelid include sebaceous glands, sweat glands, and hair follicles (see the section Topography at the beginning of the chapter). They are also referred to as *adnexal* appendages, which, in this context, refers to skin appendages that are located within the dermis but communicate through the epidermis with the surface. Although technically meibomian glands are not dermal appendages, they are modified sebaceous glands embedded in the tarsus and may give rise to some of the neoplasms discussed in the following subsections, particularly sebaceous carcinoma.

Syringoma

Syringoma, a common benign lesion derived from sweat glands, can occur in the eyelid, usually the lower eyelid, manifesting as multiple tiny flesh-colored papules. Histologically, syringomas consist of circumscribed proliferations of comma-shaped and/or ovoid ductules that are lined by columnar epithelium with pink-to-gray eosinophilic luminal cells with secretory material (Fig 12-20). Microcystic adnexal carcinoma, an infiltrative locally aggressive neoplasm, has similar histologic findings, highlighting the importance of careful clinical correlation.

Sebaceous hyperplasia

Sebaceous (gland) hyperplasia is an uncommon benign lesion of the face, eyelid, and caruncle that appears as a flesh-colored or faintly yellow lobulated nodule. Histologically, sebaceous hyperplasia consists of an enlarged sebaceous gland with an increased number of glandular lobules attached to a single central duct (Fig 12-21).

Sebaceous adenoma

Sebaceous adenoma is a rare benign lesion that can occur in the eyelid. It typically manifests as a circumscribed yellowish nodule (Fig 12-22A). Histologically, it is composed of multiple sebaceous lobules that are irregularly shaped and incompletely differentiated (Fig 12-22B).

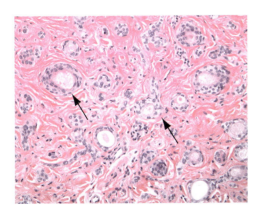

Figure 12-20 Syringoma. Histology shows ovoid and comma-shaped ductules lined by cuboidal epithelium *(arrows)* and filled with gray-pink luminal material. *(Courtesy of Nasreen A. Syed, MD.)*

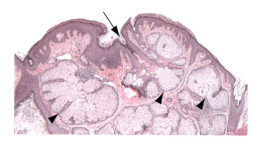

Figure 12-21 Sebaceous hyperplasia. Numerous sebaceous gland lobules *(arrowheads)* surround a central duct *(arrow)*. *(Courtesy of Nasreen A. Syed, MD.)*

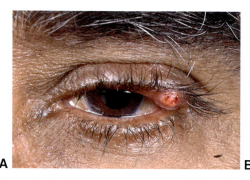

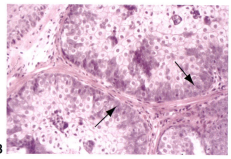

Figure 12-22 Sebaceous adenoma. **A,** Yellowish vascular nodule arising from meibomian glands at the eyelid margin. **B,** Histology shows sebaceous lobules with focal proliferations of immature basophilic (blue) sebocytes *(arrows)*. This type of sebaceous neoplasm is commonly associated with Muir-Torre syndrome. *(Part A courtesy of Swathi Kaliki, MD; part B courtesy of Nasreen A. Syed, MD.)*

The possibility of Muir-Torre syndrome (a subtype of Lynch syndrome, a hereditary cancer syndrome) should be considered when sebaceous adenoma is diagnosed, because it is the most common sebaceous neoplasm in individuals with this syndrome (see Table 12-2). Immunohistochemistry tests for DNA mismatch repair proteins may be useful in screening for cancer syndromes.

Sebaceous carcinoma

Sebaceous (gland) carcinoma is a malignant tumor that may originate in the meibomian glands, glands of Zeis, or sebaceous glands of the caruncle. It most commonly involves the upper eyelid of individuals older than 50 years, and several studies found that it is the most common primary eyelid cancer in Asian populations. The diagnosis is often missed or delayed because of this lesion's tendency to mimic other conditions (masquerade syndrome), such as a chalazion or chronic unilateral blepharoconjunctivitis (Fig 12-23).

Histologically, the well- to moderately differentiated tumors resemble sebocytes of the sebaceous gland (Fig 12-24). Poorly differentiated tumors, however, may be difficult to distinguish from other, more common malignancies, such as SCC or BCC. The use of immunohistochemical panels to diagnose sebaceous carcinoma has essentially replaced the use of special stains for lipid (eg, oil red O or Sudan black B) performed on frozen tissue sections. A variety of immunohistochemical stains have been investigated for their specificity in identifying

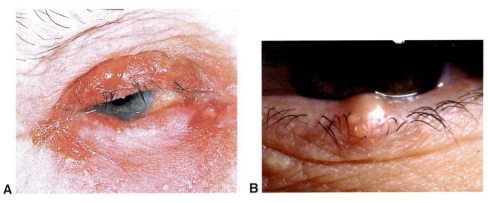

Figure 12-23 Sebaceous carcinoma, clinical appearance. **A,** This lesion mimics blepharoconjunctivitis with eyelid erythema, loss of eyelashes, ulceration, and irregular eyelid thickening. **B,** This lesion mimics a chalazion of the lower eyelid. Focal eyelash loss is present. *(Part B courtesy of Roberta E. Gausas, MD.)*

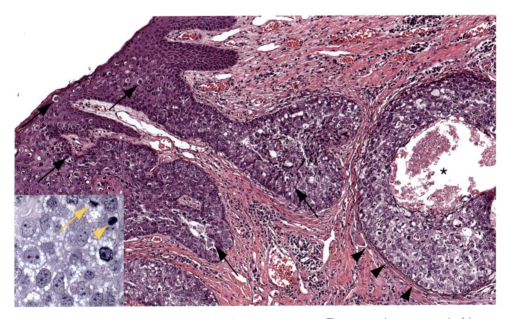

Figure 12-24 Sebaceous carcinoma, histologic appearance. The tumor is composed of basophilic cells with vacuolated cytoplasm, which form lobules with central comedonecrosis *(asterisk)*, recapitulating sebaceous holocrine secretion. Note the lack of peripheral palisading and the retraction artifact *(arrowheads)*, which are typically seen in BCC. Also note the pagetoid invasion of epidermis by individual tumor cells and small clusters of tumor cells *(arrows)*. *Inset:* Tumor cells have dark, hyperchromatic, pleomorphic nuclei with multiple small nucleoli. The cytoplasm often has a foamy or vacuolated appearance. Brisk mitotic figures *(arrow)* and apoptotic bodies *(arrowhead)* are present. *(Main image courtesy of Tatyana Milman MD; inset courtesy of Ralph C. Eagle Jr, MD.)*

sebaceous carcinoma; however, no single antibody or combination of antibodies exists that can consistently identify these tumors. An expert evaluation by an experienced pathologist may be required for an accurate diagnosis, and careful clinical correlation is essential in such cases.

A primary characteristic of sebaceous carcinoma is *pagetoid spread,* the dissemination of both individual tumor cells and small clusters of tumor cells within the epidermis or conjunctival epithelium (see Fig 12-24). The pagetoid areas do not have a direct connection to the main portion of the tumor. Another characteristic is the partial or complete replacement of conjunctival epithelium by tumor cells, or *intraepithelial sebaceous carcinoma.*

Management Treatment of sebaceous carcinoma typically involves wide local excision of the tumor; however, pagetoid and intraepithelial spread may make complete excision of sebaceous carcinoma challenging. Widespread conjunctival epithelial involvement or deeply invasive tumors may require orbital exenteration. Because it can be difficult to identify pagetoid spread or sebaceous carcinoma in situ on frozen sections, permanent sections are generally considered more reliable for evaluation of surgical resection margins than frozen sections of margins or Mohs technique. Before definitive excision, determining the extent of the tumor via routine processing of multiple small map biopsies, typically of conjunctival tissue, may provide a more accurate assessment of the extent of spread of the carcinoma, guiding management. Adjunctive therapies for sebaceous carcinoma include the use of topical chemotherapy, cryotherapy, radiotherapy, and systemic chemotherapy.

Survival rates for patients with sebaceous carcinoma are worse than those for patients with SCC, but they have improved in recent years as a result of increased physician awareness, earlier detection, more accurate diagnoses, and more appropriate treatment modalities. Typically, survival correlates with size and extent of the primary tumor. Tumor spread may be local, with direct invasion into the orbit and other adjacent structures. As metastases first involve regional lymph nodes, sentinel lymph node biopsy can be useful in tumor staging. Distant metastasis of tumor, usually to the liver and lung, may occur in rare cases.

Merkel Cell Carcinoma

Merkel cell carcinoma (MCC) is a rare neuroendocrine carcinoma that typically occurs in the head and neck skin in older adults. Infection with the Merkel cell polyomavirus infection, ultraviolet (UV) light exposure, and immunosuppression have been implicated in the pathogenesis of MCC. The tumor often presents as a dermal-based red or violaceous nodule (Fig 12-25). Histologically, the tumor is composed of monotonous round, blue cells with finely granular "salt-and-pepper" chromatin and scant cytoplasm, reflecting neuroendocrine differentiation. There are numerous apoptotic nuclei and frequent mitoses. Immunohistochemical studies show that these tumor cells stain with cytokeratin 20 antibodies and neuroendocrine markers such as synaptophysin and chromogranin A (see Fig 12-25).

MCC is managed primarily with wide local excision (with at least 5-mm margins) and biopsy of regional lymph nodes. Resection requires evaluation of surgical margins with frozen section or Mohs technique. MCC has a high mortality rate compared with other eyelid tumors. The risk of regional and distant metastasis is approximately 30%, and local recurrences

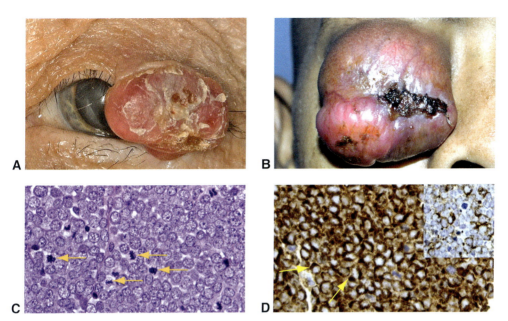

Figure 12-25 Merkel cell carcinoma (MCC). **A,** MCC presents as a reddish nodule in the upper eyelid. **B,** An aggressive form of the disease. **C,** Histology shows that the tumor is composed of blue cells with round nuclei, granular chromatin, scant cytoplasm, and frequent mitoses *(arrows)*. **D,** Immunohistochemistry with cytokeratin 20 shows the characteristic pattern of perinuclear dotlike staining *(arrows)* and immunoreactivity. *Inset:* Positivity for chromogranin A, a marker of neuroendocrine differentiation. Molecular studies for Merkel cell polyomavirus (MCPyV) DNA are positive in approximately 80% of MCCs. *(Parts A, C, and D courtesy of Tatyana Milman, MD; part B courtesy of Swathi Kaliki, MD.)*

are common. Thus, a diagnosis of MCC requires prompt and complete surgical treatment and referral to the appropriate head and neck and oncology specialists.

Melanocytic Neoplasms

Melanocytic nevus

Melanocytic nevi are benign proliferations of melanocytes that commonly occur on the eyelids. These nevi may be visible at birth or shortly after birth (congenital nevi), or they may become more obvious in adolescence or adulthood; congenital nevi tend to be larger than those appearing in later years. Congenital nevi greater than 20 cm in diameter are called *giant congenital melanocytic nevi.* The risk of congenital nevi developing into melanoma is proportional to the size of the nevus; close follow-up and/or excision of congenital nevi is warranted. Congenital nevi of the eyelid may develop in utero before the separation of the upper and lower eyelids, resulting in matching nevi on these eyelids, termed a *kissing* (or *split) nevus* (Fig 12-26). In adults, nevi typically appear as smooth, dome-shaped, sometimes hyperpigmented, lesions on the eyelid margin. Other forms of nevi can occur on the eyelid, including blue nevi, Spitz nevi, and dysplastic nevi, though only in rare cases.

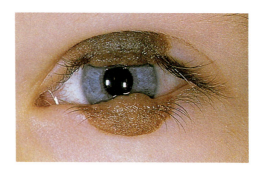

Figure 12-26 Congenital split, or kissing, nevus of the eyelid.

Histologically, common melanocytic nevi are composed of nevus cells, specialized melanocytes that have a round rather than dendritic shape and tend to cluster together in nests. The cytoplasm of the nevus cell contains a variable amount of melanin. Common nevi typically begin as macular (flat) lesions and evolve with age. In childhood, histologic examination reveals nests of nevus cells in the basal layer of the epidermis, along the dermal–epidermal junction, termed *junctional nevus* (Fig 12-27). Typically in adolescence, the junctional nests of nevus cells continue to proliferate and migrate into the superficial dermis, and the nevus becomes increasingly elevated clinically. When both junctional and intradermal components are present, the histologic classification is *compound nevus* (see Fig 12-27). Finally, sometime in adulthood, the junctional component disappears, leaving nevus cells only within the dermis, and, accordingly, the classification becomes *intradermal* or *dermal nevus* (Fig 12-28).

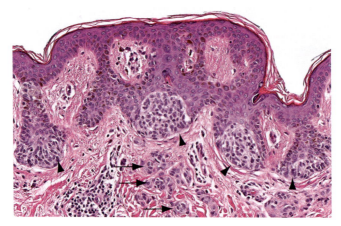

Figure 12-27 Compound nevus in an 11-year-old patient. Nests of nevus cells are visible at the dermal–epidermal junction *(arrowheads)*. A lesion with only this component would typically be classified as a junctional nevus. However, nevus cell nests are also present in the underlying dermis *(arrows)* in this lesion; thus, it is classified as compound. *(Courtesy of Tatyana Milman, MD.)*

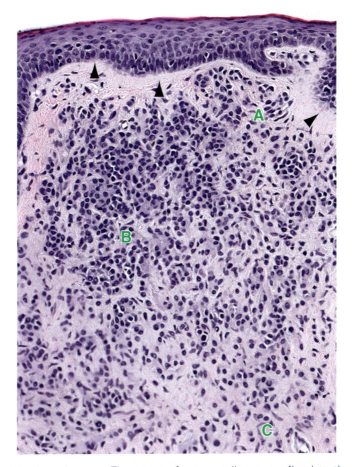

Figure 12-28 Intradermal nevus. The nests of nevus cells are confined to the dermis, and there is no junctional component. Note the collagenous layer separating the nevus cells from the epidermis (Grenz zone) *(arrowheads)* and maturation from larger type A nevus cells (A) to lymphocytoid type B nevus cells (B) and to spindle fibroblast-like or neural-like type C nevus cells (C). *(Courtesy of Tatyana Milman, MD.)*

The cytologic appearance of a common nevus evolves from type A to type C nevus cells, a process known as "maturation," which is useful for classifying melanocytic neoplasms as benign (see Fig 12-28):

- type A: round cells with round to ovoid nuclei; superficial portion of the nevus
- type B: smaller cells with less cytoplasm resembling lymphocytes; midportion of the nevus
- type C: cells with spindle configuration resembling Schwann cells of peripheral nerves; deepest portion of the nevus

Melanoma

Cutaneous melanoma (Fig 12-29) occurs on the eyelids only in rare cases. It may be associated with a preexisting nevus, develop de novo, or extend from a tumor elsewhere on the

262 • Ophthalmic Pathology and Intraocular Tumors

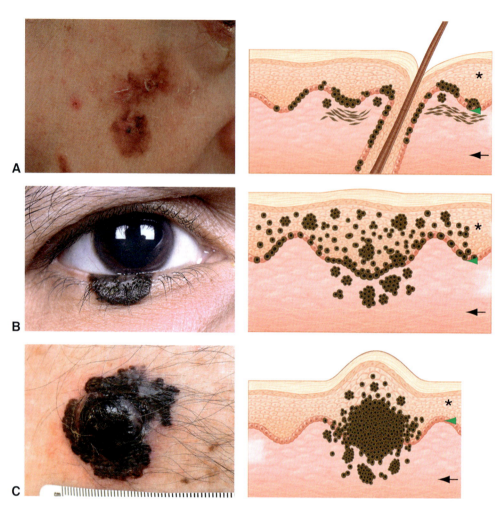

Figure 12-29 Cutaneous melanoma subtypes. **A,** Lentigo maligna melanoma manifests clinically as a variably pigmented patch on the sun-exposed cheek and lower eyelid. Illustration shows atypical melanocytes (brown cells) that proliferate predominantly in the basal layers of the epidermis in a linear or nested pattern. Note the tendency of the melanocytes to involve the outer sheaths of the hair shafts. The invasive component is seen as brown spindle and epithelioid cells in the superficial dermis. **B,** Superficial spreading melanoma presents clinically as a pigmented plaque on the lower eyelid. Illustration shows tumor cell nests at all levels of the epidermis, often in a prominent pagetoid fashion. There is a small invasive component in the dermis. Both lentigo maligna and superficial spreading melanoma spread horizontally (radial growth) through the skin. **C,** Clinical photograph of a nodular melanoma as a darkly pigmented nodule. Illustration shows a narrow intraepidermal component and more prominent vertical growth within the dermis; it is therefore more deeply invasive than the other 2 types. In all images: *asterisk* = epidermis, *arrowhead* = epidermal–dermal junction, *arrow* = dermis. *(Clinical photographs in parts A and C courtesy of Emily Chu, MD, PhD; clinical photograph in part B courtesy of Swathi Kaliki, MD. Illustrations modified with permission from Spencer WH, ed. Ophthalmic Pathology: An Atlas and Textbook. Vol 4. Saunders; 1996:2270. Illustrations by Christine Gralapp.)*

face. In a pigmented eyelid lesion, clinical features that suggest malignancy include asymmetry, border irregularity, color variegation, and diameter greater than 6 mm. Melanoma may also be heralded by a vertical (perpendicular to the skin surface) growth phase. Three main histologic subtypes of melanoma occur on the eyelids (see Fig 12-29):

- lentigo maligna melanoma
- superficial spreading melanoma
- nodular melanoma

Lentigo maligna melanoma, the most common type occurring on the eyelids, typically develops as an irregular pigmented macular lesion on the face in older adults and has a long preinvasive phase. Histologically, atypical melanocytes proliferate along the dermal–epidermal junction as single or small nests of cells in the epidermis, similar to primary acquired melanosis with atypia of the conjunctiva. Superficial invasion of the dermis is also present. *Superficial spreading melanoma,* the most common type of cutaneous melanoma, demonstrates a radial (intraepidermal) growth pattern that extends beyond the invasive component. *Nodular melanoma* is rare on the eyelids and has a significant vertical growth phase that results in a raised or indurated mass.

Clinical Pearl   When evaluating a patient with atypical pigmented lesion on the eyelid margin, it is important to carefully examine the conjunctiva for conjunctival melanoma with secondary eyelid involvement.

The characteristic histologic features of melanoma include pagetoid intraepidermal spread of atypical melanocytic nests and single cells, nuclear abnormalities, lack of maturation in the deeper portions of the mass, and atypical mitotic figures. A bandlike lymphocytic host response along the base of the mass is more common in melanoma than in benign proliferations. Prognosis is correlated with tumor thickness (Breslow thickness) in stage I (localized) disease. Metastases, when they occur, typically involve regional lymph nodes first. Frozen sections are not typically used for making a diagnosis of melanocytic lesions, as these lesions are difficult to visualize with frozen techniques.

Immunologic therapies are gaining importance in management of cutaneous melanoma. For discussion of targeted therapies for cutaneous melanoma, refer to BCSC Section 7, *Oculofacial Plastic and Orbital Surgery.*

CHAPTER **13**

Orbit and Lacrimal Drainage System

 Indicates that a supplemental case study is available in the Pathology Atlas *(aao.org/education /resident-course/pathology-atlas).*

Highlights

- Nonspecific orbital inflammation comprises a heterogeneous group of noninfectious inflammatory processes that can affect any part of the orbit.
- Lymphoproliferative lesions are among the more common infiltrative processes in the orbit and can occur within the lacrimal gland or elsewhere in the orbit.
- Rhabdomyosarcoma is the most common malignant orbital tumor in children. When this neoplasm is suspected, urgent action is required to establish a diagnosis and prevent loss of orbital and ocular function.

Topography

Bony Orbit and Soft Tissues

Seven bones form the boundaries of the orbit: the ethmoid, frontal, lacrimal, maxillary, palatine, sphenoid, and zygomatic bones. The orbital cavity contains the globe, lacrimal gland, muscles, tendons, fat, fasciae, vessels, nerves, ciliary ganglion, and cartilaginous trochlea (see Chapter 1). Inflammatory and neoplastic processes that increase the volume of the orbital contents can lead to *proptosis* (protrusion) of the globe and/or *displacement* (dystopia) from the horizontal or vertical position. The degree and direction of ocular displacement help localize the position of the mass.

The *lacrimal gland* is situated anteriorly in the superotemporal quadrant of the orbit. It is divided into orbital and palpebral lobes by the lateral portion of the aponeurosis of the levator palpebrae superioris muscle. The lacrimal gland is an eccrine gland, and the acini are round and composed of cuboidal epithelium. The nucleus is located toward the outer edge of the acinus. The ducts, which lie within the fibrovascular stroma, are lined by 2 layers: an inner, low cuboidal epithelium and an outer layer of low, flat myoepithelial cells. The histologic appearance of the lacrimal gland is very similar to that of the salivary glands.

See BCSC Section 2, *Fundamentals and Principles of Ophthalmology,* and Section 7, *Oculofacial Plastic and Orbital Surgery,* for additional discussion on the topography and anatomy of the orbit. See also Activity 1-1, Topography of the Eye and Orbit, in Chapter 1 of this volume.

Developmental Anomalies

Cysts

Orbital cysts may arise from a variety of ocular surface or orbital tissues and include cysts derived from the conjunctival or eyelid epithelium, teratomatous cysts, neural cysts, secondary cysts (mucoceles), inflammatory cysts (parasitic), and solid lesions with a cystic component. Orbital cysts can be developmental or acquired in origin. The most common type of orbital cyst, *dermoid cyst,* is a developmental lesion.

Dermoid cysts are believed to form when surface ectodermal nests become entrapped in the bony sutures during embryogenesis. Most of these cysts manifest in childhood as a unilateral mass in the lateral brow. Histologically, a dermoid cyst is lined by keratinized stratified squamous epithelium and contains keratin, sebum, and hair. Its walls contain dermal appendages, including sebaceous glands, hair follicles, and sweat glands (Fig 13-1). If the cyst wall does not have adnexal structures, it is called a *simple epithelial (epidermoid) cyst.* Simple epithelial cysts may also be lined by respiratory, conjunctival, or apocrine epithelium.

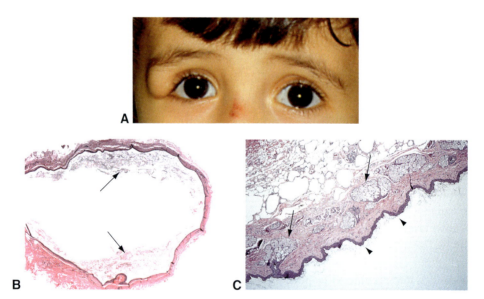

Figure 13-1 Orbital dermoid cyst. **A,** Clinical photograph of dermoid cyst of the right orbit. Note the typical superotemporal location. **B,** Low-magnification photomicrograph reveals a cyst containing keratin *(arrows).* The sebum dissolves out of the lumen during histologic processing. **C,** The cyst wall is lined by keratinized stratified squamous epithelium *(arrowheads)* and contains sebaceous glands *(arrows)* and adnexal structures. *(Part A courtesy of Sander Dubovy, MD; part B courtesy of Nasreen A. Syed, MD; part C courtesy of Hans E. Grossniklaus, MD.)*

Rupture of a dermoid cyst may cause a marked granulomatous reaction, largely due to the presence of sebum in the cyst lumen. Therefore, intact excision is preferable. See BCSC Section 7, *Oculofacial Plastic and Orbital Surgery,* for additional information.

Inflammation

Orbital inflammation can be idiopathic or secondary to a systemic inflammatory process (eg, granulomatosis with polyangiitis), retained foreign body, or infectious disease. It can be diffuse, involving multiple tissues (eg, sclerosing orbititis, diffuse anterior inflammation), or localized, involving specific orbital structures (eg, orbital myositis, optic perineuritis). Conditions masquerading as orbital inflammation include developmental orbital mass lesions and neoplastic disease, such as orbital lymphoma and rhabdomyosarcoma.

Noninfectious Inflammation

See BCSC Section 7, *Oculofacial Plastic and Orbital Surgery,* for additional information on the pathogenesis, clinical features, and treatment of the entities discussed below.

Thyroid eye disease

Thyroid eye disease (TED) (also known as *Graves disease, thyroid ophthalmopathy,* and *thyroid-associated orbitopathy*) is related to thyroid dysfunction and is the most common cause of unilateral and bilateral proptosis (exophthalmos) in adults. The signs and symptoms of TED are related to inflammation of the orbital connective tissue, alterations in the extracellular matrix of the extraocular muscles, inflammation and fibrosis of the extraocular muscles, and adipogenesis. The muscles appear firm and white, and the tendons are usually not involved. In the early stages of the disease, a cellular infiltrate of mononuclear inflammatory cells (eg, lymphocytes, plasma cells, mast cells) and fibroblasts permeates the interstitial tissues of the extraocular muscles, most commonly the inferior and medial rectus muscles (Fig 13-2). The fibroblasts synthesize hyaluronic acid (hyaluronan) and other glycosaminoglycans, resulting in enlargement of the muscles.

Clinical Pearl   The results of a thyroid function test may be normal in patients with TED.

Because orbital fibrocytes (considered precursor cells of fibroblasts) are derived from the neural crest and are pluripotent, the enhanced cell signaling that occurs in patients with TED promotes adipocyte differentiation and adipogenesis. These cellular changes lead to the characteristic features of TED.

As a result of the increased bulk within the orbit, the optic nerve may be compromised at the orbital apex, and optic nerve head swelling may result. The late stages of TED are associated with progressive fibrosis that results in restriction of ocular movement and severe eyelid retraction with resultant exposure keratitis.

Shan SJ, Douglas RS. The pathophysiology of thyroid eye disease. *J Neuroophthalmol.* 2014; 34(2):177–185.

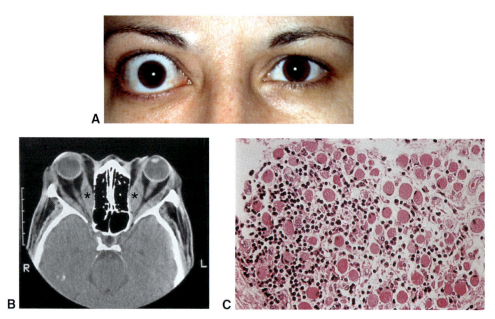

Figure 13-2 Thyroid eye disease (TED). **A,** Clinical photograph shows asymmetric proptosis and eyelid retraction, most prominently on the right. **B,** Computed tomography (CT) scan (axial view) shows fusiform enlargement of the extraocular muscles *(asterisks)* with sparing of the muscle tendons. **C,** The muscle bundles of the extraocular muscle are separated by fluid accompanied by an infiltrate of mononuclear inflammatory cells. *(Parts A and B courtesy of Sander Dubovy, MD.)*

Immunoglobulin G4–related disease

Immunoglobulin G4–related disease (IgG4-RD) is an inflammatory condition characterized by tumefactive lesions in 1 or more organs; a lymphoplasmacytic infiltrate rich in IgG4-positive plasma cells; variable degrees of fibrosis, often in a storiform pattern (whorls of cells); obliterative phlebitis; and elevated serum IgG4 levels (Fig 13-3). Orbital and ocular adnexal involvement in IgG4-RD, also known as *IgG4-related ophthalmic disease,* was initially described as bilateral and symmetric, with persistent swelling of the lacrimal glands and infiltration of IgG4 plasma cells. However, IgG4-RD can manifest not only in the lacrimal glands, but also in the extraocular muscles, orbital nerves, sclerae, and eyelids. The proposed criteria for IgG4-related ophthalmic disease include

- imaging studies showing lacrimal gland enlargement or a mass lesion involving the lacrimal gland, trigeminal nerve, or various other ophthalmic tissues
- histologic examination showing lymphoplasmacytic infiltration with associated fibrosis, and with a ratio of IgG4-positive to IgG-positive plasma cells ≥40% or >50 IgG4-positive plasma cells per high-power field (40× objective)
- serum IgG4 level ≥135 mg/dL

The diagnostic criteria for IgG4-RD and its clinical implications continue to evolve. Occasionally, extranodal marginal zone lymphoma (EMZL) of mucosa-associated lymphoid tissue (MALT) has been documented to arise in a patient with preexisting IgG4-RD.

Goto H, Takahira M, Azumi A; Japanese Study Group for IgG4-Related Ophthalmic Disease. Diagnostic criteria for IgG4-related ophthalmic disease. *Jpn J Ophthalmol.* 2015;59(1):1–7.

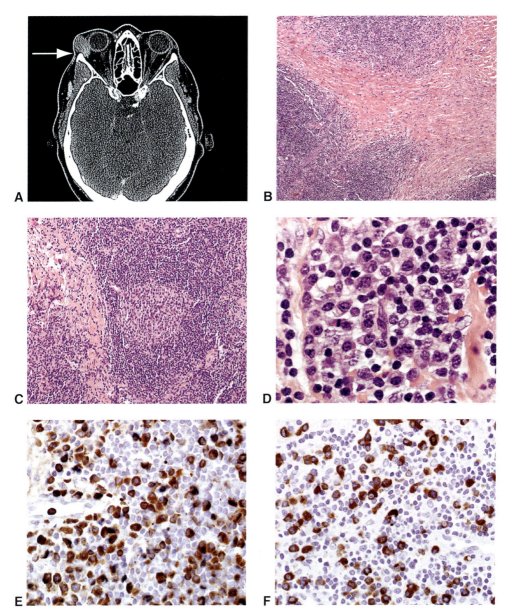

Figure 13-3 Immunoglobulin G4–related disease (IgG4-RD) in a 67-year-old patient with a 3-year history of an enlarging painless mass of the right lacrimal gland fossa. **A,** CT scan shows a homogeneously enhancing, circumscribed mass diffusely involving the right lacrimal gland *(arrow).* **B–D,** Histology demonstrates extensive collagenous fibrosis, lymphoid follicular hyperplasia, and markedly increased plasma cells. **E,** Immunohistochemistry reveals frequent IgG4-positive plasma cells, accounting for 40%–50% of total IgG-positive plasma cells. **F,** A different area of the lymphoid infiltrate stained for IgG4. A subsequent serum test showed an elevated serum IgG4 level. *(Courtesy of Kirtee Raparia, MD.)*

Nonspecific orbital inflammation

Nonspecific orbital inflammation (*NSOI;* also known as *orbital pseudotumor* or *idiopathic orbital inflammatory syndrome*) refers to a space-occupying inflammatory disorder that simulates a neoplasm but has no recognizable cause. This disorder accounts for approximately 5% of orbital lesions and can affect children and adults. Clinically, the onset is often abrupt, and patients usually report pain. The inflammatory response may be diffuse or compartmentalized. When localized to an extraocular muscle, the condition is called *orbital myositis* (Fig 13-4); when localized to the lacrimal gland, it is called *dacryoadenitis*.

In the early stages of NSOI, inflammation predominates, with a mixed inflammatory response (eosinophils, neutrophils, plasma cells, lymphocytes, and histiocytes [macrophages]) that is often perivascular and frequently infiltrates muscle and fat, causing fat necrosis. In later stages, fibrosis is the predominant feature, often with interspersed lymphoid follicles with germinal centers. The fibrosis may replace orbital fat and encase extraocular muscles and the optic nerve, restricting their function (Fig 13-5). Some cases that demonstrate significant fibrosis and deposition of collagen as the dominant histologic feature early in the course of the disorder seem to lack the inflammatory clinical signs usually associated with NSOI. Whether this "sclerosing" variant is a separate entity or a variant of NSOI remains controversial.

The differential diagnosis of NSOI includes lymphoproliferative processes such as lymphoma. Immunophenotypic and molecular genetic analyses can differentiate NSOI from lymphoid tumors based on whether the infiltrate of lymphocytes is polyclonal (NSOI) or monoclonal (lymphoma). IgG4-positive lymphoplasmacytic infiltrates are a marker for IgG4-related sclerosing disease (see the section "Immunoglobulin G4–related disease").

> Wallace ZS, Khosroshahi A, Jakobiec FA, et al. IgG4-related systemic disease as a cause of "idiopathic" orbital inflammation, including orbital myositis, and trigeminal nerve involvement. *Surv Ophthalmol.* 2012;57(1):26–33.

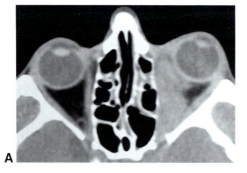 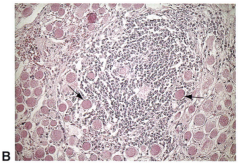

Figure 13-4 Nonspecific orbital inflammation (NSOI). **A,** CT imaging of the orbit reveals a homogeneous ill-defined mass involving the medial orbit and extending from the anterior orbit to the orbital apex. **B,** Histopathology shows skeletal muscle fibers *(arrows)* surrounded by a dense infiltrate of chronic inflammatory cells. Unlike in TED, in orbital myositis the muscle tendons are involved. *(Part A courtesy of Swathi Kaliki, MD.)*

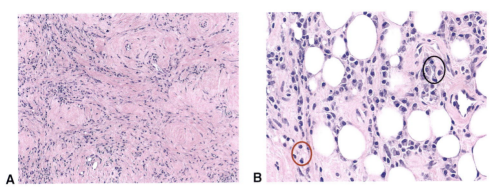

Figure 13-5 NSOI. **A,** Note the mixture of inflammatory cells in a background of dense pink fibrosis. **B,** Orbital fat infiltrated with plasma cells *(black circle)* and lymphocytes *(red circle)* in a background of fibrosis. *(Courtesy of Tatyana Milman, MD.)*

Infectious Inflammation

See BCSC Section 7, *Oculofacial Plastic and Orbital Surgery*, for additional discussion of orbital infectious diseases, and Section 8, *External Disease and Cornea*, for general discussion of microbial and parasitic infections.

Bacterial infections of the orbit

Bacterial infection of the orbit (orbital cellulitis) can occur through direct inoculation (trauma, surgery), opportunistic infection (necrotizing fasciitis, mucormycosis), spread from infection of adjacent structures (sinusitis), or spread from a distant focus (bacteremia). The most common cause of orbital cellulitis is paranasal sinus infection. Infection may be caused by a variety of organisms, including *Haemophilus influenzae, Streptococcus, Staphylococcus, Clostridium, Bacteroides, Klebsiella,* and *Proteus* species. The organism most commonly involved differs with the age of the patient. Histologically, acute inflammation, necrosis, and abscess formation may be present. Tuberculosis, which rarely involves the orbit, produces a necrotizing granulomatous reaction.

Fungal and parasitic infections of the orbit

Fungal infections of the orbit generally produce severe, insidious orbital inflammation (Fig 13-6). Rhinocerebral or rhino-orbito-cerebral *mucormycosis* usually occurs in patients with poorly controlled diabetes (especially those with ketoacidosis), solid malignant neoplasms, or extensive burns; in patients undergoing treatment with corticosteroid agents; or in patients with severe neutropenia. During the COVID-19 pandemic, there was an unprecedented resurgence of rhino-orbito-cerebral mucormycosis in those who recovered from moderate to severe infection with SARS-CoV-2. Typically, mucormycosis represents spread from an adjacent sinus infection. The specific fungal genus involved is usually *Mucor* or *Rhizopus*. On histologic examination, inflammation (acute and chronic) is present in a background of necrosis and is often granulomatous. Broad, nonseptate hyphae may be identified with hematoxylin and eosin (see Fig 13-6D), periodic acid–Schiff (PAS), and Gomori methenamine silver (GMS) stains. These fungi can invade blood vessel walls and cause a thrombotic vasculitis

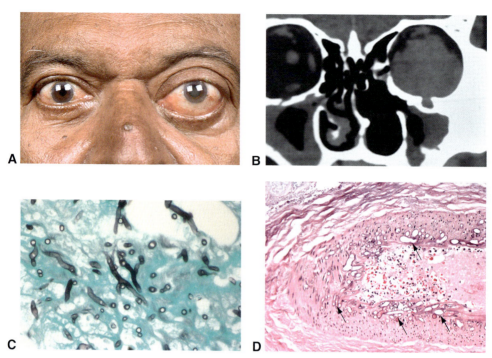

Figure 13-6 Fungal granuloma of the orbit. **A,** Clinical photograph shows left eye proptosis. **B,** CT of the orbit reveals thickened maxillary sinus mucosa and an ill-defined homogeneous lesion in the inferior orbit. **C,** Microscopic section shows branching fungal hyphae *(Aspergillus)* on Gomori methenamine silver (GMS) stain. **D,** *Mucor* hyphae are large and can often be seen on hematoxylin and eosin (H&E) stain *(arrows)*. The organisms are shown in the wall of the ophthalmic artery. *(Parts A and B courtesy of Swathi Kaliki, MD; part C courtesy of Hans E. Grossniklaus, MD; part D courtesy of Nasreen A. Syed, MD.)*

that results in ischemic necrosis. The organisms have the potential for hematogenous spread to the central nervous system (CNS), which can lead to stroke and death in the affected patient. Diagnosis is made by biopsy, often of necrotic-appearing tissues (eschar) in the nasopharynx.

Aspergillus infection of the orbit from the adjacent sinuses or hematogenous spread from other parts of the body may occur both in immunocompromised and in otherwise healthy individuals. With its slowly progressive and insidious symptoms, sino-orbital aspergillosis often goes unrecognized, resulting in a sclerosing granulomatous reaction. *Aspergillus* is often difficult to culture but may be observed in biopsied tissue as septate hyphae with 45° angle branching (see Fig 13-6C). Even with aggressive surgical therapy and adjunct therapy with antifungal agents, if extension into the brain occurs, orbital infections may be fatal.

Parasitic infections of the orbit are rare, especially in high-income countries. These infections may be caused by *Echinococcus* species (orbital hydatid cyst), *Taenia solium* (cysticercosis), and *Loa loa* (ocular filariasis [loiasis]). These infectious diseases are seen mostly in patients who come from, or have traveled to, areas where the infections are endemic. Serologic studies for specific parasites may aid diagnosis.

Infections of the lacrimal drainage system

Infections can occur in various parts of the lacrimal drainage system and may be acute or chronic. The most commonly affected areas are the canaliculus (canaliculitis) and the

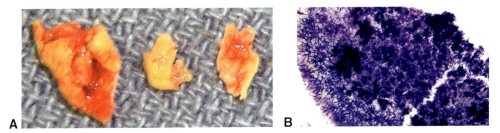

Figure 13-7 Actinomycotic dacryoliths from the lacrimal drainage system. **A,** Gross photograph of yellow sulfur granules. **B,** Histology of a sulfur granule shows a colony of gram-positive delicate branching pleomorphic filamentous bacteria, consistent with *Actinomyces*. *(Part A courtesy of Morris E. Hartstein, MD; part B courtesy of Vivian Lee, MD.)*

lacrimal sac (dacryocystitis). Obstruction or the presence of foreign material (eg, dacryolith, punctal plug) may predispose the lacrimal drainage system to infection, but infection can also develop in the absence of these factors. Bacteria, fungi, and viruses can all cause infection of the lacrimal drainage system, although the filamentous gram-positive bacterium *Actinomyces israelii* is the most common causative organism in cases of canaliculitis. This organism may form a bacterial aggregate in the lacrimal drainage system, leading to formation of a dacryolith with a characteristic yellow color, known as a "sulfur granule" (Fig 13-7).

Degenerations

Amyloid

Amyloid deposition in the orbit can be localized or occur as a manifestation of systemic amyloidosis. When amyloid deposition involves the extraocular muscles and nerves, it can cause ophthalmoplegia and ptosis. See Chapters 4, 5, 9, and 12 in this volume for more information on amyloid deposition.

Neoplasia

Neoplasms of the orbit may be primary or secondary (extensions from adjacent structures or metastatic disease). Secondary tumors are slightly more common than primary tumors (see the section Secondary Tumors at the end of this chapter). The types of orbital tumors that occur in children differ from those that occur in adults; developmental tumors are the primary orbital lesions most often encountered in children, whereas vascular and lymphoid tumors are the primary orbital lesions most often seen in adults.

In children, approximately 90% of orbital tumors are benign. Benign cystic lesions (dermoid or simple epithelial cysts) represent 50% of orbital lesions in children (see the section Developmental Anomalies earlier in this chapter). Rhabdomyosarcoma is the most common primary orbital malignant tumor in children and represents 3% of all orbital masses. The orbit may also be involved secondarily in cases of retinoblastoma, neuroblastoma, and leukemia/lymphoma.

See BCSC Section 7, *Oculofacial Plastic and Orbital Surgery,* for additional discussion on the entities described in the following subsections. Also see the Childhood Tumors of the Orbit and Eyelid Interactive Case Study in the online *Pathology Atlas.*

Lacrimal Gland Neoplasia

Because the lacrimal gland is a modified salivary gland, epithelial lacrimal gland tumors are categorized according to the World Health Organization (WHO) epithelial salivary gland tumor classification system. The most common types of epithelial lacrimal gland tumors are pleomorphic adenoma, adenocarcinoma arising from pleomorphic adenoma (carcinoma ex pleomorphic adenoma), and adenoid cystic carcinoma.

> WHO Classification of Tumours Editorial Board. *WHO Classification of Tumours of the Eye.* 5th ed. International Agency for Research on Cancer; 2023. *WHO Classification of Tumours Series*; vol. 13. Accessed November 17, 2023. https://tumourclassification.iarc.who.int/chapters/7

Pleomorphic adenoma

The most common epithelial tumor of the lacrimal gland is pleomorphic adenoma (also known as *benign mixed tumor*). It usually presents in the fourth or fifth decade of life with an indolent painless proptosis. The tumor is pseudoencapsulated and has a progressive expansive growth pattern that results in smooth bony scalloping without bone destruction. Tumor growth stimulates the periosteum to deposit a thin layer of new bone (ie, cortication) (Table 13-1).

Histologically, pleomorphic adenoma is composed of cells of varying morphologies, including epithelial, myoepithelial, and stromal cells. It has a fibrous pseudocapsule and comprises a mixture of duct-derived epithelial and stromal elements, all arising from the lacrimal glandular epithelium. The epithelial component of this neoplasm may form nests or tubules lined by 2 layers of cells, the outermost layer blending imperceptibly with the stroma (Fig 13-8). The stroma may appear myxoid and may contain heterologous elements, including cartilage and bone.

Malignant transformation may take place in a long-standing or incompletely excised pleomorphic adenoma in the form of adenocarcinoma (carcinoma ex pleomorphic adenoma), with relatively rapid growth after a period of relative quiescence. Malignancies, including adenocarcinoma and adenoid cystic carcinoma (see the following section), may also develop in pleomorphic adenomas that recur in the orbit. Treatment of lacrimal gland pleomorphic adenoma includes complete excision with a margin of normal tissue. Incomplete excision of pleomorphic adenoma may enable late tumor recurrence.

Clinical Pearl Incisional biopsy or fine-needle aspiration biopsy should be avoided in patients with pleomorphic adenoma to prevent disruption of the pseudocapsule and tumor spillage.

Table 13-1 Common Orbital Tumors

	Cavernous Venous Malformation	Schwannoma	Pleomorphic Adenoma	Adenoid Cystic Carcinoma	Ocular Adnexal Lymphoma
Age at presentation	20–40 years	20–60 years	20–50 years	40–60 years	60–70 years
Laterality	Unilateral	Unilateral	Unilateral	Unilateral	Unilateral or bilateral
Location	Mostly in the intraconal space	Mostly in the extraconal space	Orbital lobe of lacrimal gland	Orbital lobe of lacrimal gland	Intraconal and extraconal spaces
Pain	No	Some individuals experience pain, with or without paresthesia	No	Yes, with or without paresthesia	No
Orbital imaging	Well-circumscribed homogeneous mass; Mild contrast enhancement; Flow voids on MRI	Well-circumscribed oblong, elongated homogeneous lesions; Strong contrast enhancement	Well-circumscribed mass with smooth bony scalloping; Moderate contrast enhancement	Infiltrative mass with bone destruction; perineural invasion is common; Diffuse contrast enhancement	Poorly circumscribed homogeneous mass that molds around the globe and adjacent ocular structures without bony erosion
Treatment	Complete excision	Complete excision	Complete excision	Complete excision followed by radiotherapy; orbital exenteration versus intra-arterial chemotherapy in advanced cases	Radiotherapy, chemotherapy, or immunotherapy, depending on subtype; Attempts to perform complete excision may cause damage to adjacent structures
Prognosis	Good	Good	Good	Poor	Good for EMZL; poor for LPL and MCL

EMZL = extranodal marginal zone lymphoma of mucosa-associated lymphoid tissue; LPL = lymphoplasmacytic lymphoma; MCL = mantle cell lymphoma; MRI = magnetic resonance imaging.

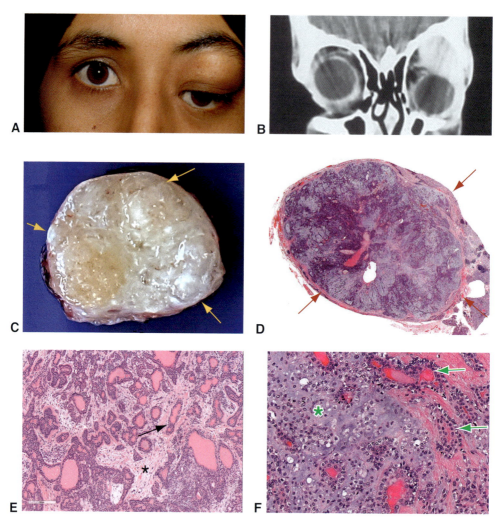

Figure 13-8 Pleomorphic adenoma (benign mixed tumor) of the lacrimal gland. **A,** Clinical photograph shows a superotemporal left orbital mass causing proptosis and inferomedial displacement of the globe. **B,** CT scan (coronal view) shows a circumscribed mass in the superotemporal orbit, without bone destruction. **C,** The mass has rounded protrusions ("bosselations"; *arrows*) and is grossly encapsulated. **D,** Low-magnification photomicrograph reveals a circumscribed mass with a pink fibrous pseudocapsule *(arrows)* formed by a rim of normal tissue. **E,** The neoplastic epithelial elements form pink ductules with proteinaceous pink luminal material *(arrow)*. Note the bluish fibromyxoid stroma *(asterisk)*. **F,** Hyaline cartilage *(asterisk)* is present in a background of pink ductules *(arrows)*. *(Parts A and B courtesy of Sander Dubovy, MD; parts C, D, and F courtesy of Tatyana Milman, MD; part E courtesy of Heather Potter, MD.)*

Adenoid cystic carcinoma

Adenoid cystic carcinoma (ACC) can develop in an individual with pleomorphic adenoma or, more commonly, arise de novo. The tumor is slightly more common in women, and the median age at presentation is about 40 years (see Table 13-1).

Unlike pleomorphic adenoma, ACC does not have a pseudocapsule; it also tends to erode bone and invade orbital nerves, which causes frequent pain and paresthesia. The tumor is grossly infiltrative. Histologically, a variety of patterns can occur; cribriform ("Swiss cheese") is the most common (Fig 13-9). Basaloid (solid) pattern and high-grade transformation have been associated with a worse prognosis. Orbital exenteration is one of the currently accepted treatments for this tumor, but some ophthalmologists have advocated for globe-sparing intra-arterial chemotherapy.

> von Holstein SL, Coupland SE, Briscoe D, Le Tourneau C, Heegaard S. Epithelial tumours of the lacrimal gland: a clinical, histopathological, surgical, and oncological survey. *Acta Ophthalmol.* 2013;91(3):195–206.

Lymphoproliferative Lesions

Ocular adnexal (conjunctival, orbit, and eyelid) lymphoproliferative lesions are traditionally divided into reactive lymphoid hyperplasia, atypical lymphoid hyperplasia, and ocular adnexal lymphoma (OAL). OALs are subtyped according to the fifth edition of the

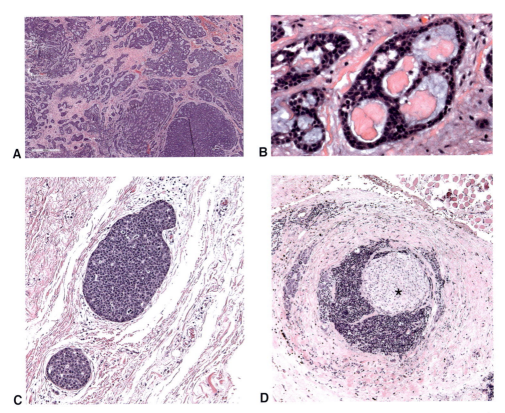

Figure 13-9 Adenoid cystic carcinoma of the lacrimal gland. **A,** Low-magnification photomicrograph shows an infiltrative basophilic tumor. **B,** Note the characteristic cribriform ("Swiss cheese") pattern of growth. **C,** Solid lobules of tumor represent the basaloid pattern, which is associated with a less favorable prognosis. **D,** Perineural invasion. Blue tumor invades the perineurium and surrounds a peripheral nerve *(asterisk)*. *(Part A courtesy of Heather Potter, MD; parts B–D courtesy of Nasreen A. Syed, MD.)*

WHO Classification of Tumours of Haematopoietic and Lymphoid Tissues. Classification schemes for lymphoid neoplasms continue to evolve with improved understanding of biology of these lesions. Classification is important for selection of treatment protocols and prognostication.

Orbital lymphoproliferative lesions present with gradual, painless unilateral or bilateral proptosis. Staging of patients with orbital lymphoproliferative lesions should be done in collaboration with a medical oncologist. Studies may include imaging with positron emission tomography (PET) or computed tomography (CT) and bone marrow biopsy.

> **Tissue Handling of Ocular Adnexal Lymphoid Lesions**
> - Before a biopsy of an orbital, conjunctival, or eyelid lymphoproliferative lesion is performed, the ophthalmologist should consult with the pathologist to determine the optimal method for tissue handling, including the volume of tissue to obtain and the type of fixative or nutrient media to use.
> - It is very important that the tissue be handled gently, because crush artifact can prevent the pathologist from rendering a diagnosis.
> - Fresh (unfixed) tissue is required for touch preparations and flow cytometry. Exposure of the biopsy specimen to air for long periods should be avoided. Tissue samples may be wrapped in saline-moistened gauze or placed in tissue culture medium to slow autolysis.
> - Molecular genetic and immunohistochemical (IHC) studies can be performed on fixed tissue.
>
> See Checklist 2-4, Ophthalmic Pathology Consultation Flow Cytometry Checklist, and Checklist 2-5, Ophthalmic Pathology Consultation Molecular Techniques and Electron Microscopy Checklist, in Chapter 2 of this volume.

Coupland SE, Heegaard S, Khoury JD. Haematolymphoid tumors. In: *WHO Classification of Tumours of the Eye.* 5th ed. International Agency for Research on Cancer; 2023. *WHO Classification of Tumours Series*; vol. 13. Accessed November 17, 2023. https://tumourclassification.iarc.who.int/chaptercontent/65/194

Lymphoid hyperplasia

Reactive lymphoid hyperplasia (RLH) is characterized histologically by prominent lymphoid follicles with germinal centers (Fig 13-10), tingible body macrophages (containing apoptotic debris), and a polymorphous population of mature lymphocytes. Other inflammatory cells may be present in small numbers in the infiltrate. *Atypical lymphoid hyperplasia (ALH)* is a diagnosis of exclusion, reserved for those lesions that do not fit into the category of a frankly reactive lymphoid hyperplasia or lymphoma after comprehensive histologic, immunophenotypic, and molecular genetic evaluation. See Chapter 2 in this volume for additional information on ancillary diagnostic methods.

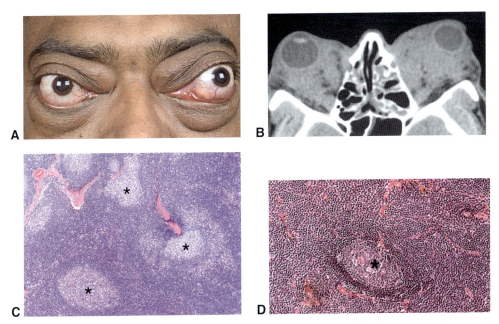

Figure 13-10 Reactive lymphoid hyperplasia. **A,** Clinical photograph of a young patient with bilateral proptosis. **B,** Orbital CT reveals bilateral ill-defined homogeneous masses. **C,** Histology demonstrates a dense infiltrate of lymphoid cells arranged in lymphoid follicles with well-formed germinal centers *(asterisks)*. A panel of immunohistochemical stains (not shown) and flow cytometry studies demonstrated a polyclonal population of lymphocytes. **D,** High-magnification image of the germinal center in a reactive follicle *(asterisk)*. *(Parts A and B courtesy of Swathi Kaliki, MD; part C courtesy of Nasreen A. Syed, MD; part D courtesy of Heather Potter, MD.)*

Lymphoma

Lymphomas of the orbit currently constitute one-half of the malignant tumors that arise in the orbit and ocular adnexa, and the incidence of orbital lymphoma is increasing. Orbital lymphomas may be a presenting manifestation of systemic lymphoma, or more commonly, they may be a primary orbital neoplasm.

Of the ocular adnexal lymphomas, 90% are mature B-cell lymphomas. EMZL is the most common type of orbital lymphoma. Other types of lymphoma, typically non-Hodgkin lymphomas such as follicular, large B-cell, and mantle cell, also occur in the orbit, but with a lower incidence. Each of these subtypes has a different prognosis for survival, and different treatment regimens tend to be used for each (see Table 13-1).

Histologically, orbital lymphomas typically demonstrate a monomorphic infiltrate of B cells, which express B-cell marker CD20 (Fig 13-11; also see Chapter 4, Fig 4-24C,D). Lymphomas can be further subclassified using immunophenotyping with different lymphoid cell markers. T-cell lymphomas of the orbit are rare, are more aggressive, and usually express T-cell marker CD3.

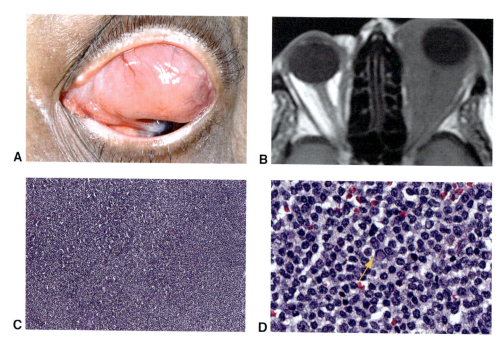

Figure 13-11 Low-grade B-cell lymphoma of the orbit. **A,** Clinical photograph of a patient with proptosis and a salmon-pink patch in the superior fornix. **B,** Orbital magnetic resonance imaging (MRI) reveals left eye proptosis with an infiltrative homogeneous mass in the intraconal space, molding around the globe. **C,** Histology shows sheets of small lymphocytes. **D,** Higher-magnification image reveals pink immunoglobulin pseudoinclusions *(Dutcher bodies)* within the nuclei *(arrow)*, typical for extranodal marginal zone lymphoma of mucosa-associated lymphoid tissue (EMZL). *(Parts A and B courtesy of Swathi Kaliki, MD; parts C and D courtesy of Tatyana Milman, MD.)*

The risk of systemic lymphoma developing in a patient with primary orbital lymphoma ranges from 30% to 40%. In contrast, the risk of secondary orbital involvement in systemic lymphoma is much lower, approximately 1%–2% of cases.

Soft-Tissue Tumors

In general, soft-tissue tumors are diagnosed both by their histologic patterns (ie, round cell, spindle cell, myxoid, epithelioid, pericytomatous, and pleomorphic) and by ancillary studies, such as IHC and molecular genetic studies. The classification of soft-tissue tumors continues to evolve as the understanding of their molecular genetics is elucidated. For an additional resource on this topic, see PathologyOutlines.com (www.pathologyoutlines.com/eye.html).

Cree IA, Milman T, Lazar AJ, et al. Soft tissue and bone tumors. In: *WHO Classification of Tumours of the Eye*. 5th ed. International Agency for Research on Cancer; 2023. WHO Classification of Tumours Series; vol. 13. Accessed November 17, 2023. https://tumourclassification.iarc.who.int/chaptercontent/65/226

Vascular Tumors

Orbital lymphatic malformations and *lymphatic-venous malformations* (previously termed *lymphangiomas*) typically present in childhood and are characterized by recurrent and fluctuating proptosis, often enlarging in individuals with upper respiratory tract infections. Histology usually reveals unencapsulated infiltrative lymphatic and venous channels and scattered lymphoid aggregates in a background of fibrosis and preexisting hemorrhage with hemosiderin deposits (Fig 13-12; also see Table 13-1).

Orbital cavernous venous malformations (previously termed *cavernous hemangiomas*) are typically located intraconally and are encapsulated, consisting of large, expanded venous channels with serum–red blood cell separation, occasional thrombosis, and calcification (Fig 13-13). In contrast, *infantile (capillary) hemangiomas* are unencapsulated and more cellular, often with a cutaneous component, and are composed of capillary-sized vessels (see Chapter 12). See BCSC Section 7, *Oculofacial Plastic and Orbital Surgery*, for additional information on vascular lesions of the orbit.

> International Society for the Study of Vascular Anomalies (ISSVA) classification for vascular anomalies. ISSVA website. Revised May 2018. Accessed November 14, 2023. www.issva.org/classification
>
> Nassiri N, Rootman J, Rootman DB, Goldberg RA. Orbital lymphaticovenous malformations: current and future treatments. *Surv Ophthalmol.* 2015;60(5):383–405.

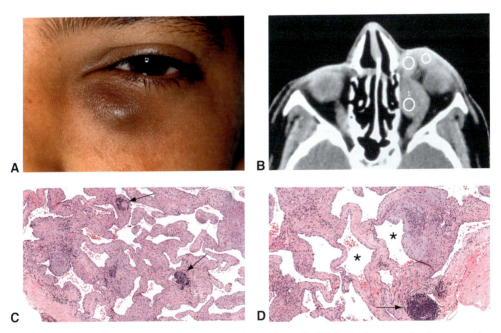

Figure 13-12 Orbital lymphatic venous malformation. **A,** Clinical photograph shows an inferior orbital lesion extending anteriorly and nasally below the left lower eyelid of a young patient. **B,** CT scan (axial view) depicts a multilobulated, infiltrative mass *(white circles)* in the left orbit. **C,** Histology shows numerous irregular lymphoid channels and lymphoid follicles *(arrows).* **D,** Higher-magnification image demonstrates endothelium-lined channels *(asterisks)* and a lymphoid follicle *(arrow)* in a background of fibrosis. *(Parts A and B courtesy of Sander Dubovy, MD; parts C and D courtesy of Heather Potter, MD.)*

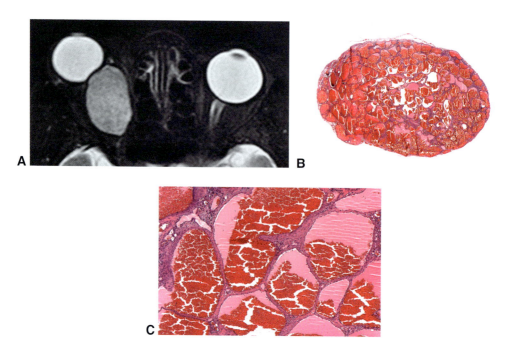

Figure 13-13 Orbital cavernous venous malformation (cavernous hemangioma). **A,** MRI scan (axial view) shows a well-circumscribed retrobulbar intraconal mass. **B,** Low-magnification histology demonstrates an encapsulated ovoid mass. **C,** Higher-magnification image shows the large venous channels lined with flat endothelial cells and smooth muscle, filled with red blood cells with serum–red blood cell separation, consistent with a low-flow lesion. *(Part A courtesy of Swathi Kaliki, MD; parts B and C courtesy of Tatyana Milman, MD.)*

Tumors With Fibrous Differentiation

Solitary fibrous tumor

Solitary fibrous tumor (SFT) is the most common mesenchymal tumor of the orbit in adults. The superonasal orbit is a common site. The tumor typically presents in the fifth decade but can occur in younger or older individuals as well. Signs and symptoms include proptosis, pain, diplopia, blurred vision, and epiphora.

Several studies have demonstrated that other soft-tissue tumors (eg, hemangiopericytomas, fibrous histiocytomas, and giant cell angiofibromas of the orbit) share common histologic, immunohistochemical, and molecular genetic characteristics; thus, these tumors have been reclassified as SFTs. Histologic examination reveals a circumscribed mass, composed of a variably cellular proliferation of spindle cells in a background of collagenous stroma and characteristic branching "staghorn" blood vessels (Fig 13-14). STAT6 nuclear positivity on IHC studies is highly sensitive and specific for SFTs, which reflects underlying *STAT6* gene rearrangement. Larger tumor size, older patient age, increased mitotic activity, and necrosis are associated with recurrence and metastasis.

> Demicco EG, Harms PW, Patel RM, et al. Extensive survey of STAT6 expression in a large series of mesenchymal tumors. *Am J Clin Pathol.* 2015;143(5):672–682.

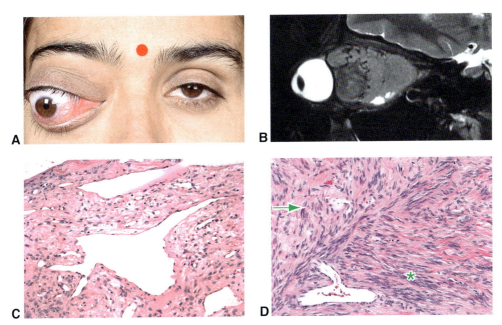

Figure 13-14 Solitary fibrous tumor. **A,** Clinical photograph of severe proptosis of the right eye. **B,** MRI reveals a well-defined heterogeneous retrobulbar mass. **C,** Histology shows a spindle cell neoplasm with a characteristic slitlike, branching (staghorn) vascular pattern. **D,** Alternating close-packed *(asterisk)* and less cellular *(arrow)* proliferation of spindle cells in a pink collagenous background. Note the branching vascular channel on the lower left. *(Parts A and B courtesy of Swathi Kaliki, MD; part C courtesy of Nasreen A. Syed, MD; part D courtesy of Tatyana Milman, MD.)*

Mitamura M, Kase S, Suzuki Y, et al. Solitary fibrous tumor of the orbit: a clinicopathologic study of two cases with review of the literature. *In Vivo.* 2020;34(6):3649–3654.

Tumors With Muscle Differentiation

Rhabdomyosarcoma

Rhabdomyosarcoma is the most common primary malignant orbital tumor of childhood with an average age of onset at 5–7 years. The typical presentation in children is rapid-onset, progressive unilateral proptosis. There is often reddish discoloration of the eyelids that is *not* accompanied by local heat (calor) or systemic fever, as is common in cellulitis (Fig 13-15A,B).

Clinical Pearl   Patients with suspected rhabdomyosarcoma require immediate attention, with urgent imaging and biopsy, due to the extremely rapid growth of this tumor.

Rhabdomyosarcoma arises from primitive mesenchymal cells that differentiate toward skeletal muscle. There are 4 types of orbital rhabdomyosarcoma:

- embryonal (most common, usually excellent prognosis)
- alveolar (unfavorable prognosis)

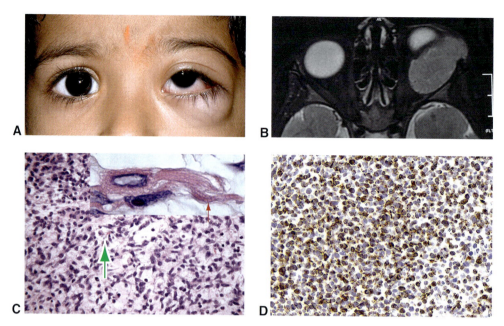

Figure 13-15 Rhabdomyosarcoma. **A,** Child with left proptosis and an inferior orbital mass. **B,** MRI scan (axial view) shows a large, well-circumscribed orbital tumor and proptosis. **C,** Embryonal rhabdomyosarcoma. Primitive ovoid and spindle cells with eccentric pink cytoplasmic tails and mitotic figures *(green arrow)* loosely arranged in a myxoid stroma. *Inset:* Cross-striations *(red arrow)* represent the Z bands of actin–myosin complexes within the cytoplasm of a tumor cell. **D,** Neoplastic cells diffusely express desmin, a marker of muscle differentiation. *(Parts A and B courtesy of Swathi Kaliki, MD; parts C and D courtesy of Tatyana Milman, MD.)*

- pleomorphic (exceedingly rare, adults, unfavorable prognosis)
- spindle cell (rare, excellent prognosis)

Embryonal rhabdomyosarcoma (ie, *botryoid variant*) may develop in the conjunctival stroma and may present as grapelike submucosal clusters. Histologically, spindle cells are arranged in a loose syncytium with occasional elongated cells demonstrating cytoplasmic cross-striations (strap cells). These cross-striations are found in approximately 60% of cases of embryonal rhabdomyosarcoma (Fig 13-15C). Immunohistochemically, rhabdomyosarcoma is typically positive for desmin, muscle-specific actin, and myogenin (Fig 13-15D).

> Molecular genetic studies are important for identifying genetic translocations that have prognostic and therapeutic significance in patients with sarcoma.

Orbital rhabdomyosarcoma has a better prognosis (overall 5-year survival rate of about 90%) than does rhabdomyosarcoma occurring in other body sites. *PAX3-FOXO1* and *PAX7-FOX1* gene rearrangements that are found in individuals with alveolar rhabdomyosarcoma are associated with unfavorable outcomes. See BCSC Section 6, *Pediatric Ophthalmology and Strabismus,* for additional discussion of rhabdomyosarcoma.

Tissue Handling of Sarcoma
- Before a biopsy of a suspected sarcoma is performed, the ophthalmologist should consult with the pathologist to determine the optimal method for tissue handling, including the volume of tissue to obtain and the type of fixative or nutrient media to use.
- Fresh (unfixed) tissue is required for touch preparations and cytogenetic studies. Exposure of the biopsy specimen to air for long periods should be avoided. Tissue samples may be wrapped in saline-moistened gauze or placed in tissue culture medium to slow autolysis.
- Molecular genetic and IHC studies can be performed on fixed tissue.

Also see Table 2-1 and Checklist 2-5 in Chapter 2 of this volume.

Hibbitts E, Chi YY, Hawkins DS, et al. Refinement of risk stratification for childhood rhabdomyosarcoma using *FOXO1* fusion status in addition to established clinical outcome predictors: A report from the Children's Oncology Group. *Cancer Med.* 2019;8(14):6437–6448.

Peripheral Nerve Sheath and Central Nervous System Tumors

Neurofibroma

Neurofibroma, the most common peripheral nerve sheath tumor, is a slow-growing tumor that consists of a mixture of endoneurial fibroblasts, Schwann cells, and axons. Neurofibromas may be circumscribed but are not encapsulated. They are firm and rubbery. Microscopically, the spindle-shaped cells have slender, wavy nuclei. These nuclei are arranged in ribbons and cords in a matrix of myxoid tissue and collagen with entrapped mast cells that contains axons.

Neurofibromas can occur sporadically or in association with neurofibromatosis 1 (NF1). The diffuse and plexiform type of neurofibroma is considered pathognomonic for NF1, presenting as an uncircumscribed thick and irregular lesion (Fig 13-16). *Plexiform* refers to an intricate network, or *plexus*, classically described as a "bag of worms." Eyelid plexiform neurofibroma typically causes an S-shaped eyelid deformity. NF1-associated

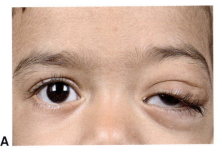
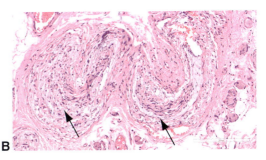

Figure 13-16 Plexiform neurofibroma. **A,** Typical S-shaped deformity of the upper eyelid. **B,** Histology shows thickened, tortuous nerves with proliferation of endoneurial fibroblasts and Schwann cells *(arrows)*. *(Part A courtesy of Swathi Kaliki, MD; part B courtesy of Saumya Jakati, MD.)*

neurofibromas can transform into malignant peripheral nerve sheath tumor, a highly aggressive sarcoma.

Schwannoma

Schwannomas (also known as *neurilemomas*) arise from Schwann cells of peripheral nerves and are the most common nerve sheath tumors found in the orbit of adults. Slow growing and encapsulated, these tumors may contain cystic spaces and areas of hemorrhagic necrosis (see Table 13-1). A schwannoma may be solitary or occur in association with a genetic syndrome such as neurofibromatosis or schwannomatosis. Histologically, schwannoma can demonstrate various growth patterns. The typical schwannoma is characterized either by slender spindle cells arranged in a palisaded Antoni A pattern, forming Verocay bodies (collections of fibrils resembling sensory corpuscles), or by loosely arranged cells in myxoid stroma (Antoni B pattern) (Fig 13-17). Axons are usually absent. Schwannomas typically demonstrate a diffuse strong positivity for S-100 protein.

Meningioma

Meningiomas are derived from the meninges and as such are found in the CNS. Meningiomas that affect the orbit are typically primary tumors of the intracranial cavity that invade through the orbital bones, usually the sphenoid bone, and behave as an infiltrative mass lesion in the orbit. A minority of meningiomas found in the orbit arise primarily from the optic nerve sheath. These tumors tend to stay within the sheath, resulting in compression of the optic nerve. For further discussion of meningioma and other CNS tumors occurring in the orbit, see Chapter 14.

Adipocytic Tumors

Lipomas are exceptionally rare in the orbit. Their pathologic characteristics include encapsulation and a distinctive lobular appearance. Like lipomas, *liposarcomas* are rare in the orbit. Liposarcomas are malignant tumors with adipocytic differentiation, frequently featuring *lipoblasts*. Several liposarcoma types have been recognized. Cytogenetic and/or molecular studies for chromosome translocations and alterations in several genes, including *MDM2* amplification, are increasingly used in the diagnosis of liposarcomas.

> Because lipomas histologically resemble normal or prolapsed fat and atypical lipomatous tumor/well-differentiated liposarcoma, their incidence has historically been overestimated.

Bony Lesions of the Orbit

Fibrous tumors of the bone

Fibrous dysplasia of bone may involve 1 bone (monostotic) or more than 1 (polyostotic). When the orbit is affected, the condition is usually monostotic; however, the tumor may cross suture lines to involve multiple orbital bones. Patients often present during the first 3 decades of life with symptoms related to globe displacement and narrowing of the optic canal and lacrimal drainage system. Plain radiographic studies show a ground-glass

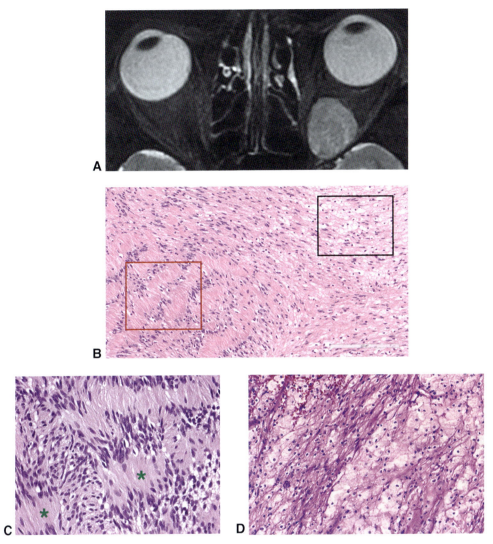

Figure 13-17 Schwannoma. **A,** MRI shows a well-defined heterogeneous mass in the orbit. **B,** Histology reveals spindle cells arranged in palisaded Antoni A *(red box)* and loose Antoni B *(black box)* patterns. **C,** Antoni A pattern: spindle cell nuclei are arranged in linear palisades with intervening pink cytoplasmic processes. Palisading of nuclei may form a Verocay body *(asterisks)*. **D,** Antoni B pattern: loosely arranged cells in a myxoid stroma. *(Part A courtesy of Swathi Kaliki, MD; part B courtesy of Saumya Jakati, MD; parts C and D courtesy of Nasreen A. Syed, MD.)*

appearance with lytic foci. Fluid-containing cysts may also be present. As a result of arrest in the maturation of bone, trabeculae are composed not of lamellar bone but instead of woven bone with a fibrous stroma that is highly vascularized. Histologically, the bony trabeculae often have a C-shaped appearance and lack appreciable osteoblastic rimming (Fig 13-18A). *Fibro-osseous dysplasia (juvenile ossifying fibroma)* is characterized histologically by spicules of bone rimmed by osteoblasts (Fig 13-18B). At low magnification, ossifying fibroma may be confused with a psammomatous meningioma.

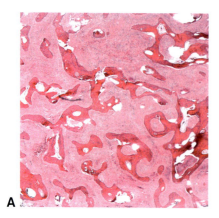
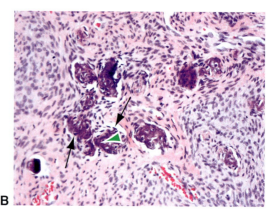

Figure 13-18 Osseous tumors. **A,** Fibrous dysplasia. The bony trabeculae are often C-shaped, composed of immature woven bone, and surrounded by a fibrous stroma. **B,** Fibro-osseous dysplasia (juvenile ossifying fibroma). Bone spicules, reminiscent of psammoma bodies, are set in a cellular fibrous stroma. Unlike psammoma bodies, bone spicules contain osteocytes *(arrowhead)* and are rimmed by osteoblasts *(arrows)*. *(Part A courtesy of Nasreen A. Syed, MD; part B courtesy of Tatyana Milman, MD.)*

Osteogenic and chondrogenic tumors of the orbit are rare; of these, *osteoma* is the most common. Most commonly, an osteoma arises from the frontal sinus as a slow-growing, well-circumscribed mass, composed of mature bone. Other rare osteogenic and chondrogenic orbital tumors include both benign entities (eg, osteoblastoma) and sarcomas (eg, osteosarcoma, Ewing sarcoma, mesenchymal chondrosarcoma).

Lacrimal Sac Neoplasia

Lacrimal sac neoplasms are rare and may mimic dacryocystitis clinically. In 1 study of patients undergoing dacryocystorhinostomy or chronic nasolacrimal duct obstruction, neoplasm was the cause in only 5% of cases. Most lacrimal sac neoplasms are *papillomas* and *squamous cell carcinomas*.

> Krishna Y, Coupland SE. Lacrimal sac tumors—a review. *Asia Pac J Ophthalmol (Phila)*. 2017; 6(2):173–178.

Secondary Tumors

Secondary malignant orbital tumors are lesions that invade the orbit by direct extension from adjacent structures, such as the paranasal sinus, intracranial cavity, eye, eyelids, or ocular surface. *Metastatic* tumors are malignant lesions that have spread from a distant primary site, usually via a hematogenous route. The most common primary tumor sites that result in orbital metastasis are the breast in women and the prostate in men. In children, neuroblastoma is the most common primary tumor metastatic to the orbit.

CHAPTER **14**

Optic Nerve

 This chapter includes a related video. Go to aao.org/bcscvideo_section04 or scan the QR code in the text to access this content.

Highlights

- The optic nerve consists of retinal ganglion cell axons and glial cells.
- Because the optic nerve is contiguous with the brain, many of the conditions that affect the optic nerve are like those that affect the central nervous system.
- The optic nerve is vulnerable to disease processes extending from adjacent structures, including infections and neoplasms.
- If giant cell arteritis is suspected, corticosteroid treatment should be initiated immediately.

Topography

The optic nerve, which is embryologically derived from the optic stalk, is continuous with the optic tract in the brain. Therefore, many diseases of the optic nerve reflect those of the central nervous system (CNS). The optic nerve measures 35–55 mm, extending from the eye to the optic chiasm, where the fibers decussate; from there, the fibers continue until they synapse in the lateral geniculate nucleus. The optic nerve is divided into 4 topographic areas (the length of each is given in parentheses):

- intraocular (0.7–1.0 mm)
- intraorbital (25–30 mm, with curvature and slack to accommodate eye movement)
- intracanalicular (4–10 mm)
- intracranial (~10 mm)

The clinically visible portion of the optic nerve inside the eye is known as the *optic disc*. The portion of the optic nerve inside the eye and anterior to the lamina cribrosa is known as the *optic nerve head (ONH)*. These terms are often used interchangeably.

The optic nerve consists of retinal ganglion cell (RGC) axons and glial cells (Fig 14-1). Glial cells (*glia* = glue), including oligodendrocytes, astrocytes, and microglial cells, make up the supportive tissue of the CNS. Their functions are listed in Table 14-1.

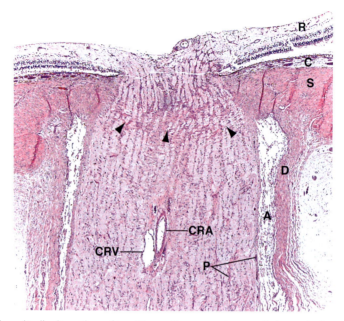

Figure 14-1 Longitudinal section of healthy optic nerve. Axons of the retinal ganglion cells (R) travel in the nerve fiber layer toward the optic nerve head (ONH) and make a 90° turn posteriorly to become the axonal fibers of the optic nerve. Optic nerve axons pass through the fenestrations in the lamina cribrosa *(arrowheads)*, a perforated area in the posterior sclera (S), and become myelinated, increasing the diameter of the retrolaminar nerve. Sclera surrounding the lamina cribrosa is continuous with the dura (D) of the optic nerve. A = arachnoid; C = choroid; CRA = central retinal artery; CRV = central retinal vein; P = pial septa. *(Courtesy of Tatyana Milman, MD.)*

Table 14-1 Supporting Cells in the Central Nervous System

Cell Type	Function
Astrocytes	Provide support and nutrition for neurons like ganglion cells
Microglial cells	Perform phagocytic function similar to that of histiocytes
Oligodendrocytes	Produce and maintain myelin sheath of optic nerve

The optic nerve becomes myelinated by oligodendrocytes just posterior to the lamina cribrosa of the sclera, making it larger in diameter than the optic nerve head. The optic nerve is encased in a meningeal sheath that consists of the following:

- the external dense connective tissue sheath, or *dura* (which merges with the sclera anteriorly and the dura of the brain posteriorly)
- the cellular *arachnoid sheath* composed of meningothelial cells (which forms part of the internal sheath of the optic nerve and is the continuation of the arachnoid mater around the brain)
- the fibrovascular *pial sheath* (which also forms part of the internal sheath and is the continuation of the pia mater around the brain)

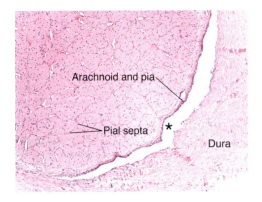

Figure 14-2 Cross section through a healthy optic nerve. The axons of the optic nerve are segregated into fascicles by the delicate, fibrovascular pial septa. The nuclei of oligodendrocytes, astrocytes, and microglia are visible between the eosinophilic axons. The subdural space *(asterisk)* is relatively narrow in the typical optic nerve. *(Courtesy of Tatyana Milman, MD.)*

The pial vessels and connective tissue extend into the optic nerve and divide the nerve fibers into fascicles. The subarachnoid space of the optic nerve sheath contains cerebrospinal fluid (Fig 14-2; also see Fig 14-1).

The vascular supply of the optic nerve stems predominantly from pial vessels, which are branches of the ophthalmic and superior hypophyseal arteries; the short posterior ciliary arteries mainly supply the optic nerve head. See BCSC Section 2, *Fundamentals and Principles of Ophthalmology*, and Section 5, *Neuro-Ophthalmology*, for additional discussion of the optic nerve and its vascular supply.

Developmental Anomalies

The numerous developmental anomalies of the optic nerve include optic nerve hypoplasia, optic nerve colobomas, optic nerve head pits, morning glory disc anomaly, and Bergmeister papilla. Only those entities that have been well characterized histologically are discussed in this section. See BCSC Section 5, *Neuro-Ophthalmology*, and Section 6, *Pediatric Ophthalmology and Strabismus*, for additional discussion of developmental anomalies of the eye, including the optic nerve.

Colobomas

Colobomas of the optic nerve result from incomplete closure of the embryonic fissure. They are often inferonasal and may be associated with colobomatous defects of the retina and choroid, ciliary body, and iris (Fig 14-3A). Histologically, there is a large defect in the optic nerve; atrophic, gliotic retina lines the defect. The sclera is commonly ectatic and bowed posteriorly (Fig 14-3B). The defect wall may contain adipose tissue and even smooth muscle (Video 14-1).

 VIDEO 14-1 Disorders of the optic nerve.
Courtesy of Nora V. Laver, MD, and Teresa Horan, MD.
Available at: aao.org/bcscvideo_section04

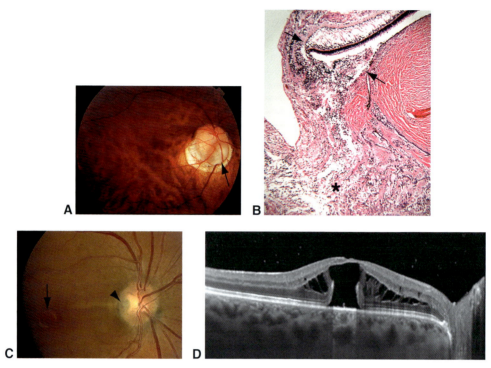

Figure 14-3 Optic nerve coloboma and pit. **A,** Fundus photograph of the right eye shows a colobomatous defect in the inferonasal optic nerve *(arrow).* **B,** Photomicrograph shows gliotic, disorganized retina *(asterisk)* that prolapses into the ONH defect, which is lined by excavated sclera. Unaffected retina, retinal pigment epithelium, and choroid terminate at the edge of the colobomatous defect *(between arrows).* **C,** Fundus photograph (right eye, different patient) shows an optic nerve pit *(arrowhead)* with associated macular edema *(arrow).* **D,** Optical coherence tomography (OCT) image from the same patient as in part C shows an optic pit–associated maculopathy with intraretinal cystoid edema and subretinal fluid. *(Parts A and B courtesy of Tatyana Milman, MD; parts C and D courtesy of Benjamin J. Kim, MD.)*

Optic Nerve Pits

An optic nerve pit is another developmental defect that is likely caused by incomplete embryonic fissure closure (Fig 14-3C). Clinically and histologically, there is a small depression in the optic disc that is associated with a defect in the lamina cribrosa. Histologically, herniation of malformed (abnormal) retina into the defect is typically found. Associated shallow serous retinal detachments with macular schisis can be seen in 25%–75% of eyes with inferotemporal pits (Fig 14-3D; also see Video 14-1).

Inflammation

Inflammation can affect the optic nerve directly or indirectly via many mechanisms. *Optic neuropathy* may present as sudden or gradual progressive vision loss; the optic nerve may appear swollen, normal, or pale (optic atrophy). Mass effect from orbital or intracranial infection or inflammation can also cause optic neuropathy. Some systemic inflammations and infections cause occlusive vasculitis, resulting in ischemic optic neuropathy.

Optic neuritis is an all-encompassing term referring to inflammation of the optic nerve, which can result from infectious or noninfectious etiologies. Neuritis may be isolated or part of a constellation of findings and may involve either the anterior or posterior segment of the eye. *Neuroretinitis* is characterized as acute vision loss with associated optic nerve and macular edema with exudates in a "star" pattern. *Optic perineuritis* represents inflammation of the optic nerve sheath with sparing of the optic nerve. Table 14-2 summarizes the various forms of inflammation that can affect the optic nerve.

Infections That Cause Optic Neuropathy

Infectious agents may cause direct necrosis of nerve structures or demyelination of the optic nerve due to an immune response to localized or systemic infection. Histiocytes and microglia remove the damaged myelin, and astrocytic proliferation ultimately produces a glial scar *(plaque)*. Infectious optic neuritis is discussed further in BCSC Section 5, *Neuro-Ophthalmology.*

Bacterial or parasitic infections Infections of the optic nerve can occur because of systemic infection or, much less commonly, from spread of infection from adjacent anatomical structures (eg, sinusitis). Common causative agents of these infections include the following:

- optic neuritis: *Treponema pallidum, Mycobacterium tuberculosis*
- neuroretinitis: *Bartonella (henselae, quintana), T pallidum, M tuberculosis, Toxoplasma gondii, Borrelia burgdorferi*
- optic perineuritis: *T pallidum*

Viral infections The optic nerve may be infected by viral pathogens, including human herpes simplex virus types 1 and 2 and varicella-zoster virus. These infections may manifest as optic neuritis, ischemic optic neuropathy caused by occlusive vasculitis, or immune-mediated demyelination. Acute disseminated encephalomyelitis (ADEM) is an immune-mediated demyelinating disease that often follows bacterial or viral infection. Postviral or postvaccination optic neuritis is a rare but established cause of autoimmune optic neuropathy.

Fungal infections Mucormycosis, cryptococcosis, aspergillosis, and coccidioidomycosis are some of the fungal infections that can involve the optic nerve. *Mucormycosis* (previously called *zygomycosis*) generally results from direct extension from nearby structures, usually a contiguous sinus infection. It is associated with diabetes and other systemic conditions that can cause an immunocompromised state, including long-term use of corticosteroids. It may affect the optic nerve via direct infiltration, occlusive vasculitis, focal necrosis, or mass effect. *Cryptococcosis* generally begins as a pulmonary infection, which can disseminate to the brain. Optic nerve involvement generally occurs via direct spread from the intracranial cavity and is commonly associated with multiple foci of necrosis with little inflammatory reaction (Fig 14-4). *Aspergillosis* may cause compressive optic neuropathy due to mass effect or ischemic optic neuropathy resulting from occlusive vasculitis. Like cryptococcosis, *coccidioidomycosis* also begins as a primary pulmonary infection and can disseminate to other areas of the body, including the optic nerve and eye, producing necrotizing granulomas.

Table 14-2 Inflammation Affecting the Optic Nerve

Inflammation	Mechanisms	Example
Optic neuritis	Demyelination, necrosis of astrocytes or glial elements	Acute demyelinating encephalomyelitis (ADEM), multiple sclerosis, neuromyelitis optica (NMO), myelin oligodendrocyte glycoprotein (MOG) disease, postinfectious optic neuritis (eg, from COVID-19), syphilis
Optic perineuritis	Infiltration of the leptomeninges by polymorphonuclear leukocytes	Granulomatosis with polyangiitis, immunoglobulin G4–related disease (IgG4-RD), MOG disease, sarcoidosis, syphilis
Neuroretinitis	Inflammation of the optic nerve and retina	*Bartonella* infection, Lyme disease, sarcoidosis, syphilis, toxoplasmosis, tuberculosis, viral infection
Meningitis	Increased intracranial pressure or secondary to optic neuritis	Cryptococcosis, coccidioidomycosis, Lyme disease, tuberculosis, viral infection

Courtesy of Kevin Lai, MD.

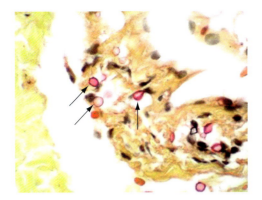

Figure 14-4 Cryptococcosis of the optic nerve in an immunocompromised patient. The dura is infiltrated by cryptococcal organisms *(arrows)*. This yeast has a mucopolysaccharide capsule that stains red with mucicarmine stain. No inflammatory infiltrate is visible. *(Courtesy of Tatyana Milman, MD.)*

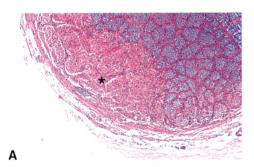
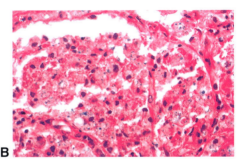

Figure 14-5 Demyelination of the optic nerve. **A,** Luxol fast blue stain for myelin. The blue-stained area indicates normal myelin. Note the sectoral absence of myelin in the lower left corner of the optic nerve *(asterisk),* corresponding to a focal area of demyelination. **B,** Higher magnification. The blue material (myelin) is engulfed by histiocytes (macrophages).

Noninfectious Inflammations That Affect the Optic Nerve

Noninfectious inflammatory disorders of the optic nerve include classic optic neuritis in individuals with *multiple sclerosis (MS), giant cell arteritis (GCA),* and *sarcoidosis.* Further discussion of the conditions in this section can be found in BCSC Section 5, *Neuro-Ophthalmology.*

Multiple sclerosis   MS is a common inflammatory demyelinating disease of the CNS that causes optic neuritis. The histologic findings of optic neuritis caused by MS are similar to those of ADEM, with loss of myelin in the retrolaminar optic nerve and sectoral atrophy of the ganglion cells in more advanced cases (Fig 14-5).

Giant cell arteritis   Although GCA does not cause direct inflammation of the optic nerve, it is a systemic inflammatory disorder that can cause optic nerve ischemia that results in profound vision loss. GCA is characterized by inflammation that affects medium to large arteries. Histologically, a chronic inflammatory infiltrate is seen in the vessel wall, often centered on the internal elastic lamina, resulting in its destruction. The inflammation is granulomatous; epithelioid histiocytes and sometimes multinucleated giant cells are present, as well as lymphocytes. The intima is usually thickened and fibrotic, with broad disruption of the internal elastic lamina; the lumen may be thrombosed and subsequently recanalized (Fig 14-6).

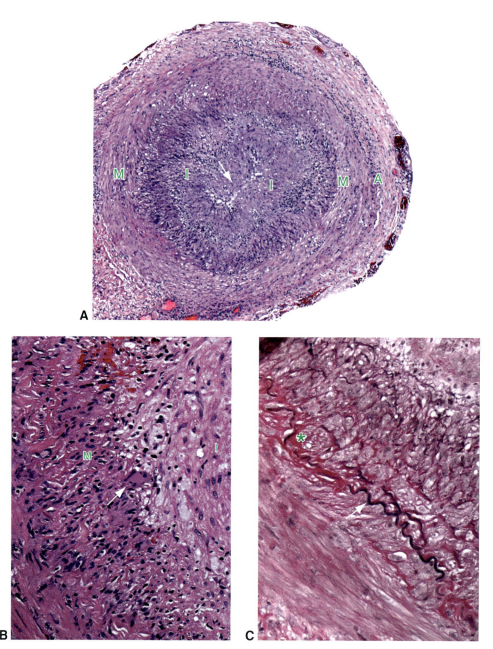

Figure 14-6 Temporal artery biopsy in giant cell arteritis. **A,** Vascular lumen *(arrow)* is markedly narrowed by intimal hyperplasia and inflammation. A prominent transmural inflammatory infiltrate involves the intima (I), media (M), and adventitia (A). **B,** The inflammatory infiltrate is centered at the level of internal elastic lamina, between the intima (I) and the media (M). Note the multinucleated giant cell *(arrow)* and numerous small lymphocytes and histiocytes. Internal elastic lamina is destroyed. **C,** Verhoeff–van Gieson elastic stain shows segmental loss of the internal elastic lamina *(asterisk)*. A short segment of the wavy internal elastic lamina remains *(arrow)*. *(Courtesy of Nora V. Laver, MD.)*

These same inflammatory features can affect the posterior ciliary arteries, resulting in their occlusion and in liquefactive necrosis of the optic nerve. When the inflammation subsides, there may be scarring in the vessel wall, primarily in the intima and at the level of destroyed elastic lamina, with focal loss of the muscularis layer (transmural scarring). This can be a primary finding in a biopsy specimen ("healed arteritis") rather than active inflammation.

When GCA is suspected, treatment with corticosteroid therapy should be initiated immediately. Because corticosteroid treatment can diminish inflammation, temporal artery biopsy should be performed within 10–14 days from initiation of treatment. Bilateral temporal artery biopsies are useful only in rare cases, increasing the yield at most by 2%–5%. Typically, contralateral biopsies are employed when findings of the initial temporal artery biopsy are negative or atypical and there is high clinical suspicion for GCA. See Chapter 2 in this volume for discussion of temporal artery biopsy specimen handling.

Clinical Pearl

- The presence of giant cells is not required to establish a diagnosis of GCA.
- It is important to inform the pathologist of any corticosteroid treatment so that the findings can be interpreted appropriately.
- In the event of an unexpected biopsy result, a second expert opinion may be helpful.

Sarcoidosis Another systemic disorder that can involve the optic nerve, sarcoidosis is often associated with retinal, vitreal, and uveal lesions (Fig 14-7; see also Chapter 11, Fig 11-9). Unlike the characteristic noncaseating granulomas in the eye, optic nerve lesions may demonstrate necrosis. Refer to Section 9, *Uveitis and Ocular Inflammation*, for further discussion.

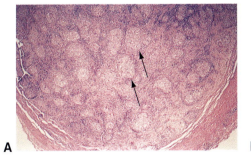 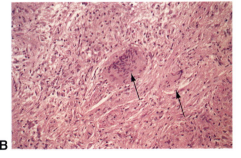

Figure 14-7 Sarcoidosis of the optic nerve. **A,** Low-magnification photomicrograph shows a cross section of the optic nerve with discrete noncaseating granulomas *(arrows)*. **B,** Higher magnification shows multinucleated giant cells *(arrows)* in the granulomas. *(Courtesy of Hans E. Grossniklaus, MD.)*

Degenerations

Optic Atrophy

Although the etiology varies, the sequence of events that leads to optic atrophy is uniform: injury to the retinal ganglion cells (RGCs) and the axons of the anterior optic nerve (the portion of the nerve near the globe) results in axonal swelling, clinically apparent as ONH edema (Fig 14-8). Axonal swelling and loss of RGCs are followed by retrograde degeneration of axons (ie, ascending atrophy, or Wallerian degeneration) toward the lateral geniculate body. Pathologic processes within the cranial cavity or orbit result in descending atrophy toward the RGC bodies (see BCSC Section 5, *Neuro-Ophthalmology*, for more on optic atrophy). Loss of myelin and oligodendrocytes accompanies the axonal degeneration. The optic nerve also shrinks, despite the proliferation of astrocytes and fibroconnective tissue (gliosis) in the pial septa (Fig 14-9).

Glaucoma is a group of diseases characterized by optic neuropathy, resulting in optic atrophy. Histologically, there is early loss of RGC axons, blood vessels, and glial cells, particularly at the level of the lamina cribrosa. As the disease advances, the ONH becomes excavated, with posterior bowing of the lamina cribrosa (see Fig 14-9D). Evidence of optic nerve atrophy may precede detectable functional vision loss. See BCSC Section 10, *Glaucoma*, for further discussion.

Another example of optic atrophy is Schnabel cavernous optic atrophy. Although this condition was initially observed in glaucomatous eyes after acute intraocular pressure elevation, it has been increasingly identified in elderly patients without glaucoma who have generalized arteriosclerotic disease. Schnabel cavernous optic atrophy is characterized microscopically by large cystoid spaces in the nerve posterior to the lamina cribrosa (Fig 14-10A).

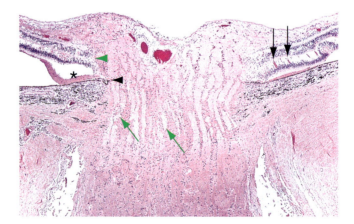

Figure 14-8 ONH edema. Swollen intralaminar axons demonstrate vacuolar alteration with pale staining *(green arrows)* and displace the retina laterally *(green arrowhead)* from its normal termination just above the end of Bruch membrane *(black arrowhead)*. Juxtapapillary serous intraretinal fluid *(black arrows)* and serous subretinal fluid *(asterisk)* are also present. *(Courtesy of Tatyana Milman, MD.)*

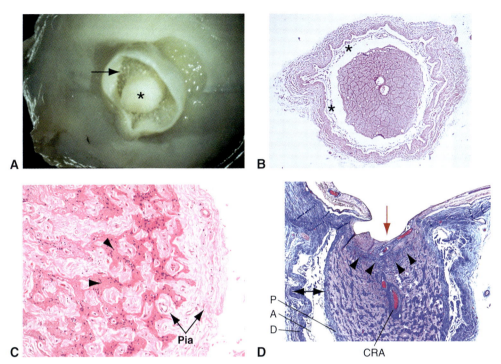

Figure 14-9 Optic nerve atrophy. **A,** Gross appearance of an optic nerve *(asterisk)* with widened subdural space *(arrow)* due to shrinkage of the nerve. **B,** Low-magnification photomicrograph also shows a widened subdural space *(asterisks)*. **C,** Cross section of an atrophic nerve shows loss of axons *(arrowheads)*, accompanied by glial proliferation and widening of fibrovascular pial septa *(arrows)*. **D,** Glaucomatous optic atrophy. Masson trichrome stains the collagen of the sclera, lamina cribrosa, and meninges dark blue and the axonal fascicles pink. The optic nerve demonstrates advanced cupping *(red arrow)*, accompanied by posterior bowing of the lamina cribrosa *(arrowheads)*. Axonal atrophy and thickening of pial septa are present. The subdural and subarachnoid spaces are widened due to severe optic nerve atrophy *(double-ended arrow)*. A = arachnoid sheath; CRA = central retinal artery; D = dural sheath; P = pia. *(Part A courtesy of Debra J. Shetlar, MD; parts C and D courtesy of Tatyana Milman, MD.)*

These spaces contain mucopolysaccharides, which stain with Alcian blue (Fig 14-10B). The source of these mucopolysaccharides was originally thought to be vitreous, forced into the ischemic necrosis–induced cavernous spaces by elevated intraocular pressure; however, the mucopolysaccharides are more likely produced in situ, within the atrophic spaces of the optic nerve.

Optic Nerve Head Drusen

Drusen of the ONH are calcific bodies embedded within the parenchyma of the optic nerve. Their etiology is unclear, but evidence suggests that abnormal axonal metabolism leads to mitochondrial calcification and drusen formation. Drusen are usually bilateral and associated with small, crowded ONHs with abnormal vasculature. When superficial, drusen

300 • Ophthalmic Pathology and Intraocular Tumors

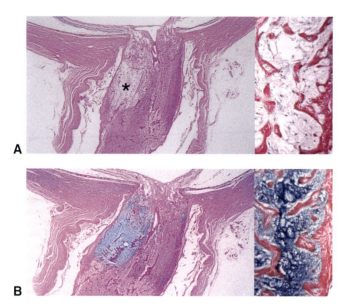

Figure 14-10 Schnabel cavernous optic atrophy. **A,** Photomicrograph shows atrophy resulting in cystoid spaces *(asterisk)* within the optic nerve. *Right inset:* Higher magnification of the cystoid spaces filled with a myxoid material. **B,** Cystic spaces are filled with Alcian blue–positive material. *Right inset:* Higher magnification of Alcian blue–positive material. *(Low-magnification images courtesy of Hans E. Grossniklaus, MD; higher-magnification right insets courtesy of Nora V. Laver, MD.)*

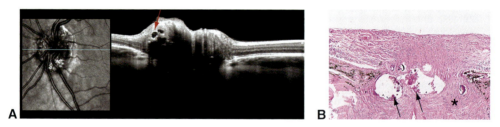

Figure 14-11 ONH drusen. **A,** OCT cross section through the ONH shows an elevated disc surface and drusen visualized as optically empty cavities *(arrow),* with a reflection from the posterior surface. **B,** Histologically, ONH drusen appear as discrete basophilic calcified deposits *(arrows)* just anterior to the lamina cribrosa *(asterisk).* The clear spaces in the ONH are histologic sectioning artifacts due to dropout of hard calcific material. *(Part A courtesy of Laurel N. Vuong, MD.)*

appear on the optic disc as refractile, rounded pale-yellow or white deposits (Fig 14-11A). ONH drusen may cause visual field defects; in rare cases, they can cause anterior ischemic optic neuropathy, resulting in significant vision loss. Most ONH drusen are located anterior to the lamina cribrosa.

ONH drusen are usually seen in otherwise healthy eyes. Less frequently, ONH drusen can be associated with the following:

- angioid streaks
- papillitis

- optic atrophy
- long-term glaucoma
- vascular occlusions

Histologically, ONH drusen appear as basophilic, irregular, calcified acellular deposits (Fig 14-11B) that contain mucopolysaccharides, amino acids, DNA, RNA, and iron. For more information, see BCSC Section 5, *Neuro-Ophthalmology,* and Section 6, *Pediatric Ophthalmology and Strabismus.* Also see Video 14-1.

> Hamann S, Malmqvist L, Costello F. Optic disc drusen: understanding an old problem from a new perspective. *Acta Ophthalmol.* 2018;96(7):673–684.

Neoplasia

Tumors may affect the ONH (eg, melanocytoma, peripapillary choroidal melanoma, choroidal osteoma, and hemangioma) or the retrobulbar portion of the optic nerve (eg, glioma and meningioma). Invasion of the optic nerve can occur through direct extension of orbital or CNS tumors (eg, leptomeningeal carcinomatosis). Direct infiltration of the optic nerve may occur in hematologic malignancies (eg, leukemia). The discussion in the following sections focuses on the histologic features of the more common optic nerve neoplasms. See BCSC Section 5, *Neuro-Ophthalmology,* and Section 7, *Oculofacial Plastic and Orbital Surgery,* for more information on these entities.

Melanocytoma

Melanocytoma of the ONH is a benign, heavily pigmented (dark-brown to jet-black) melanocytic tumor located eccentrically on the ONH and adjacent choroid (Fig 14-12A). It may be elevated and extend into the adjacent retina or extend posteriorly into the optic nerve. Melanocytomas are slow-growing, and malignant transformation to melanoma is rare. Histologically, melanocytoma is a magnocellular nevus, composed of closely packed, heavily pigmented, plump polyhedral melanocytes. Because the dense pigment obscures nuclear detail (Fig 14-12B,C), melanin bleach preparations (Fig 14-12D) are necessary to reveal the tumor's bland cytologic features, such as abundant cytoplasm, small nuclei with finely dispersed chromatin, and inconspicuous nucleoli. Necrosis and histiocytic infiltration are sometimes observed within melanocytoma but are not necessarily indicative of aggressive behavior. See also Chapters 11 and 16.

Glioma

Gliomas (astrocytomas) may arise in any part of the visual pathway, including the ONH and optic nerve. *Pilocytic astrocytoma* is frequently associated with neurofibromatosis 1 (NF1). These tumors are low-grade circumscribed astrocytic gliomas (CNS WHO grade 1) and commonly present in the first decade of life. When the dura mater remains intact, the nerve exhibits fusiform or sausage-shaped enlargement within the sheath (Fig 14-13A).

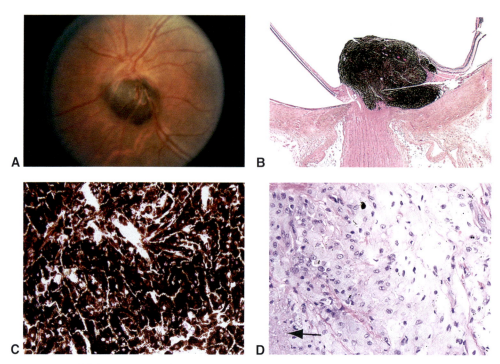

Figure 14-12 Melanocytoma of the optic nerve. **A,** Fundus photograph shows a dark mass on the inferior edge of the ONH. **B,** Low-magnification photomicrograph of melanocytoma shows a dome-shaped, jet-black mass involving the prelaminar optic nerve. The tumor also involves the juxtapapillary choroid and retina. **C,** Higher magnification shows darkly pigmented polyhedral melanocytes with dense intracytoplasmic pigment obscuring nuclear detail. **D,** Melanin bleach preparation shows the bland nuclear morphology and abundant cytoplasm of the melanocytoma cells. Note the area of necrosis within the tumor *(arrow)*. *(Part A courtesy of Robert H. Rosa Jr, MD; parts B–D courtesy of Tatyana Milman, MD.)*

Biopsy of these lesions is generally not required when neuroimaging is diagnostic. Histologic examination of pilocytic astrocytoma shows proliferation of spindle-shaped astrocytes with delicate, hairlike (pilocytic) cytoplasmic processes that expand the optic nerve parenchyma (Fig 14-13B,C). The nuclei are round to elongated; mitotic figures are rare. Enlarged, strongly eosinophilic filaments, known as *Rosenthal fibers,* may be found in these tumors and represent degenerating cell processes (see Fig 14-13C). In addition, calcification and foci of microcystoid degeneration can be seen; the pial septa may be thickened; and the meninges may demonstrate reactive hyperplasia and astrocyte infiltration. See Chapter 2, Table 2-3, for the immunohistochemical profile of optic nerve glioma.

High-grade gliomas (WHO CNS grade 4; also known as *glioblastoma multiforme*) rarely involve the optic nerve and are increasingly classified according to key molecular changes such as *IDH* pathogenic variation. When optic nerve involvement occurs, it is usually due to primary brain tumor invasion of the optic nerve rather than gliomas arising in the nerve. Primary malignant gliomas of the anterior visual pathway occur mainly

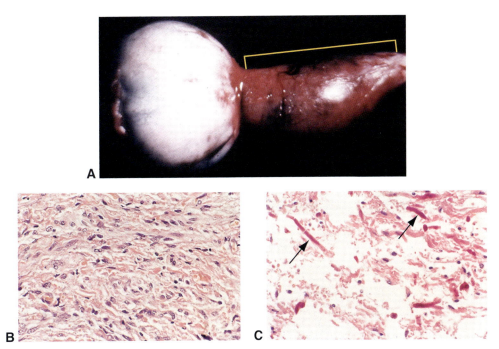

Figure 14-13 Astrocytoma of the optic nerve. **A,** Macroscopic examination of an optic nerve glioma exhibiting fusiform or sausage-like enlargement within the optic nerve sheath *(bracket)*. **B,** Histologically, in pilocytic astrocytoma neoplastic glial cells are elongated to resemble hairs. **C,** Degenerating eosinophilic filaments, aggregates of glial fibrillary acidic protein known as *Rosenthal fibers (arrows)*, may be observed in these tumors. *(Part A courtesy of Nora V. Laver, MD; part B courtesy of Anat Stemmer-Rachamimov, MD.)*

in adults. They are characterized histologically by nuclear pleomorphism, high mitotic activity, and necrosis.

Meningioma

Primary optic nerve sheath meningiomas arise from the arachnoid layer of the optic nerve sheath, usually involve the intraorbital optic nerve (92%), and display a slow, circumscribed growth (Fig 14-14). They are less common than secondary orbital meningiomas, which extend from a primary intracranial site, usually through the sphenoid bone. Most cases are sporadic, but some arise in individuals with neurofibromatosis 2 (NF2), particularly children. Primary optic nerve sheath meningiomas may invade the nerve and eye and, in rare cases, may extend through the dura to invade the orbit and extraocular muscles.

Histologically, most of these tumors are benign, low grade (WHO CNS grade 1 or 3), and lacking in atypical features or aggressive growth. *Meningothelial meningioma* is a common subtype composed of plump cells with indistinct cytoplasmic margins (also called a *syncytial growth pattern*) arranged in whorls (see Fig 14-14C,D). *Psammoma bodies,* extracellular

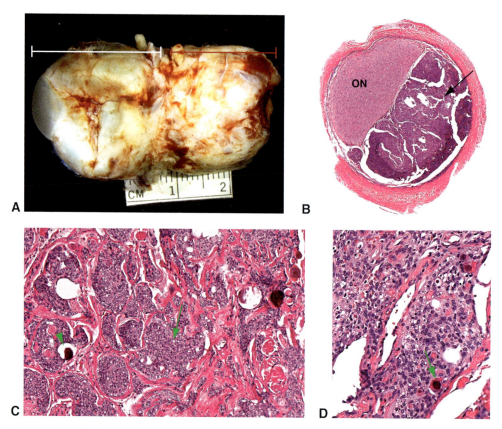

Figure 14-14 Optic nerve sheath meningioma. **A,** Gross photograph showing a globe *(white bracket)* with massive thickening *(red bracket)* of the optic nerve and sheath just posterior to the sclera, secondary to meningioma. **B,** Meningioma *(arrow)* growth compressing and deforming the optic nerve (ON). **C,** Meningioma with meningothelial growth pattern showing characteristic whorls *(arrow)* and psammoma bodies *(arrowhead)*. **D,** Higher magnification of meningioma with calcified psammoma bodies adjacent to a whorl *(arrow)*. *(Part A courtesy of Nasreen A. Syed, MD; parts B–D courtesy of Tatyana Milman, MD.)*

rounded calcifications surrounded by a cluster of meningioma cells, are variably present (see Fig 14-14C,D). See Chapter 2, Table 2-3, for the immunohistochemical profile of meningioma.

> Louis DN, Perry A, Wesseling P, et al. The 2021 WHO Classification of Tumors of the Central Nervous System: a summary. *Neuro Oncol.* 2021;23(8):1231–1251.

PART II

Intraocular Tumors: Clinical Aspects

CHAPTER **15**

Introduction to Part II

Part II of this volume covers the clinical diagnostic and prognostic aspects of and therapeutic options for intraocular tumors. Intraocular tumors make up a broad spectrum of benign and malignant lesions that can lead to loss of vision, loss of the eye, and/or loss of life. Effective management of these lesions depends on accurate diagnosis; a main goal of the content in Part II is to enable comprehensive ophthalmologists to accurately make diagnoses, including

- melanocytic tumors (Chapter 16)
- vascular tumors (Chapter 17)
- retinoblastoma (Chapter 18)
- ocular involvement from systemic malignancies (Chapter 19)

When evaluating a patient with a tumor, an ophthalmologist should have sufficient knowledge either to make an accurate diagnosis or at least to develop a differential diagnosis. There should be a low threshold for referral to a specialist when the diagnosis is uncertain, or when the potential treatment involves complex therapies and/or a multispecialty approach. Given the specialized expertise required in most cases, ophthalmologists with specific training in ocular oncology will need to manage these conditions.

Since the 1980s, significant advances have been made in understanding the biology of intraocular tumors and in managing these lesions with an emphasis on globe salvage. The Collaborative Ocular Melanoma Study (COMS), funded by the National Institutes of Health, was one of the largest clinical trials in ocular oncology. The COMS gathered important information concerning the most common primary intraocular malignant tumor in adults, choroidal melanoma. The COMS reported outcomes for enucleation versus brachytherapy for the treatment of medium-sized tumors. The results confirmed that eye-sparing plaque brachytherapy performed in well-selected cases does not adversely affect melanoma-related morbidity or mortality. Based on these results, the most common treatment for uveal melanoma is now eye-sparing radiation instead of enucleation.

As in other oncology specialties, ocular oncology is making a shift toward molecular diagnosis and prognosis, with the goal of implementing personalized medicine for these lesions. For uveal melanoma, researchers have identified key cytogenetic aberrations that are associated with metastatic disease, including monosomy of chromosome 3, especially with gains in chromosome 8. Gene expression profile testing, another molecular technique, is highly predictive for late metastasis in uveal melanoma. Both forms of prognostic testing require tumor sampling obtained through fine-needle aspiration biopsy (FNAB) of the tumor or evaluation of paraffin-embedded tissue. Information gained from FNAB is useful for tumor prognostication and identification of patients at high risk for distant metastasis. This is reviewed in detail in Part I: Ophthalmic Pathology in this volume.

As with uveal melanoma, advances in understanding the molecular genetics of retinoblastoma also continue to evolve. Retinoblastoma, the most common primary intraocular cancer in children, is most often caused by a pathogenic variant in the *retinoblastoma tumor suppressor gene (RB1)*, which was isolated, cloned, and sequenced in the 1980s (the first tumor suppressor gene ever sequenced). Although tumor biopsy is contraindicated for retinoblastoma, the aqueous humor is a high-yield source of cell-free tumor DNA; thus, aqueous fluid can be used as a liquid biopsy. This 2017 discovery led to the ability to molecularly profile the genetic and genomic alterations in the tumor, even in the absence of tumor tissue, and opened the door for clinical testing to identify both diagnostic and prognostic biomarkers. Further, evaluation of the aqueous can facilitate the identification of the *RB1* pathogenic variant driving the tumorigenesis, which enhances clinicians' ability to screen for the mutation in the blood, identify germline disease, and provide appropriate genetic counseling to the patient and family (see Chapter 18). Treatment of retinoblastoma has also evolved; like choroidal melanoma treatment, treatment of retinoblastoma has transitioned toward globe-conserving therapy with ever more localized forms of chemotherapy and other treatments, including laser therapy and cryotherapy. Historically, external beam radiotherapy was a foundational treatment for retinoblastoma; however, now it is very rarely used, and then usually only as a last resort for treating active disease in a remaining eye. This change in treatment approach is due, in part, to the recognition of the potential risk for increasing the incidence of second nonocular malignancies in children who harbor a germline pathogenic variation in *RB1*. In addition, the development of safe intravitreal injections of chemotherapy revolutionized ophthalmologists' ability to manage vitreous retinoblastoma seeding, which was previously the most common reason for intraocular tumor relapse.

In the United States and Europe, most malignancies are staged using the classification system developed by the American Joint Committee on Cancer (AJCC), which stages cancer in patients based on tumor size, lymph node status, and distant metastasis. Both clinical and pathologic data may be used to clinically stage a tumor. For retinoblastoma, the role of germline predisposition is recognized by incorporating category "H" for "hereditary retinoblastoma" into the AJCC classification. It is an important distinction that the patients themselves—not just a single organ, such as the eye—are staged.

As noted, intraocular tumors may result in progressive and irreversible vision loss, loss of the eye, and loss of life, requiring a multidisciplinary approach to patient care. It is important for the physician to recognize when their patient has low vision so that patient education and, if appropriate, referral for multidisciplinary vision rehabilitation can be considered before loss of function and independence occur. The American Academy of Ophthalmology's Initiative in Vision Rehabilitation page on the ONE Network (aao.org/education/low-vision-and-vision-rehab) and Technology Tools for Children with Low Vision (aao.org/eye-health/tips-prevention/technology-apps-devices-children-blind-low-vision) provide resources for low vision management, including patient handouts and information about additional vision rehabilitation opportunities and technology tools for the pediatric population beyond those provided by the ophthalmologist.

CHAPTER **16**

Melanocytic Tumors

 This chapter includes related videos. Go to aao.org/bcscvideo_section04 or scan the QR codes in the text to access this content.

Highlights

- Uveal melanomas may develop in the iris, ciliary body, or choroid. Ciliary body and choroidal melanomas have a worse prognosis than iris melanomas because of their substantially higher risk for metastasis.
- Signs suggestive of iris melanoma include large size, prominent ectropion uveae, intratumoral vascularity, sectoral cataract, secondary glaucoma, seeding of the iris stroma and peripheral angle structures, extrascleral extension, and documented progressive growth.
- Posterior uveal melanomas arising from the ciliary body and choroid are associated with a high mortality rate. Referral to an ocular oncologist should be considered for patients with tumors displaying features suggestive of malignancy.
- Features suggestive of choroidal melanoma include large size, presence of subretinal fluid, surface lipofuscin, vision symptoms, and documented growth.
- Uveal melanomas may be treated with enucleation, brachytherapy or proton beam therapy, or excision, depending on tumor size and location.

Introduction

Intraocular melanocytic tumors develop from uveal melanocytes in the iris, ciliary body, and choroid. The 2 main groups of melanocytic tumors of the uveal tract (uvea) are benign nevi and melanomas. In contrast to melanocytic cancers of the skin and mucosal membranes, which usually initially spread through the lymphatics, melanocytic malignancies of the uvea typically exhibit hematogenous metastasis. Pigmented intraocular tumors that originate from the pigmented epithelium of the iris, ciliary body, and retina constitute another group of melanin-containing tumors of neuroepithelial origin. These rare tumors are discussed separately at the end of this chapter (see also Chapter 11).

Iris Nevus

An iris nevus is a variably pigmented lesion of the iris stroma that causes minimal distortion of the iris architecture. It is a benign tumor, likely congenital in origin, that contains increased numbers of specialized melanocytes (nevus cells). Many of these lesions are small, produce no symptoms, and are recognized incidentally during routine ophthalmic examination. Their prevalence is uncertain, although iris nevi may occur more frequently in patients with neurofibromatosis type 1.

Iris nevi should be distinguished from iris freckles (Fig 16-1A), which are flat lesions (rather than tumors) associated with an increased amount of intracellular melanin. Iris freckles may be associated with ultraviolet (UV) light exposure and are more prevalent in older adults. Although iris freckles have no malignant potential, numerous iris freckles may be associated with increased risk for cutaneous melanoma, which is similarly associated with increased lifetime exposure to UV light. Individuals with multiple iris freckles may benefit from routine skin evaluation by a dermatologist.

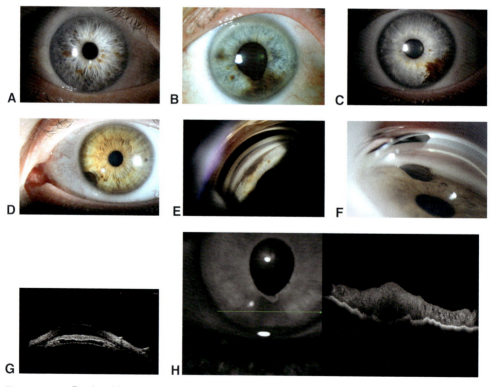

Figure 16-1 Benign iris melanocytic lesions, clinical appearance. **A,** Iris freckles are flat and often multiple. **B–D,** Iris nevi have a variable appearance and may be flat **(B, C)** or nodular **(D).** They may cause ectropion uveae **(B). C–H,** The slit-lamp **(C, D),** gonioscopic **(E, F),** ultrasound biomicroscopic (UBM) **(G),** and optical coherence tomography (OCT) **(H)** appearances of chronic iris nevi are shown. *(Parts A and C–G courtesy of Alison Skalet, MD, PhD; part B courtesy of Tero Kivelä, MD; part H courtesy of Jesse L. Berry, MD.)*

Ophthalmoscopically, iris nevi present in 2 forms: (1) *circumscribed iris nevi,* which are flat to nodular, solitary or multiple, and involve a discrete portion of the iris; and (2) *diffuse iris nevi,* which may involve an entire sector or, in rare instances, the entire iris. Iris nevi may cause ectropion uveae (Fig 16-1B) and, occasionally, a sectoral cataract.

Iris nevi are best evaluated by slit-lamp biomicroscopy coupled with gonioscopy. It is important to carefully assess lesions involving the angle to rule out a ciliary body tumor because the most important differential diagnosis is iris or ciliary body melanoma. High-frequency ultrasound biomicroscopy (UBM) is helpful when evaluating lesions that involve the angle because it can reveal a ciliary body component. Figure 16-1 shows examples of the clinical appearance of iris freckles and nevi.

Iris nevi usually do not require treatment beyond observation, including photographic documentation.

Iris Melanoma

Iris melanomas constitute 3%–5% of all uveal melanomas (Fig 16-2). Small melanomas of the iris may be challenging to clinically distinguish from benign iris nevi.

Iris melanomas range in appearance from amelanotic (off-white) to dark-brown lesions, and three-quarters of them involve the inferior iris (see Fig 16-2A, C, D). In rare cases, their growth pattern is diffuse, resulting in unilateral acquired hyperchromic heterochromia (darker iris) and secondary glaucoma. One subtype grows in a pattern that resembles tapioca pudding (see Fig 16-2D, F).

Clinical evaluation of iris melanoma is identical to evaluation of iris nevi. Signs suggesting malignancy include large size, prominent ectropion uveae and intratumoral vascularity (see Fig 16-2D), sectoral cataract, secondary glaucoma, seeding of the iris stroma (see Fig 16-2B) and peripheral angle structures, extrascleral extension, and documented progressive growth. The differential diagnosis of iris melanoma is listed in Table 16-1 and pictured in Figure 16-3.

Advances in high-frequency ultrasonography (echography) enable excellent characterization of iris tumor size and anatomical relationship to normal ocular structures (see Figs 16-1G, H and 16-2G, H). Iris fluorescein angiography may document intrinsic vascularity; however, this finding has limited value in narrowing the differential diagnosis. Biopsy may be considered when the diagnosis is unclear.

In cases of documented growth or secondary glaucoma, diagnostic/therapeutic excision of an iris melanoma is indicated. Alternatively, brachytherapy (radioactive plaque) or proton beam therapy may be used, particularly for larger lesions and lesions with extensive angle involvement.

The prognosis for most patients with iris melanoma is excellent; the mortality rate is low (1%–4%), possibly because the tumor is usually small and likely because its biological behavior is distinct from the behaviors of ciliary body and choroidal melanomas. The main risk factor for metastatic death is invasion of the anterior chamber angle, which may present as poorly controlled glaucoma, mimicking pigmentary glaucoma.

Cherkas E, Kalafatis NE, Marous MR, Shields CL. Iris melanoma: review of clinical features, risks, management, and outcomes. *Clin Dermatol.* Published online: October 21, 2023. doi:10.1016/j.clindermatol.2023.10.009

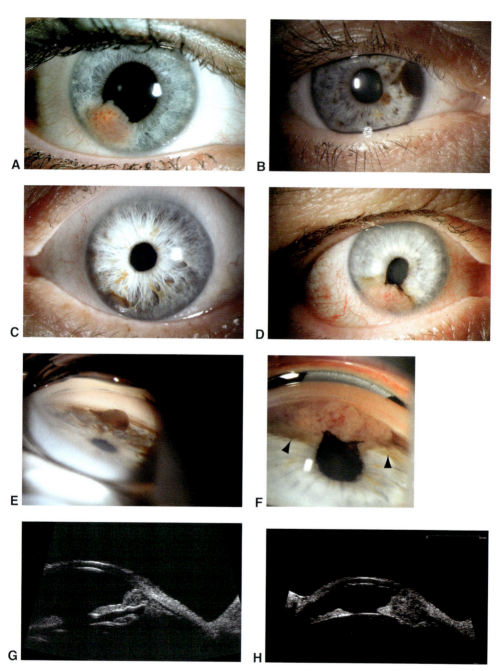

Figure 16-2 Iris melanoma, clinical appearance. **A,** The lesion can be amelanotic with visible intrinsic vascularity. **B,** Alternatively, it may be densely pigmented, obscuring any blood vessels (note dispersed pigment on the iris stroma). **C–H,** The slit-lamp **(C, D)**, gonioscopic **(E, F)**, and UBM **(G, H)** appearances of 2 iris melanomas are shown. The melanoma shown in parts C, E, and G is a small nodular tumor involving the anterior chamber angle; fine-needle aspiration biopsy revealed a melanoma mainly composed of epithelioid cells. The tumor shown in parts D, F, and H is a large amelanotic melanoma with prominent vascularity. Note the flat pigmented portion of the tumor (**F,** *arrowheads*) along the edges of the mass surrounding the amelanotic portion. *(Part A courtesy of Tero Kivelä, MD; parts B–H courtesy of Alison Skalet, MD, PhD.)*

Table 16-1 Differential Diagnosis of Iris Melanoma

Iris freckle (see Fig 16-1A)
Iris nevus (see Fig 16-1B–H)
Primary iris cyst (pigment epithelial or stromal) (see Fig 16-3A)
Iris melanocytoma
Lisch nodules (in neurofibromatosis, variably pigmented, multiple, small, flat, or nodular lesions) (see Fig 16-3B)
Congenital ocular or oculodermal melanocytosis (diffuse iris nevus) (see Figs 16-3D and 16-4G, H)
Iridocorneal endothelial (ICE) syndrome (Cogan-Reese iris nevus type)
Iris pigment epithelial proliferation (epithelial downgrowth after trauma or surgery)
Iris foreign body (secondarily pigmented)
Juvenile xanthogranuloma (amelanotic or tan-colored)
Retained lens material simulating iris nodule (amelanotic)
Metastatic carcinoma to the iris (amelanotic) (see Fig 16-3C)

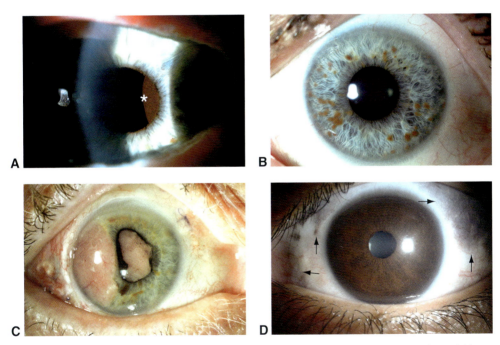

Figure 16-3 Differential diagnosis of iris melanoma. **A,** A pigment epithelial cyst *(asterisk)* can bow the iris forward focally. The cyst is visible after dilation. **B,** Multiple Lisch nodules (melanocytic hamartomas, typically tan to golden brown) in neurofibromatosis. **C,** Metastasis from a pulmonary carcinoma visible as an amelanotic mass on the temporal half of the iris and inside the pupil. The tumor distorts the pupil shape. **D,** Congenital ocular melanocytosis can cause a diffuse iris nevus but is associated with pigmented patches on the episclera and sclera *(arrows)*. Note the deeply pigmented, velvety stromal thickening in the iris. *(Parts A and B courtesy of Tero Kivelä, MD; parts C and D courtesy of Alison Skalet, MD, PhD.)*

Khan S, Finger PT, Yu GP, et al. Clinical and pathologic characteristics of biopsy-proven iris melanoma: a multicenter international study. *Arch Ophthalmol.* 2012;130(1):57–64.

Laino AM, Berry EG, Jagirdar K, et al. Iris pigmented lesions as a marker of cutaneous melanoma risk: an Australian case-control study. *Br J Dermatol.* 2018;178(5):1119–1127.

Popovic M, Ahmed IIK, DiGiovanni J, Shields CL. Radiotherapeutic and surgical management of iris melanoma: a review. *Surv Ophthalmol.* 2017;62(3):302–311.

Ciliary Body and Choroidal Nevi

Nevi of the ciliary body are rare, mostly small, and often first identified during histologic examination of globes enucleated for other reasons. Choroidal nevi (Fig 16-4) may occur in up to 8% of White individuals. Similar to iris nevi, most choroidal nevi cause no symptoms and are recognized incidentally on routine ophthalmic examination. Ophthalmoscopically, the typical choroidal nevus appears as a flat or minimally elevated, pigmented (gray to brown) choroidal lesion with soft margins (see Fig 16-4A–E). Some nevi are amelanotic (see Fig 16-4F).

Choroidal nevi are often associated with overlying retinal pigment epithelium (RPE) disturbance and drusen (see Fig 16-4A, D). These features are characteristic of a chronic quiescent lesion. A minority of choroidal nevi develop atypical features such as localized serous retinal detachment over and around the nevus, surface lipofuscin (see Fig 16-4E, F), or choroidal neovascular membranes. These atypical nevi may result in reduced vision, metamorphopsia, and visual field defects. Although these clinical features can occur in the context of a benign lesion, they should also raise suspicion for malignant transformation; careful follow-up for progression and lesion growth is indicated.

In the choroid, congenital ocular melanocytosis is similar in appearance to a diffuse nevus (see Fig 16-4G). This condition increases the lifetime risk for ciliary body and choroidal melanoma (1 in 400 compared with 1 in 180,000 for the general population).

Clinical Pearl Congenital ocular melanocytosis carries a 1 in 400 lifetime risk for uveal melanoma and an increased risk for glaucoma. It is important to recognize that individuals with this condition can have a spectrum of increased pigmentation and may display some or all features. Features can include increased cutaneous periocular pigment, deep scleral pigment, iris heterochromia, and partial or diffuse choroidal melanocytosis. Careful examination involving comparison to the contralateral iris and choroid is important when diagnosing this condition. Lifelong routine ophthalmic surveillance, including ciliary body imaging, is indicated to monitor melanoma development (see Fig 16-4G, H).

Findings on fluorescein angiography usually are not helpful for diagnosis of choroidal nevi; these lesions may demonstrate either hypofluorescence or hyperfluorescence. Nevi are distinguished from choroidal melanomas and other pigmented fundus lesions by clinical evaluation and multimodal imaging, as described in the section Melanoma of the Choroid and Ciliary Body.

The management of choroidal nevi includes photographic documentation of all lesions; ultrasonographic measurement of lesions thicker than 1 mm; and lifelong periodic reassessment to detect signs of growth or change consistent with transformation into choroidal

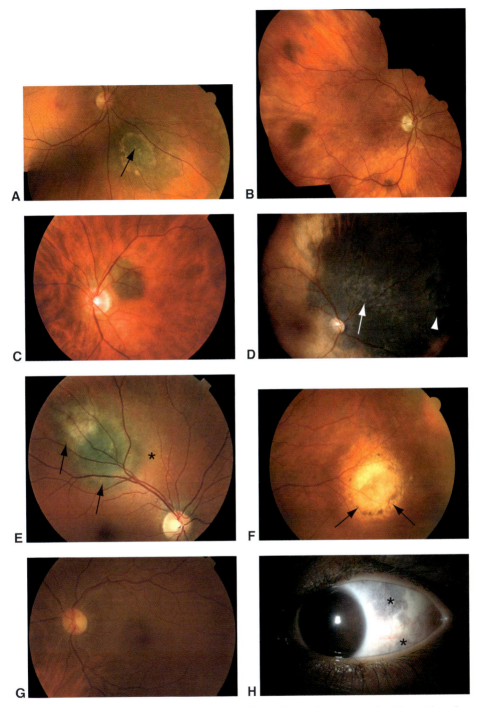

Figure 16-4 Choroidal nevi, clinical appearance. Choroidal nevi are generally thinner than 2 mm and variably gray to brown. They may be solitary (**A**) or multiple (**B**). Nevi may demonstrate drusen on their surface (**A,** *arrow*). **C,** Small nevi lack changes in retinal pigment epithelium (RPE). **D,** Large nevi usually exhibit changes in RPE (note the drusen *[arrow]* and focal RPE hyperplasia *[arrowhead]*). **E–F,** Some nevi display surface lipofuscin, which appears as orange pigment on dark tumors (**E,** *arrows*) and pigmented melanolipofuscin on amelanotic tumors (**F,** *arrows*); it can be associated with subretinal fluid (**E,** *asterisk*). **G,** Congenital ocular melanocytosis has a diffuse nevuslike dark choroidal appearance. **H,** Appearance of patchy gray sclera *(asterisks)* and diffuse iris pigmentation associated with ocular melanocytosis. All lesions in this figure were followed for several years without evidence of growth. *(Parts A, B, F, and H courtesy of Alison Skalet, MD, PhD; parts C–E and G courtesy of Tero Kivelä, MD.)*

melanoma (Fig 16-5). Optical coherence tomography (OCT) can help to exclude the presence of subclinical subretinal fluid.

Benign nevi may increase in diameter in the absence of malignant transformation. In a long-term study of choroidal nevi, nevi enlarged a median of 1 mm overall; however, the median yearly rate of enlargement was less than 0.1 mm, and none of the enlarging nevi developed new orange pigment or subretinal fluid. The frequency of enlargement was reportedly 54% in patients younger than 40 years and 19% in patients older than 60 years. If rapid or more extensive enlargement is documented, especially in patients older than 40 years, malignant transformation should be suspected (Fig 16-6).

> Mashayekhi A, Siu S, Shields CL, Shields JA. Slow enlargement of choroidal nevi: a long-term follow-up study. *Ophthalmology.* 2011;118(2):382–388.
> Shields CL, Dalvin LA, Ancona-Lezama D, et al. Choroidal nevus imaging features in 3806 cases and risk factors for transformation into melanoma in 2355 cases: the 2020 Taylor R. Smith and Victor Curtin Lecture. *Retina.* 2019;39(10)1840–1851.

Melanoma of the Choroid and Ciliary Body

Choroidal and ciliary body melanomas (posterior uveal melanomas) are the most common primary intraocular malignancies in adults. Approximately 6700–7100 new cases of uveal melanomas are reported annually worldwide, of which 65% affect non-Hispanic White individuals; 87,000–106,000 survivors are under follow-up care. The incidence varies according to age, ethnicity, and latitude. Ethnicity-specific incidences range from 0.4 cases per million people of Asian descent to 1.7 cases per million in Hispanic individuals and 6.0 cases per million in non-Hispanic White individuals. Among White individuals, the incidence is higher in populations living in higher-latitude regions. From south to north, the incidence increases from 4.6 to 7.5 cases per million, respectively, in the United States and from 2.6 to 8.4 cases per million, respectively, in Europe.

Fewer than 1% of choroidal and ciliary body melanomas are diagnosed in children younger than 18 years. Approximately 80% of choroidal and ciliary body melanomas are detected in adults between 45 and 80 years of age. In the United States and Europe, the mean age at diagnosis is 60–65 years; in Asia, it is 45–50 years.

Additional risk factors for posterior uveal melanoma include the following:

- light complexion (light skin, blue eyes, blond hair)
- ocular melanocytic abnormalities, such as nevi and congenital ocular and oculodermal melanocytosis (lifetime risk of melanoma in these patients = 1 in 400)
- dysplastic nevus syndrome (threefold-increased risk of melanoma)
- germline *BAP1* variation or other genetic predisposition

The role of UV radiation as a risk factor for posterior melanoma remains unclear, although most studies indicate that UV light does not play a significant role.

> Krantz BA, Dave N, Komatsubara KM, Marr BP, Carvajal RD. Uveal melanoma: epidemiology, etiology, and treatment of primary disease. *Clin Ophthalmol.* 2017;11:279–289.

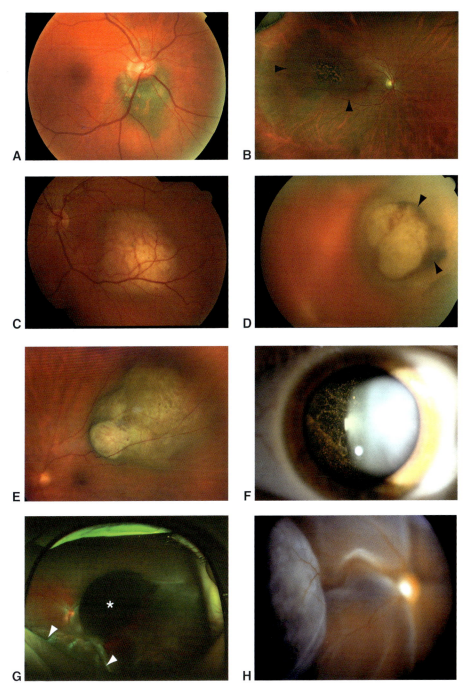

Figure 16-5 Choroidal melanoma, clinical appearance. **A, B,** Choroidal melanomas may be quite thin. Note the prominent surface lipofuscin in each case and the large area of flat involvement surrounding the elevated portion centrally in part B *(arrowheads)*; however, they are more commonly elevated (>2 mm in height). Melanomas are usually pigmented **(A, B, E, F)** or, less commonly, amelanotic **(C, D).** Smaller melanomas typically have a dome shape, whereas larger tumors that have broken through Bruch membrane display a collar-button shape **(D, E).** Melanoma formation is often accompanied by subretinal hemorrhage **(D,** *arrowheads)*. **F,** Retinal invasion and vitreous seeding may occur. **G, H,** Very large tumors may be associated with large areas of serous retinal detachment. In part G, the tumor apex is darkly pigmented *(asterisk)*, and retinal detachment is visible at the lower left *(arrowheads)*. *(Parts A and H courtesy of Tero Kivelä, MD; parts B–D and G courtesy of Alison Skalet, MD, PhD; parts E and F courtesy of Elaine M. Binkley, MD.)*

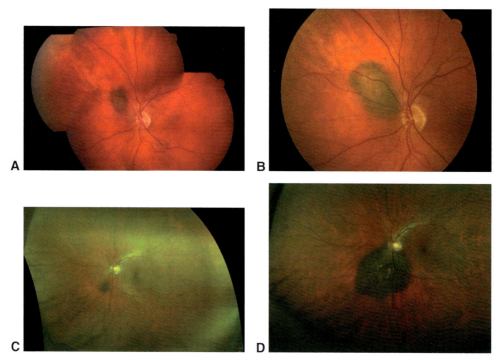

Figure 16-6 Malignant transformation of choroidal nevus to melanoma. **A,** Small choroidal nevus. **B,** Over an observation period of 13 months, the nevus expanded its borders and acquired surface lipofuscin. **C,** A different patient with a small peripapillary choroidal nevus. **D,** The nevus shown in part C demonstrated substantial growth and emergence of surface lipofuscin over an observation period of 6.5 years. *(Courtesy of Alison Skalet, MD, PhD.)*

Clinical Characteristics

The typical *choroidal melanoma* is a variably pigmented, elevated, dome-shaped mass (see Fig 16-5). Initial symptoms and signs may deceptively resemble manifestations of vitreous detachment; however, metamorphopsia, reduced vision, and a visual field defect from direct tumor growth or secondary retinal detachment may eventually develop, depending on tumor location. In many patients, choroidal melanomas are asymptomatic and are identified incidentally on routine dilated eye examination. Significant growth of a preexisting choroidal nevus or the emergence of surface lipofuscin or subretinal fluid should lead to suspicion of malignant transformation into melanoma (see Fig 16-6).

The degree of pigmentation ranges from amelanotic (off-white) to dark brown. At the RPE level, clumps of lipofuscin may be present on the surfaces of smaller tumors (see Figs 16-5A, B and 16-6B, D). Surface lipofuscin appears orange on pigmented tumors and dark on amelanotic tumors. Localized subretinal fluid is common in cases of melanoma, and larger tumors may be associated with more extensive serous detachment of the neurosensory retina (see Fig 16-5G, H). Over time, 50% of tumors erupt through Bruch membrane and assume a mushroom or collar-button shape (see Fig 16-5D, E). This process may be associated with subretinal hemorrhage. Some tumors also erode through the retina, causing vitreous hemorrhage or vitreous seeding of a tumor (see Fig 16-5F). If extensive retinal detachment develops, anterior displacement of the lens–iris diaphragm and secondary angle-closure glaucoma occasionally occur. Neovascularization of the iris may occur with larger tumors.

Because they are located posterior to the iris, *ciliary body melanomas* often remain asymptomatic until they become rather large (Fig 16-7A). Symptoms and signs eventually include dilated, often tortuous, episcleral vessels (sentinel vessels) in the region of the tumor (Fig 16-7B);

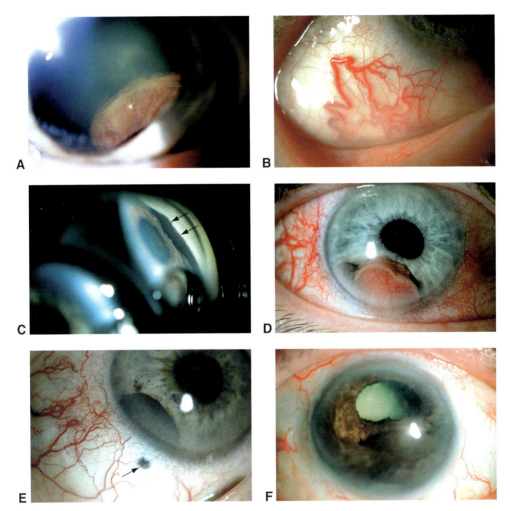

Figure 16-7 Ciliary body melanoma, clinical appearance. **A,** Ciliary tumors often are not evident unless the pupil is widely dilated. They may indent the lens. **B,** Sentinel episcleral vessels. **C,** Anterior extension of a ciliary body melanoma may be detected only by gonioscopy *(arrows)*. **D,** The tumor may invade the anterior chamber. **E,** The tumor may extend through the sclera *(arrow)* via emissary channels. **F,** Ring melanomas grow circumferentially within the ciliary body and may extend into the anterior chamber. *(Courtesy of Tero Kivelä, MD.)*

reduced vision from induced astigmatism or cataract when the tumor makes contact with the lens; photopsia and visual field alterations from associated retinal detachment in more advanced cases; and, in rare cases, secondary glaucoma.

Ciliary body melanomas usually are not visible unless the pupil is widely dilated. Some erode through the iris root into the anterior chamber and become visible during gonioscopy (Fig 16-7C) or external examination (Fig 16-7D). Infrared transillumination can be used to identify the anterior border of these tumors. Eventually, the tumor extends through the sclera along aqueous drainage channels (Fig 16-7E), producing an epibulbar nodule. Some ciliary body melanomas assume a diffuse growth pattern and extend up to 360° around the eye; in this case, they are known as *ring melanomas* (Fig 16-7F).

Diagnostic Evaluation

Clinical evaluation of suspected posterior uveal melanomas includes obtaining a history (eg, personal and family histories of cancer), performing a full ophthalmic examination, and ordering multiple types of imaging studies (multimodal imaging) (Figs 16-8, 16-9). When used appropriately, the tests described in this chapter enable accurate diagnosis of most melanocytic tumors. Atypical lesions may require characterization through other testing modalities, including intraocular biopsy (see discussion later in this chapter and in Chapter 2); alternatively, when appropriate, these lesions may be closely observed for characteristic changes in clinical behavior to establish a correct diagnosis.

The most important diagnostic technique for evaluating intraocular tumors is *indirect ophthalmoscopy*. It provides stereopsis, a wide field of view, and visualization of the peripheral fundus, particularly when performed in conjunction with scleral depression. Indirect ophthalmoscopy and wide-field fundus photography enable clinical assessment of tumor size and surface features. *Slit-lamp biomicroscopy* in combination with *gonioscopy* is the best method for clinically establishing the presence of the tumor and extent of its anterior involvement (see Fig 16-7C), although high-frequency UBM also allows excellent visualization of anterior ocular structures (see Figs 16-1, 16-2). In addition, slit-lamp biomicroscopy enables a detailed assessment of the surface features of posterior tumors, including whether lipofuscin and subretinal fluid are present and whether there is any retinal tumor invasion or vitreous involvement.

Multimodal imaging is the standard of care in the diagnosis and ongoing management of melanocytic tumors. *Fundus photography* is valuable for documenting the appearance and basal dimensions of a choroidal tumor, along with identification of gradual changes in its shape (see Fig 16-6). Fundus photographs (see Figs 16-8A, B and 16-9A, B) can reveal the full extent of many tumors and document their relationships with intraocular landmarks. Comparison with the optic disc can help to approximate tumor size. The relative positions of retinal blood vessels may be helpful markers of changes in lesion size. Fundus photographs also allow clinicians to use intrinsic scales to measure the basal diameter of a choroidal melanoma.

Fundus autofluorescence (FAF) imaging helps to highlight lipofuscin, which is brightly autofluorescent (see Fig 16-9C, D). In addition, recent leakage of subretinal fluid produces increased autofluorescence, whereas persistent or past leakage may result in decreased

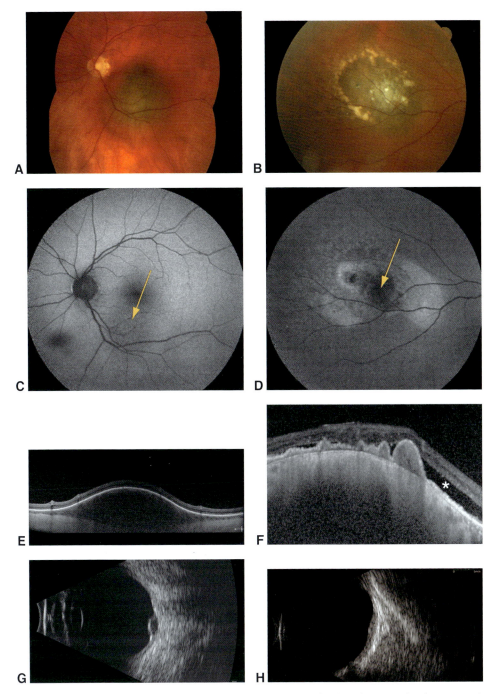

Figure 16-8 Multimodal imaging of choroidal nevi. **A, B,** Color fundus photographs document the tumor borders and surface appearance of 2 thin choroidal nevi. **C,** Fundus autofluorescence (FAF) reveals minimal RPE disturbance in the area of the choroidal lesion *(arrow)*. **D,** FAF shows centrally decreased autofluorescence because of RPE loss *(arrow)* and increased autofluorescence associated with more recent leakage, creating the appearance of a fluid gutter. **E,** Enhanced depth imaging OCT (EDI-OCT) reveals no subretinal fluid associated with the lesion shown in parts A and C. **F,** EDI-OCT shows that the lesion depicted in parts B and D has both numerous surface drusen and mild subretinal fluid *(asterisk)*. **G, H,** B-scan ultrasonography reveals that both lesions are thin. *(Courtesy of Alison Skalet, MD, PhD.)*

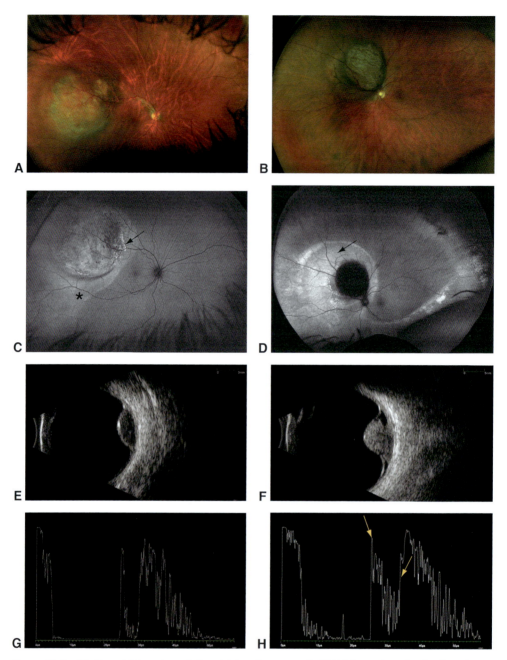

Figure 16-9 Multimodal imaging of choroidal melanomas. **A, B,** Wide-angle color fundus photographs document the tumor borders and surface appearance of 2 choroidal melanomas. **C,** FAF image of the lesion shown in part A reveals increased diffuse autofluorescence associated with subretinal fluid *(asterisk)* adjacent to the variably autofluorescent tumor. Increased autofluorescence is associated with lipofuscin *(arrow)*. **D,** FAF image of the lesion shown in part B. The highly elevated tumor blocks underlying autofluorescence. Diffusely increased autofluorescence is associated with subretinal fluid adjacent to the tumor *(arrow)*. **E,** B-scan ultrasonography reveals the dome shape of the tumor shown in parts A and C. **F,** B-scan ultrasonography reveals the collar-button shape of the tumor shown in parts B and D. Images obtained from B-scan ultrasonography are helpful in measuring tumor size. **G, H,** Corresponding A-scan ultrasonographic images reveal low internal reflectivity associated with each melanoma. Part H shows characteristic angle kappa with decreasing internal reflectivity from the lesion apex to its base *(arrows* at apex and base). *(Courtesy of Alison Skalet, MD, PhD.)*

autofluorescence from secondary RPE atrophy. *Enhanced depth imaging OCT* or *swept-source OCT* is helpful when developing the differential diagnosis because they can reveal degenerative RPE and photoreceptor changes in chronic lesions, which are less likely to be small melanomas, as well as lipofuscin and subretinal fluid in suspicious melanocytic choroidal tumors.

Fluorescein angiography findings are not pathognomonic for choroidal melanoma but can help to distinguish between tumors and hemorrhagic processes that may mimic tumors. *Indocyanine green angiography* is not more accurate than fluorescein angiography for diagnosis, but it often shows altered choroidal blood flow in the region of the tumor. However, neither technique is commonly used to diagnose melanoma.

Standardized ultrasonography is the most important ancillary tool for evaluating ciliary body and choroidal melanomas (see Fig 16-9E–H). The growth and regression of an intraocular tumor can be documented with serial examinations. B-scan ultrasonography provides information about the size (thickness and basal diameter), general shape, and location of intraocular tumors (see Figs 16-8G, H and 16-9E, F). This type of ultrasonography typically shows a dome-shaped (see Fig 16-9E) or collar button/mushroom–shaped (see Fig 16-9F) choroidal mass with acoustic hollowness and choroidal excavation. Serous retinal detachment is often associated with larger tumors. B-scan ultrasonography is also the best technique for detection of posterior extrascleral extension. Standardized A-scan ultrasonography (see Fig 16-9G, H) usually reveals a solid tumor pattern with low- to medium-amplitude internal reflections (low to medium internal reflectivity) and a characteristic feature called angle kappa, in which the internal reflectivity decreases from the apex to the base of the lesion because of sound attenuation through the tumor (see Fig 16-9H). Intrinsic vascularity is visible in many cases.

The anterior location of ciliary body melanomas makes standard ultrasonography more difficult to perform. In contrast, high-frequency UBM, which lacks these limitations, enables excellent imaging of the anterior segment and ciliary body (see Fig 16-2G, H). In addition, although ultrasonography is generally considered highly reliable in the differential diagnosis of posterior uveal melanomas, it may be difficult or impossible to distinguish a necrotic melanoma from a subretinal hemorrhage or a melanoma from an atypical metastatic tumor using this technology.

When high-frequency ultrasonography is unavailable, *transillumination* may help the clinician to assess the degree of pigmentation and determine the basal diameters of suspected ciliary body or anterior choroidal melanomas. The shadow of a tumor is visible with a bright, focused light source (eg, high-intensity fiber-optic device) placed either on the surface of the topically anesthetized eye in a quadrant opposite the lesion or directly on the cornea by means of a dark corneal cap. Fiber-optic transillumination is also routinely used to locate the uveal melanoma and delineate its borders during surgery for radioactive plaque insertion (Fig 16-10A). B-scan ultrasonography can be used after plaque placement to confirm appropriate positioning (Fig 16-10B).

Although *computed tomography (CT)* and *magnetic resonance imaging (MRI)* are not widely used to assess uncomplicated intraocular melanocytic tumors, they are useful for identifying tumors in eyes with opaque media and possibly for determining extrascleral

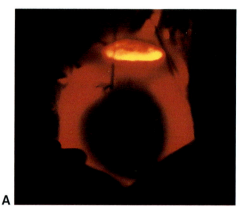
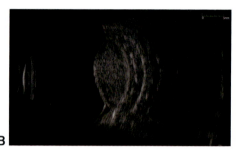

Figure 16-10 Intraoperative localization of melanoma for treatment purposes. **A,** Transillumination of the eye reveals a shadow at the site of a choroidal melanoma. This technique can be used to mark the tumor base for accurate radioactive plaque placement. **B,** B-scan ultrasonography after radioactive plaque placement confirms optimal positioning; the metal of the plaque is highly reflective on ultrasonography and can be detected traversing the entire diameter of the tumor. *(Part A courtesy of Tero Kivelä, MD; part B courtesy of Alison Skalet, MD, PhD.)*

extension and the involvement of other organs. MRI may also help to distinguish intraocular hemorrhage and atypical vascular lesions from melanocytic tumors.

Differential Diagnosis

This section describes the most common lesions considered in the differential diagnosis of posterior uveal melanoma.

Accurate diagnosis of a *choroidal nevus*, discussed earlier in this chapter, is associated with clinical experience and availability of ancillary testing modalities. For the evaluation and management of posterior pigmented lesions with characteristics predictive of growth, patients may be referred to ocular oncology centers. No single clinical factor is pathognomonic for benign versus malignant choroidal melanocytic lesions. Fewer than 10% of benign choroidal nevi have surface lipofuscin, and 15% or fewer are associated with subretinal fluid (see Fig 16-8B, D, F). In addition, 11%–58% of choroidal nevi have overlying drusen, a frequency that increases with the patient's age. The presence of surface drusen reflects the chronicity of a melanocytic choroidal tumor but can also be detected in melanomas that have transformed from formerly quiescent nevi. More than 20% of choroidal melanocytic tumors thicker than 3 mm are melanomas; far fewer than 1% of such tumors thinner than 1 mm are melanomas. Tumors 1–3 mm in thickness are more difficult to definitively classify on the basis of clinical evaluation alone; therefore, close surveillance for growth is often warranted. The risk of malignancy substantially increases for lesions with basal diameters larger than 6 mm.

Risk factors for the growth of small choroidal melanocytic lesions are well characterized; they include 5 clinical features that have given rise to the mnemonic "*t*o *f*ind *s*mall *o*cular *m*elanomas *d*oing *im*aging (see sidebar).

A mnemonic to remember risk factors for growth of choroidal nevi based on imaging is: *"to find small ocular melanomas doing imaging (TFSOM-DIM)"*:

- **T**hickness of the tumor >2 mm (ultrasound)
- **F**luid under the retina (optical coherence tomography)
- **S**ymptoms (visual acuity)
- **O**range pigmentation (lipofuscin) overlying the tumor (autofluorescence)
- **M**elanoma hollow (acoustic hollowness on ultrasound)
- **D**iameter (>5 mm on photography)

The MOLES scoring system can also be used to predict the likelihood of a lesion representing a melanoma. Lesions are assigned points (0 = absent, 1 = borderline, 2 = present), with a score >3 indicating probable melanoma:

- **M**ushroom shape
- **O**range pigment (lipofuscin)
- **L**arge size (base >4 disc diameters or thickness >2 mm)
- **E**nlargement
- **S**ubretinal fluid

The following factors also suggest the presence of melanoma:

- larger size at presentation
- juxtapapillary location
- absence of drusen or degenerative RPE changes
- homogeneous low internal reflectivity on ultrasonography
- hot spots on fluorescein angiography

To document growth of the tumor, the clinician may periodically photograph it and perform OCT and/or B-scan ultrasonography. Slow growth does not necessarily suggest or confirm malignancy. In a study of 284 benign choroidal nevi, 31% showed slow, progressive enlargement (median increase in diameter = 1 mm) over a long observation period (7 years or more). The frequency of enlargement may be higher in patients younger than 40 years (54%) than in patients older than 60 years (19%). Enlarging nevi may not develop any new lipofuscin or subretinal fluid suggestive of malignant change. Thus, when rapid or progressive growth occurs or new risk factors appear, definitive treatment should be considered.

When risk factors for growth are identified, transscleral or transvitreal fine-needle aspiration biopsy (FNAB) for cytology and molecular testing is an option prior to definitive treatment. Cytologic evaluation of cells obtained by FNAB of a small melanocytic tumor requires an experienced cytopathologist because the FNAB specimen may have low cellularity, and diagnosis based on such samples is typically challenging. The risks of biopsy include vitreous hemorrhage, retinal breaks, and theoretical tumor seeding outside of the eye. The decision to biopsy (rather than observe or treat) the lesion involves a careful analysis of the tumor and discussion of the risks and benefits with the patient.

Melanocytoma (magnocellular nevus) of the choroid or optic nerve head typically appears as a dark-brown to black elevated lesion. Optic nerve melanocytoma is usually located eccentrically over the optic nerve head and may be elevated. It often has fibrillary or feathery margins caused by extension into the nerve fiber layer (see Chapter 14, Fig 14-12). Because a melanocytoma rarely transforms into melanoma, it is important to distinguish between the 2 entities. However, choroidal melanocytomas, particularly when large, can be challenging to distinguish from choroidal melanomas without biopsy. In cases of indeterminate diagnosis or lesion growth, biopsy should be considered.

Congenital hypertrophy of the RPE (CHRPE) refers to sharply defined, flat, very darkly pigmented lesions that range from 1 mm to more than 10 mm in diameter. Patients are asymptomatic, and the lesion can be noted at any age. In younger patients, CHRPE often appears homogeneously black (Fig 16-11A); in older individuals, foci of depigmentation (lacunae) often develop (Fig 16-11B), and the lesion may slowly enlarge. The histologic findings are identical to findings in *grouped pigmentation of the retina*, also known as *bear tracks* or *grouped CHRPE* (Fig 16-11C). In patients with *Gardner syndrome,* a subtype of *familial*

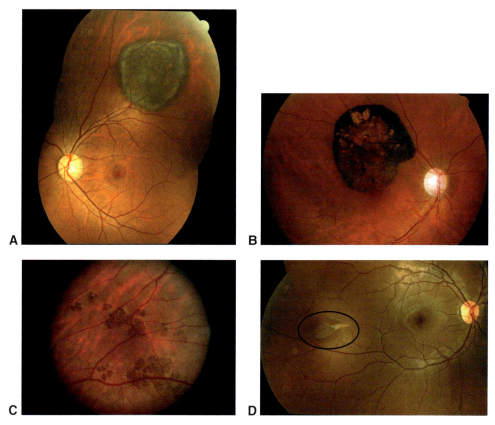

Figure 16-11 Congenital hypertrophy of the RPE (CHRPE), various clinical appearances. **A,** Large, homogeneously black CHRPE lesion. **B,** CHRPE with atrophic lacunae. **C,** Grouped pigmentation of the RPE represents a variant of CHRPE. **D,** Appearance of the RPE hamartoma associated with familial adenomatous polyposis. Note the depigmented margins and pisciform shape *(oval)*.
(Parts A and D courtesy of Alison Skalet, MD, PhD; parts B and C courtesy of Tero Kivelä, MD.)

adenomatous polyposis, the presence of multiple atypical CHRPE-like patches is a putative marker for colon cancer. These lesions are distinct from multifocal CHRPE in that they lack sectoral distribution and exhibit irregular depigmented margins, often with a pisciform shape (Fig 16-11D). OCT shows abrupt outer retinal loss and choroidal thinning with thickened and irregular RPE.

Patients with *age-related macular degeneration (AMD)* may present with macular or extramacular subretinal neovascularization, hemorrhage, and fibrosis, accompanied by varying degrees and patterns of pigmentation (Fig 16-12A). Hemorrhage, a finding commonly associated with neovascular (exudative) AMD, usually does not occur with melanomas unless the tumor has broken through Bruch membrane. Clinical evaluation of the fellow eye is helpful in documenting AMD. OCT shows predominantly subretinal and intraretinal abnormalities. Ultrasonography reveals high or heterogeneous reflectivity rather than low internal reflectivity, along with a lack of intrinsic vascularity. When in doubt, the clinician may use fluorescein angiography to help reveal early hypofluorescence secondary to hemorrhage-related blockage, which is often followed by late hyperfluorescence distributed in the choroidal neovascular membrane (Fig 16-12B). Serial observations show involutional alterations of the evolving disciform lesion.

Choroidal detachments can be hemorrhagic or serous. They are often associated with hypotony and may develop after ophthalmic surgery in the early postoperative period. Hemorrhagic detachments are often dome-shaped, involve multiple quadrants, and may be associated with breakthrough vitreous bleeding. Ultrasonographic findings may closely resemble findings in melanoma but may reveal the absence of intrinsic vascularity and involution of the hemorrhage over time. Observational management is indicated in most cases.

Peripheral exudative hemorrhagic chorioretinopathy (PEHCR) is a spontaneously developing, often asymptomatic, peripheral lesion in older adults that resembles choroidal detachment. It is often linked to suprachoroidal or subretinal bleeding and lipid exudation (Fig 16-12C); associated retinal detachment is uncommon. PEHCR is considered analogous to AMD, and the fellow eye often shows similar or a nonexudative chorioretinal degeneration. PEHCR almost always undergoes spontaneous involution.

Choroidal osteomas are benign, presumably acquired, bony tumors that typically arise from the juxtapapillary choroid in young adults (more commonly in women) and are bilateral in 20%–25% of cases. The characteristic lesion appears yellow to orange and has well-defined margins (Fig 16-12D). Ultrasonography reveals a high-amplitude echo corresponding to the bony plate and the loss of normal orbital echoes behind the lesion (acoustic shadowing). CT can reveal calcification but is not needed for diagnosis. Choroidal osteomas typically enlarge slowly over many years and can decalcify over time. If they involve the macula, vision is generally impaired. Subretinal neovascularization is a common complication. The etiology of these lesions is unknown, but chronic low-grade choroidal inflammation may be a contributing factor (see Chapter 11 for discussion of the pathology of choroidal osteoma).

Choroidal hemangiomas (see Chapters 11 and 17) resemble the surrounding fundus in color and may appear lightly pigmented or orange. When a slit beam is passed over the lesion, it can appear to glow. Over time, serous retinal detachment may develop. These lesions, which are often associated with overlying cystic retinal degeneration, are hyperechogenic on ultrasonography; they show characteristic vascular patterns on fluorescein angiography and indocyanine green angiography.

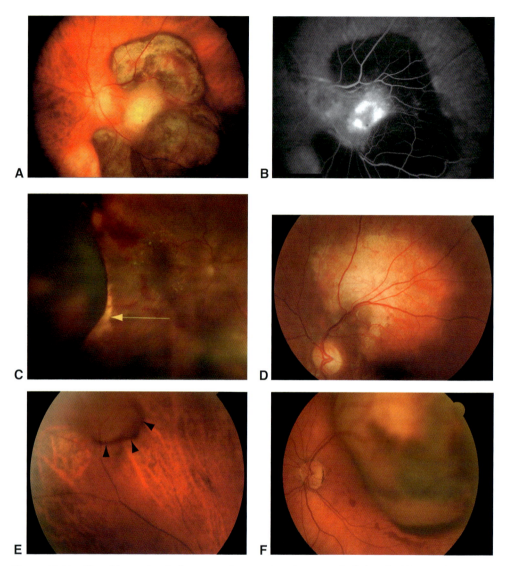

Figure 16-12 Conditions simulating posterior uveal melanoma. **A,** Subretinal hemorrhage secondary to neovascular (exudative) macular degeneration. **B,** Fluorescein angiography (same patient as in part A) reveals hyperfluorescence and late fluorescein leakage in the central macula associated with the choroidal neovascular membrane, and hypofluorescence associated with subretinal blood–induced blockage of fluorescein transmission. **C,** Peripheral exudative hemorrhagic chorioretinopathy (PEHCR); note the semitranslucent, sharply demarcated hemorrhagic pigmented epithelial detachment nasally along with surrounding subretinal hemorrhage and lipid exudates at the base *(arrow)*. **D,** Choroidal osteoma with yellow-orange color and well-defined pseudopod-like margins. **E,** Varix of the vortex vein *(arrowheads)*. This lesion is more likely to be developmental than degenerative. **F,** Metastasis to the choroid from lung cancer. Note the subretinal hemorrhage (patchy dark areas on lesion surface). *(Parts A, B, D, and E courtesy of Tero Kivelä, MD; part C courtesy of Elaine M. Binkley, MD; part F courtesy of Alison Skalet, MD, PhD.)*

Varix of the vortex vein (Fig 16-12E) is predominantly found in the nasal quadrants and can reach 4–5 mm in diameter. When filled with blood, it appears dark. The clinician can diagnose this condition by observing its coincidence with the vortex vein ampulla and by gently compressing the eye during indirect ophthalmoscopy or ultrasonography, which causes the varix to deflate.

Intraocular metastases (Fig 16-12F; see also Chapter 19) are generally amelanotic and thus pale or yellowish, unless they originate from a cutaneous melanoma. Most show medium to high or heterogeneous reflectivity on ultrasonography. Table 16-2 lists additional factors to consider in cases with amelanotic choroidal masses.

Roelofs KA, O'Day R, Harby LA, et al. The MOLES system for planning management of melanocytic choroidal tumors: is it safe? *Cancers (Basel)*. 2020;12(5):1311.

Shields CL, Dalvin LA, Yu MD, et al. Choroidal nevus transformation into melanoma per millimeter increment in thickness using multimodal imaging in 2355 cases: the 2019 Wendell L. Hughes Lecture. *Retina*. 2019;39(10):1852–1860.

Classification

Although it would be logical to classify choroidal and ciliary body melanomas according to tumor volume, no simple and reliable classification method has been developed. Instead, several different systems are used to categorize these melanomas by size. The *Collaborative Ocular Melanoma Study (COMS)* classified posterior uveal melanomas as small, medium, or large according to thickness and basal diameter (Table 16-3). The tumor, node, metastasis (TNM) staging system developed by the American Joint Committee on Cancer (AJCC) is a classification method often used in clinical practice. This system categorizes posterior uveal melanomas as small (T1), medium (T2), large (T3), or very large (T4) according to tumor thickness and basal diameter. These tumor categories, together with the presence or absence of ciliary body involvement, extrascleral extension, and systemic involvement, are used to assign melanomas to 7 stages that differ according to prognosis; stage IV tumors have the worst prognosis.

Metastatic Evaluation

The incidence of metastatic uveal melanoma may reach 50% at 25 years after treatment for ciliary body or choroidal melanoma. The COMS showed that the incidences of metastatic

Table 16-2 Differential Diagnosis of Amelanotic Choroidal Mass

Amelanotic melanoma
Chorioretinal granuloma
Choroidal detachment
Choroidal hemangioma
Choroidal metastasis
Choroidal osteoma
Posterior scleritis
Sclerochoroidal calcification

Modified from Shields JA, Shields CL. *Intraocular Tumors: A Text and Atlas*. Saunders; 1992:137–153.

Table 16-3 Collaborative Ocular Melanoma Study (COMS) Tumor Size Criteria

COMS Tumor Size	Thickness (mm)	Basal Dimensions (mm)
Small	<2.5	≤16
Medium	2.5 to ≤10.0	≤16
Large	>10.0	>16

Note: Lesions >50% in the ciliary body and some juxtapapillary lesions were excluded from the COMS.

Table 16-4 Imaging Options for Staging and Surveillance of Metastases in Uveal Melanoma

Initial Staging
CT of the chest/abdomen/pelvis with IV contrast material
Noncontrast CT of the chest; MRI of the abdomen with gadolinium contrast
Chest x-ray and MRI of the abdomen with gadolinium contrast

Posttreatment Surveillance	
Liver Imaging	Lung Imaging
MRI of the abdomen with gadolinium contrast	Chest CT scan
CT scan with IV contrast material	2-view chest x-ray
Abdominal ultrasonography	

CT = computed tomography; IV = intravenous; MRI = magnetic resonance imaging.

Note: Options for imaging studies at initial staging and during surveillance after treatment of the primary uveal melanoma are shown. For lung and liver imaging, options are listed in the order of most to least sensitive. Decisions regarding imaging technique are multifactorial.

disease after initial treatment were 25% at 5 years and 34% at 10 years. However, metastatic disease at the time of initial presentation is rare (<2% of patients). It is likely that some patients have undetectable micrometastases at the time of primary treatment.

The liver is the primary organ involved in metastatic uveal melanoma; in 90% of patients, liver involvement is the first manifestation of metastatic disease. Other relatively frequent sites—generally after liver metastasis—include the lungs, bones, and skin. Among patients with metastases who were autopsied, liver involvement was identified in 100%, whereas lung involvement was identified in 50%.

All patients benefit from image-based evaluation of metastasis before definitive treatment of intraocular melanoma (Table 16-4). The purpose of this evaluation is twofold:

1. To determine whether the patient has any other medical conditions that contraindicate surgical management or require treatment. For example, the COMS and smaller studies revealed a second primary cancer in approximately 10% of patients. If there is any suspicion that a lesion in the eye is a metastatic tumor, the clinician should ensure a thorough medical evaluation to identify the site of primary malignancy.
2. To rule out the possibility of detectable metastatic melanoma in the eye, especially for larger and higher-stage tumors. When metastatic disease is clinically present

during the pretreatment evaluation, treatment of the primary intraocular tumor will depend on patient and physician preference.

The initial staging evaluation for uveal melanoma should include a comprehensive physical examination and imaging of the lungs and liver. The extent of disease can be evaluated by chest/abdominal/pelvic CT with intravenous contrast material or, alternatively, by MRI of the abdomen with gadolinium contrast or liver ultrasonography, combined with chest imaging comprising CT or an x-ray. Liver imaging is the most important component of the staging evaluation. Lung imaging is also usually performed at the time of diagnosis, although its yield is low. A positron-emission tomography (PET) scan typically is not performed for uveal melanoma staging or surveillance because these tumors may not be fluorodeoxyglucose-avid; thus, this imaging modality has low sensitivity.

To detect early metastatic disease in patients with uveal melanoma, serial surveillance imaging is often performed over time. Strategies vary, such that some centers image only the liver and others recommend imaging both the liver and lungs. Imaging modalities used in the initial staging may also be used in surveillance imaging, with the recognition that exposure to ionizing radiation (ie, CT scans) should be minimized. Liver function tests can be considered; however, they are not widely used in the modern era of uveal melanoma management because of low sensitivity and specificity. Possible novel blood markers for the early detection of metastatic uveal melanoma are being explored.

In 2018, the first National Comprehensive Cancer Network (NCCN) clinical practice guidelines for uveal melanoma were published. The NCCN guidelines recommend that surveillance imaging be considered for 10 years after treatment of the intraocular tumor and then as clinically indicated. Systemic imaging recommendations were stratified according to the expected risk of distant metastasis (see Chapter 11). For patients with a high risk for metastasis (eg, AJCC T4, gene expression profiling class 2), imaging is recommended every 3–6 months for 5 years, and then every 6–12 months for 10 years. For patients with intermediate risk (eg, AJCC T2 and T3, class 1B), imaging is recommended every 6–12 months for 10 years. For patients with low risk (eg, AJCC T1, class 1A), surveillance imaging once every 12 months should be considered up to 5 years posttreatment and as clinically indicated. Some patients may choose to decline asymptomatic surveillance imaging because of the limited treatment options for advanced uveal melanoma and the anxiety caused by serial imaging.

If a lesion of concern is identified on surveillance imaging, a biopsy of the liver or other organ may confirm metastatic disease. Biopsy is appropriate before initiating treatment for metastatic disease.

The interval between the diagnosis of primary uveal melanoma and onset of metastasis depends on many clinical, histologic, cytogenetic, and molecular genetic factors. It varies from a few months to more than 25 years. When metastatic disease is diagnosed at a sufficiently early stage, treatment options include surgical resection; chemotherapy, such as intra-arterial hepatic chemotherapy and chemoembolization; immunotherapy or biological therapy; and hepatic selective internal radiation therapy (SIRT, also known as intrahepatic radioembolization). In 2021, the US Food and Drug Administration (FDA) approved tebentafusp, a biologic medication that can improve survival among individuals with metastatic uveal melanoma. Studies of potential adjuvant therapies to prevent the development of metastatic disease are ongoing.

> AJCC Ophthalmic Oncology Task Force. International validation of the American Joint Committee on Cancer's 7th edition classification of uveal melanoma. *JAMA Ophthalmol.* 2015;133(4):376–383. Published correction appears in *JAMA Ophthalmol.* 2015;133(9):1096.
> Nathan P, Hassel JC, Rutkowski P, et al; IMCgp100-202 Investigators. Overall survival benefit with tebentafusp in metastatic uveal melanoma. *N Engl J Med.* 2021;385(13):1196–1206.
> NCCN Clinical Practice Guidelines in Oncology: Melanoma: Uveal. Version1.2024. National Comprehensive Cancer Network website. Accessed November 4, 2024. www.nccn.org/guidelines/guidelines-detail?category=1&id=1488

Treatment

For many years, the management of posterior uveal melanomas was controversial for 2 reasons: (1) data were limited regarding the natural history of untreated patients with posterior uveal melanoma; and (2) there were insufficient data concerning patients who were matched for known and unknown risk factors and managed by different therapeutic techniques to compare the effectiveness of those techniques. Currently, both surgical and radiotherapeutic techniques are used to treat posterior uveal melanoma. Treatment selection depends on 4 factors:

1. size, location, and extent of the tumor
2. vision statuses of the affected and fellow eyes
3. age and general health of the patient
4. patient and physician preference

Research has suggested that non-White and socioeconomically disadvantaged individuals with uveal melanoma are more likely to undergo primary enucleation. Further studies are needed to understand the reasons for this trend and improve access to all treatment modalities for these patients. For more information on social determinants of health, see Chapter 1 in BCSC Section 1, *Update on General Medicine*.

Observation

There is substantial controversy regarding the diagnosis and management of small choroidal melanomas. Treatment should be considered for lesions with any of the 5 main risk factors for growth (thickness greater than 2 mm, subretinal fluid, symptoms, lipofuscin, or tumor margin in contact with the optic nerve head) and for all lesions with documented growth. Short-term observation to verify growth of a suspected small uveal melanoma is considered appropriate conventional management, especially when the tumor is located in the macular area. As mentioned earlier, FNAB can be an alternative but is technically challenging for small tumors and carries a risk of vision loss. Observations of active and larger melanomas may be appropriate in older adults and individuals with systemic illness who are poor candidates for any therapeutic intervention.

Enucleation

Historically, enucleation has been the gold standard for treatment of malignant intraocular tumors. An early hypothesis suggested that surgical manipulation of eyes containing a melanoma would lead to tumor dissemination and increased mortality; this perspective is no longer accepted. Enucleation remains appropriate for some small to medium (T1 and T2) and many large (T3) and very large (T4) choroidal melanomas, especially when useful vision has been lost, the patient declines other treatments, or the patient's ability to attend follow-up is limited. The COMS showed no difference in survival for patients with medium-sized melanomas who received brachytherapy compared with enucleation. The COMS also revealed no evidence that pre-enucleation external beam radiotherapy improved 5-year survival among patients with large choroidal melanomas. However, local orbital recurrence was more frequent after enucleation alone.

> Hawkins BS; Collaborative Ocular Melanoma Study Group. The Collaborative Ocular Melanoma Study (COMS) randomized trial of pre-enucleation radiation of large choroidal melanoma: IV. Ten-year mortality findings and prognostic factors. COMS report number 24. *Am J Ophthalmol.* 2004;138(6):936–951.
>
> Rajeshuni N, Zubair T, Ludwig CA, Moshfeghi DM, Mruthyunjaya P. Evaluation of racial, ethnic, and socioeconomic associations with treatment and survival in uveal melanoma, 2004–2014. *JAMA Ophthalmol.* 2020;138(8):876–884.

Brachytherapy with a radioactive plaque

The application of a radioactive plaque to the sclera overlying an intraocular tumor is the most common globe-sparing treatment for uveal melanoma. This technique, which has been widely available since the 1950s, allows a very high dose of radiation to be delivered to the tumor (typically 80–100 gray [Gy] at the tumor apex and up to 1000 Gy at the tumor base); a comparatively lower dose is delivered to the surrounding normal structures of the eye. Although various isotopes can be used (eg, cobalt 60, strontium 90, iridium 192, and palladium 103), the most common isotopes are iodine 125 and ruthenium 106. In the United States, iodine 125 is the isotope most frequently used in the treatment of uveal melanomas of any size; in Europe, ruthenium 106 is preferred for smaller melanomas. Advances in intraoperative localization, especially the use of ultrasonography (see Fig 16-10B), have increased local tumor control rates; currently, they are often greater than 90%. In most patients, the tumor size decreases, sometimes with regression to a flat scar (Fig 16-13). Other patients exhibit less change in tumor thickness; however, ultrasonographic changes such as increased reflectivity and decreased vascularity, along with clinical features such as subretinal fluid resolution, suggest appropriate involution of the tumor. Although rare, local recurrence may occur; therefore, it is important to monitor the treatment response by serial imaging, including photography and ultrasonography. Regrowth may occur at the tumor margin or more diffusely.

> American Brachytherapy Society–Ophthalmic Oncology Task Force. The American Brachytherapy Society consensus guidelines for plaque brachytherapy of uveal melanoma and retinoblastoma. *Brachytherapy.* 2014;13(1):1–14.

Charged-particle radiation

High–linear energy transfer radiation with charged particles (protons or helium ions) is effective in the management of ciliary body and choroidal melanomas, with local tumor control rates reportedly reaching 98%. The tumor response is similar to the response observed after brachytherapy. In this technique, tantalum clips are surgically attached to the

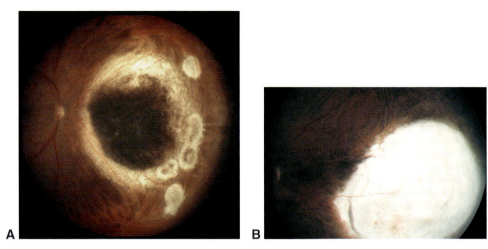

Figure 16-13 Choroidal melanoma, treated. **A,** Mildly elevated remnant of a melanoma surrounded by atrophic chorioretinal scarring nasal to the optic nerve head after plaque brachytherapy. **B,** After transscleral resection of a choroidal melanoma located temporal to the macula, the RPE and choroid are absent (and the outer retina is likely atrophic), but blood vessels indicate that the inner retina is present. *(Part A courtesy of Jacob Pe'er, MD; part B courtesy of Tero Kivelä, MD.)*

scleral surface before delivery of the first radiation fraction; these clips allow tumor localization with MRI and CT guidance. Compared with a radioactive plaque, the charged-particle beams deliver a more homogeneous dose of radiation energy to a tumor, and the lateral spread of radiation energy is less extensive. This type of therapy requires a specific charged-particle accelerator and is not available in every treatment center.

Radiation-associated complications

Depending on tumor size and location, after treatment with either plaque brachytherapy or charged-particle radiation, more than 50% of patients experience vision-limiting radiation-related adverse effects, especially optic neuropathy and maculopathy. These effects are often associated with radiation-induced damage to the microvasculature. Although they may or may not respond to intravitreal anti–vascular endothelial growth factor (anti-VEGF) treatment, patients are typically offered a trial of anti-VEGF therapy. Future studies are needed to determine the optimal patient selection criteria and treatment interval for anti-VEGF therapy. After initial radiotherapy, large tumors may develop "toxic tumor syndrome," in which an inflammatory reaction and exudative retinal detachment can develop because of the necrotic tumor. Neovascular glaucoma may also develop as part of this syndrome or because of radiation retinopathy; it can be treated with conservative therapies. Eyes with neovascular glaucoma sometimes require secondary enucleation. Chronic dry eye may develop with either form of radiation. Charged-particle radiation may also be associated with cicatricial changes to the eyelid margins. When the tumor is anteriorly located, radiation cataract is common and can be managed with routine cataract extraction; care is needed to avoid incisions in areas of irradiated sclera or cornea. Radiation retinopathy appears to be dose-dependent and typically develops 1 to several years after brachytherapy.

Archer DB, Amoaku WM, Gardiner TA. Radiation retinopathy—clinical, histopathological, ultrastructural and experimental correlations. *Eye (Lond)*. 1991;5(Pt 2):239–251.

Romano MR, Catania F, Confalonieri F, et al. Vitreoretinal surgery in the prevention and treatment of toxic tumour syndrome in uveal melanoma: a systematic review. *Int J Mol Sci*. 2021;22(18):10066.

External beam radiotherapy

Conventional external beam radiotherapy is ineffective for uveal melanoma. In recent years, some centers have used fractionated stereotactic radiotherapy and gamma knife radiosurgery as the primary treatment. Further studies of these methods are warranted, but the published results and adverse effects are similar to the outcomes of other irradiation methods.

Alternative treatments

Transpupillary thermotherapy and photodynamic therapy In the past, laser photocoagulation played a limited role in the treatment of melanocytic tumors. Selected small choroidal melanomas are currently managed by transpupillary thermotherapy (TTT), in which a long-duration, large-spot-size, relatively low-energy infrared diode laser raises the temperature of the choroid. More frequently, TTT is performed to augment plaque brachytherapy or control local recurrence at the tumor margin. Compared with brachytherapy, TTT alone may be associated with a higher rate of local tumor recurrence; some of these recurrences are extraocular. Photodynamic therapy has also been used for small tumors, but it exhibits limited efficacy and increased recurrence risk. Therefore, it is generally reserved for cases in which alternative options are unavailable.

Surgical excision Surgical transscleral resection or endoresection during vitrectomy has been successfully performed in eyes with malignant and benign intraocular tumors (see Fig 16-13B). Concerns regarding surgical excision include the inability to evaluate tumor margins for residual disease, the high incidence of pathologically recognized scleral and retinal involvement in medium and large choroidal melanomas, and the possibility of spreading the tumor intraocularly and extraocularly. The surgical techniques are generally quite demanding; they require an experienced surgeon with specialized training. Local excision of a uveal melanoma is currently coupled with adjuvant radiotherapy, such as brachytherapy or proton beam therapy, to reduce local recurrence rates to levels comparable with the levels after radiotherapy.

Chemotherapy Currently, chemotherapy is not effective in the treatment of primary uveal melanoma, and it is not routinely used in the treatment of metastatic disease.

Immunotherapy Immunotherapy involves using systemic cytokines, immunomodulatory agents, or vaccine therapy to attempt activation of a tumor-directed T-cell immune response. This treatment is theoretically appropriate for uveal melanoma because primary tumors arise in an immune-privileged organ and may express antigens to which the host lacks tolerance. However, immunotherapy currently is not available for treatment of primary uveal melanoma. Immunotherapy for metastatic disease has been used with limited success.

Exenteration In the past, exenteration was recommended for patients with extrascleral extension of a posterior uveal melanoma, but it is rarely used today. Unless orbital invasion is very advanced, the current approach comprises more conservative treatment for these patients: enucleation plus limited tenonectomy, modified plaque brachytherapy, or proton beam therapy.

Prognosis and Prognostic Factors

There are 5 main clinical risk factors for melanoma-related mortality:

- larger tumor size
- ciliary body extension
- extraocular extension
- older age
- tumor regrowth after globe-conserving therapy, especially radiotherapy

The most important histologic parameter in uveal melanoma metastasis risk stratification is cell type (a component of AJCC tumor grading). Molecular profiling of uveal melanoma has emerged as the most powerful predictor of patient survival. See Chapter 11 for a more detailed discussion of the histologic and molecular prognostic factors in uveal melanoma.

Dogrusöz M, Jager MJ. Genetic prognostication in uveal melanoma. *Acta Ophthalmol.* 2018;96(4):331–347.

Fine-needle aspiration biopsy

Intraocular fine-needle aspiration biopsy (FNAB) is not routinely used in the diagnosis of uveal tumors because examination and use of noninvasive imaging techniques can accurately identify most tumors. FNAB can be used in cases of diagnostic uncertainty or when genetic prognostic testing is needed. The procedure is performed under direct visualization through a dilated pupil, transvitreally (Video 16-1) or transsclerally (Video 16-2). Iris tumors may be accessible for FNAB through a transcameral approach. Cells obtained through FNAB can be evaluated for cytologic features to assist in diagnosis. FNAB is more commonly performed for prognostic purposes in tumors clinically diagnosed as uveal melanomas. In this clinical scenario, cells obtained through FNAB are processed to extract RNA or DNA for molecular testing and assessment of metastasis risk. Various techniques may be used, including chromosomal analysis and gene expression profiling (see Chapters 2 and 11).

 VIDEO 16-1 Transvitreal fine-needle aspiration biopsy.
Courtesy of Thomas Aaberg Jr, MD.
Available at: aao.org/bcscvideo_section04

 VIDEO 16-2 Transscleral fine-needle aspiration biopsy.
Courtesy of Thomas Aaberg Jr, MD.
Available at: aao.org/bcscvideo_section04

Intraocular FNAB may allow tumor cells to exit the eye, although this concept is controversial. In general, properly performed FNAB does not carry a high risk of tumor seeding.

However, retinoblastoma is a notable exception. If a retinoblastoma is suspected, FNAB should be avoided.

Ongoing work is addressing the role of aqueous biopsy in uveal melanoma prognostication; this approach may play a role in future clinical management.

> Finn AP, Materin MA, Mruthyunjaya P. Choroidal tumor biopsy: a review of the current state and a glance into future techniques. *Retina*. 2018;38 Suppl 1:S79–S87.
>
> McCannel TA, Chang MY, Burgess BL. Multi-year follow-up of fine-needle aspiration biopsy in choroidal melanoma. *Ophthalmology*. 2012;119(3):606–610.
>
> Wierenga APA, Cao J, Mouthaan H, et al. Aqueous humor biomarkers identify three prognostic groups in uveal melanoma. *Invest Ophthalmol Vis Sci*. 2019;60(14):4740–4747.

Collaborative Ocular Melanoma Study

Data from the prospective, randomized, COMS trial provide an additional framework for patient discussions concerning long-term survival and the rates of globe conservation with enucleation and iodine 125 brachytherapy. See the sidebar Collaborative Ocular Melanoma Study (COMS) for details.

> Collaborative Ocular Melanoma Study (COMS). National Eye Institute. ClinicalTrials.gov. Last update posted June 2, 2006. Accessed January 15, 2024. https://clinicaltrials.gov/ct2/show/NCT00000124

COLLABORATIVE OCULAR MELANOMA STUDY (COMS)

Large Choroidal Melanoma Study Arm

- evaluated 1003 patients with choroidal melanomas >16 mm in basal diameter and/or >10 mm in apical height (>8 mm if peripapillary)
- compared enucleation alone with enucleation preceded by external beam radiotherapy
- showed no significant difference in 5-year and 10-year all-cause mortality rates (approximately 40% and 60%, respectively)
- indicated that adjunctive radiotherapy did not improve overall survival but reduced the risk of orbital recurrence
- established the appropriateness of primary enucleation alone in managing large choroidal melanomas not amenable to globe-conserving therapy

Medium Choroidal Melanoma Study Arm

- evaluated 1317 patients with choroidal melanomas 6–16 mm in basal diameter and/or 2.5–10 mm in apical height (up to 8 mm if peripapillary)
- compared enucleation with iodine 125 brachytherapy
- showed no significant difference in 5-year and 10-year all-cause mortality rates (approximately 20% and 35%, respectively)
- showed no significant difference in 5-year and 10-year frequencies of histologically confirmed metastases (approximately 10% and 18%, respectively)

- revealed the following ancillary findings: (1) only 2 of 660 enucleated eyes were misdiagnosed and did not have choroidal melanoma; (2) at 5 years, the local tumor recurrence rate was 10% and the secondary enucleation rate was 13%; and (3) at 3 years, there was a decline in visual acuity to 20/200 in approximately 40% of patients, while the visual angle quadrupled (ie, there were 6 lines of vision loss) in approximately 50% of patients

Small Choroidal Melanoma Study

- observed 204 patients with tumors measuring 4–8 mm in basal diameter and/or 1.0–2.4 mm in apical height, but many of the tumors were nongrowing

Table 16-5 Pigmented Tumors in the Differential Diagnosis of Choroidal Melanoma

Melanocytoma
Adenoma/adenocarcinoma of the retinal pigment epithelium (RPE)
Congenital hypertrophy of the RPE (CHRPE)
Simple hamartoma of the RPE
Combined hamartoma of the retina and RPE
Metastasis from cutaneous melanoma

Table 16-5 lists other pigmented tumors in the differential diagnosis of choroidal melanoma.

Melanocytoma of the Iris, Ciliary Body, and Choroid

Melanocytomas (magnocellular nevi) are rare tumors composed of characteristically large, polyhedral melanocytic cells that have small, bland nuclei and abundant cytoplasm filled with large melanin granules (see Chapter 14, Fig 14-12). Iris melanocytoma cells may seed the anterior chamber angle, causing glaucoma. Melanocytomas of the ciliary body usually are not clinically detectable because of their peripheral location. In some cases, extrascleral extension of a melanocytoma along an emissary canal appears as a darkly pigmented, fixed subconjunctival mass. Melanocytomas of the choroid appear as elevated, pigmented tumors, similar to a nevus or a melanoma. Malignant changes have been identified in some melanocytomas.

When a melanocytoma is suspected, photographic and ultrasonographic studies are appropriate. If growth is documented, biopsy should be considered to exclude melanoma.

Shields CL, Kaliki S, Hutchinson A, et al. Iris nevus growth into melanoma: analysis of 1611 consecutive eyes: the ABCDEF guide. *Ophthalmology*. 2013;120(4):766–772.

Shields JA, Shields CL, Eagle RC Jr. Melanocytoma (hyperpigmented magnocellular nevus) of the uveal tract: the 34th G. Victor Simpson lecture. *Retina*. 2007;27(6):730–739.

Epithelial Tumors of the Uveal Tract and Retina

Adenoma and Adenocarcinoma

Benign adenomas of the nonpigmented and pigmented ciliary epithelium may appear clinically indistinguishable from amelanotic and pigmented melanomas arising in the ciliary body. Benign adenomas of the RPE are rare. These lesions are oval, deeply pigmented tumors that abruptly arise from the RPE. Adenomas rarely enlarge and seldom undergo malignant change. Adenocarcinomas of the RPE are also very rare; only a few cases have been reported. These lesions typically have feeder retinal vessels and may be associated with yellowish lipid exudates. Despite the presence of malignant features on histologic examination, metastatic potential is minimal. Adenomas and adenocarcinomas show high internal reflectivity on ultrasonography.

Hyperplasia of the ciliary epithelium or RPE usually develops in response to trauma, inflammation, or other ocular insults (Fig 16-14A). Because of their location, ciliary body lesions often do not become clinically evident. However, they may occasionally become sufficiently large to simulate a ciliary body melanoma. Posteriorly located lesions may be more commonly recognized and can lead to diagnostic uncertainty. Early management of these

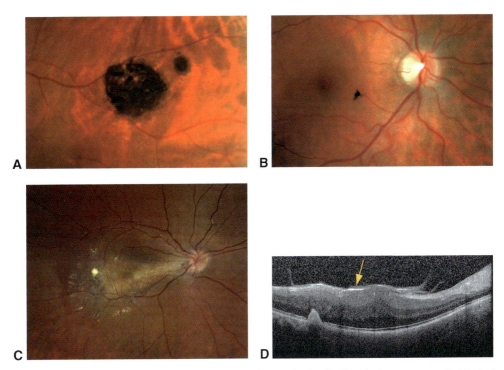

Figure 16-14 Lesions of the RPE. **A,** Reactive hyperplasia. **B,** Simple hamartoma. **C,** Clinical appearance of a combined hamartoma of the retina and RPE. Note the slight elevation, fine granular pigment, and semitranslucent membrane over the lesion surface. **D,** OCT examination of the lesion shows a thick epiretinal membrane *(arrow)* and disorganized retinal laminations. *(Parts A and B courtesy of Tero Kivelä, MD; parts C and D courtesy of H. Culver Boldt, MD.)*

atypical lesions typically comprises observation to document their stability. In rare cases, adenomatous hyperplasia may mimic a choroidal melanoma.

Simple Hamartoma

Simple hamartoma of the RPE is a small (≤1 mm), sharply demarcated, pigmented transretinal lesion that is located near the center of the macula, arising from the RPE (Fig 16-14B). This type of lesion is benign and does not change over time.

Combined Hamartoma

Combined hamartoma of the RPE and retina is a rare disorder that most frequently occurs near the optic nerve head margin, although it may also be detected in the peripheral fundus. Typically, the hamartoma appears as a pigmented, slightly elevated lesion with vitreoretinal traction and tortuous retinal vessels (Fig 16-14C, D; see also Chapter 10, Fig 10-46). Glial cells within this lesion may contract, producing clinically visible traction lines in the retina. Exudative complications associated with the vascular component of the lesion may develop. This type of lesion has been mistaken for melanoma because of its pigmentation, slight elevation, and propensity to change in young individuals. Combined hamartoma of the RPE and retina is associated with neurofibromatosis type 2 (NF2); children with these lesions should be screened for NF2, particularly when the lesions are bilateral.

> Naseripour M, Hemmati S, Aghili SS, et al. Congenital simple hamartoma of the retinal pigment epithelium: 4 cases with multimodal imaging. *Ophthalmic Genet.* Published online: May 3, 2023. doi:10.1080/13816810.2023.2206889
>
> Shields CL, Thangappan A, Hartzell K, Valente P, Pirondini C, Shields JA. Combined hamartoma of the retina and retinal pigment epithelium in 77 consecutive patients: visual outcome based on macular versus extramacular tumor location. *Ophthalmology.* 2008;115(12):2246–2252.e3.

CHAPTER 17

Vascular Tumors

Highlights

- Although vascular tumors do not have malignant potential, they can cause serious ocular morbidity that leads to permanent vision loss.
- Vascular tumors can be grouped by their primary location in the choroid or the retina.
- Prenatal (eg, congenital) retinal vascular tumors have tight junctions and do not have associated leakage or exudation.
- Vascular tumors may be associated with systemic disorders such as Sturge-Weber, Wyburn-Mason, and von Hippel–Lindau syndromes.

Introduction

Vascular tumors (also called *angiomatous tumors*) are benign lesions that can develop in the retina and/or choroid. Some of the vascular lesions are not true neoplasms but rather are hamartomatous lesions or vascular malformations. Some are associated with systemic disorders. Although these lesions do not have malignant potential, they can cause serious ocular morbidity, leading to permanent vision loss. Tumors in this category include choroidal hemangiomas and retinal vascular tumors, such as retinal cavernous hemangioma, retinal arteriovenous malformations, retinal (capillary) hemangioblastoma, and retinal vasoproliferative tumors.

Choroidal Vascular Tumors

Choroidal Hemangiomas

Hemangiomas of the choroid occur in circumscribed and diffuse forms.

Circumscribed choroidal hemangiomas A *circumscribed choroidal hemangioma* typically occurs sporadically (ie, without any systemic association) (Fig 17-1). This dome-shaped, often inconspicuous vascular hamartoma is generally located posterior to the equator, often in the macular area (see Fig 17-1A, B; see also Chapter 11, Fig 11-21). Because it blends with the adjacent normal choroid, initially it may be difficult to distinguish this tumor from the surrounding fundus. Eventually, degenerative changes occur in the overlying retinal pigment epithelium (RPE), making the tumor more visible on clinical examination and fundus

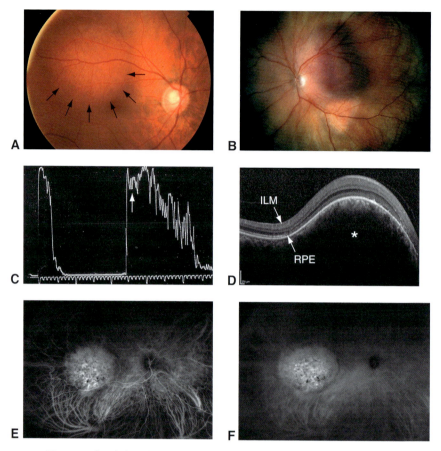

Figure 17-1 Circumscribed choroidal hemangioma. **A,** Dome-shaped tumor (inferior edge outlined by *arrows*) is similar in color to that of the surrounding fundus. **B,** Wide-angle fundus photograph better highlights the reddish color of the hemangioma. **C,** A-scan ultrasonographic image shows characteristic high internal reflectivity *(arrow).* **D,** Optical coherence tomography (OCT) reveals a dome-shaped lesion with very low signal intensity *(asterisk).* ILM = internal limiting membrane; RPE = retinal pigment epithelium. **E, F,** Indocyanine green angiography demonstrates early hypercyanescence (E), which is due to the choroidal location; during the angiogram, the cyanescence increases in intensity with a "delayed washout phenomenon" (F). *(Parts A and B courtesy of Tero Kivelä, MD; part D courtesy of Robert H. Rosa Jr, MD; parts E and F courtesy of Elaine M. Binkley, MD.)*

photography. These tumors also cause cystoid degeneration in the overlying outer retinal layers, and in some cases, they cause a secondary exudative retinal detachment that often extends into the foveal region, resulting in blurred vision and metamorphopsia.

Circumscribed choroidal hemangioma may be difficult to diagnose because it can resemble other choroidal lesions, including

- amelanotic choroidal melanoma
- choroidal osteoma
- carcinoma metastatic to the choroid
- granuloma of the choroid

Diffuse choroidal hemangiomas *Diffuse choroidal hemangioma* generally occurs in individuals with encephalofacial angiomatosis (also known as Sturge-Weber syndrome). In rare cases, it may occur in individuals with congenital ocular melanocytosis (phakomatosis pigmentovascularis). Diffuse choroidal hemangioma produces diffuse homogeneous reddish-orange coloration of the fundus, resulting in an ophthalmoscopic pattern referred to as *"tomato ketchup" fundus* (Fig 17-2). Secondary glaucoma and exudative retinal detachment often develop in eyes with this lesion. For more information on encephalofacial angiomatosis, see BCSC Section 6, *Pediatric Ophthalmology and Strabismus*.

Diagnosis Ancillary diagnostic studies are helpful in evaluating both types of choroidal hemangiomas. A-scan ultrasonography (echography) shows a high-amplitude initial echo and high-amplitude broad internal echoes (high internal reflectivity; see Fig 17-1C). B-scan ultrasonography reveals localized or diffuse choroidal thickening with prominent internal reflections but without choroidal excavation or acoustic shadowing. Optical coherence tomography (OCT) of circumscribed lesions typically demonstrates minimal internal signal (see Fig 17-1D), a smooth surface, and tapered borders. In the early choroidal filling phase, fluorescein angiography (FA) reveals hyperfluorescence of large choroidal vessels; the fluorescence increases throughout the angiogram, with late staining of the tumor and late leakage or pooling in the cystoid spaces of the overlying retina. Indocyanine green (ICG) angiography, the preferred modality for imaging choroidal vascular lesions, demonstrates early hypercyanescence because of the intrinsic vascularity of these lesions (see Fig 17-1E, F). This hypercyanescence peaks at approximately 3–4 minutes, and there is a classic "washout" of the dye in later frames, leaving a persistently hypercyanescent rim. If this pattern is not seen, infiltrative lesions should be considered in the differential diagnosis.

Treatment Asymptomatic choroidal hemangiomas require no treatment. The most common indication for treatment is exudative retinal detachment with subretinal fluid tracking toward the fovea and subsequent cystoid macular edema (CME).

The current treatment of choice for symptomatic circumscribed choroidal hemangioma is photodynamic therapy (PDT; see Therapeutic considerations sidebar). Most choroidal

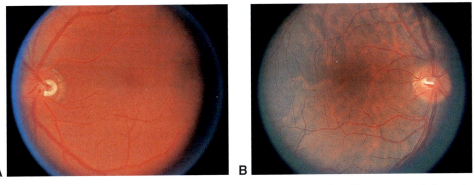

Figure 17-2 Diffuse choroidal hemangioma, clinical photographs. The saturated "tomato ketchup" red-orange color of the affected left fundus **(A)** contrasts markedly with the color of the unaffected right fundus **(B)** of the same patient.

hemangiomas respond to PDT, with resolution of the subretinal fluid and partial regression of the lesion, often with associated improvement in vision. However, CME may persist, particularly if it is chronic, and any degenerative changes in the overlying RPE may limit visual recovery; PDT may need to be repeated. Transpupillary thermotherapy (TTT) has also been used to effectively treat circumscribed choroidal hemangiomas and is the primary treatment modality in countries where PDT is not available. See BCSC Section 12, *Retina and Vitreous*, for further discussion of choroidal hemangioma.

Therapeutic considerations Photodynamic therapy (PDT) involves intravenous (IV) infusion of a photosensitive dye, verteporfin, which is activated with application of an infrared diode laser at 689-nm wavelength through the pupil, focused on the fundus. Once activated, the dye causes the release of free radicals, leading to vasoconstriction and thrombosis, which in turn induce regression of aberrant blood vessels. PDT was initially used to treat age-related macular degeneration (AMD) in the 1999 Treatment of Age-Related Macular Degeneration With Photodynamic Therapy (TAP) trial and the 2001 Verteporfin in Photodynamic Therapy (VIP) trial.

Standard-fluence ("full-fluence") PDT refers to an energy of 50 J/cm^2 and light intensity of 600 mW/cm^2 over 83 seconds. For treatment of circumscribed choroidal hemangioma, PDT may be performed either using the same standard laser parameters as those used for neovascular (exudative) AMD or for double the duration (166 seconds). Verteporfin is slowly administered via IV infusion, followed by direct application of the laser to the tumor. Unlike procedures using a diode laser, PDT is not painful.

After the procedure, patients should wear dark glasses and protective clothing and avoid direct sunlight, because the verteporfin results in temporary photosensitivity of the skin and eyes.

Low-dose radiation (via brachytherapy or external radiotherapy methods such as charged-particle, stereotactic, or external beam) has also been successfully used to treat choroidal hemangiomas, including those unresponsive to PDT. All of these radiation methods can be used to treat patients with circumscribed choroidal hemangioma; for diffuse choroidal hemangioma, because of the extensive involvement of the choroid, external beam radiotherapy techniques are often used, but plaque brachytherapy may be used in some cases. Complications associated with radiation include dry eye, cataract, and radiation retinopathy. These complications, in addition to the exudative retinal detachment caused by the hemangioma, may limit recovery of vision. In addition, fibrotic changes can occur over the lesion, affecting vision.

To date, little published evidence has supported the use of vascular endothelial growth factor (VEGF) inhibitors to treat choroidal hemangioma. Oral β-blockers have also been tried with variable efficacy.

Arevalo JF, Arias JD, Serrano MA. Oral propranolol for exudative retinal detachment in diffuse choroidal hemangioma. *Arch Ophthalmol*. 2011;129(10):1373–1375.

Boixadera A, García-Arumí J, Martínez-Castillo V, et al. Prospective clinical trial evaluating the efficacy of photodynamic therapy for symptomatic circumscribed choroidal hemangioma. *Ophthalmology*. 2009;116(1):100–105.

Gunduz AK, Mirazayev I, Tetik D, Ates FS. Circumscribed choroidal hemangioma: comparative efficacy of transpupillary thermotherapy, indocyanine green–enhanced transpupillary thermotherapy, and photodynamic therapy and analysis of baseline clinical features effecting treatment outcomes. *Photodiagnosis Photodyn Ther*. 2021;36:102529.

Retinal Vascular Tumors

Retinal vascular tumors include 4 distinct clinical entities in 2 subcategories (Table 17-1):

- *prenatal origin*; tumors maintain tight vascular junctions (ie, they do not leak) and do not present with subretinal fluid or exudation:
  - retinal cavernous hemangioma
  - retinal arteriovenous malformations
- *postnatal origin*; associated with exudative retinal detachments and visual impairment:
  - retinal (capillary) hemangioblastoma (RH)
  - retinal vasoproliferative tumors (also called nodular retinal gliosis)

Prenatal Retinal Vascular Tumors: Nonleaking Lesions

Retinal cavernous hemangioma

Cavernous hemangioma of the retina is an uncommon lesion that resembles a cluster of grapes (Fig 17-3). These lesions may also occur on the optic nerve head (ONH). In rare cases, retinal cavernous hemangioma may be associated with similar cavernomatous lesions of the skin and central nervous system (CNS) that are caused by a pathogenic variant in the gene *KRIT1* (also referred to as *CCM1*). Patients with intracranial lesions may experience associated seizures. Given that these lesions are prenatal in origin, cavernous hemangiomas are not typically associated with exudation; thus, treatment is rarely required. However, small hemorrhages as well as gliotic and fibrotic areas may appear on the surface of the lesion. FA may reveal plasma–erythrocyte separation within the vascular spaces of the lesion manifesting as fluorescent caps over dark, sedimented erythrocytes without leakage; this separation is virtually diagnostic of cavernous hemangioma. In contrast to hemangioblastomas, retinal cavernous hemangiomas fill very slowly. The fluorescein remains in the vascular spaces for an extended period without leakage (see BCSC Section 12, *Retina and Vitreous*).

Choquet H, Pawlikowska L, Lawton MT, Kim H. Genetics of cerebral cavernous malformations: current status and future prospects. *J Neurosurg Sci*. 2015;59(3):211–220.

Gass JD. Cavernous hemangioma of the retina. A neuro-oculo-cutaneous syndrome. *Am J Ophthalmol*. 1971;71(4):799–814.

Retinal arteriovenous malformations

Congenital retinal arteriovenous malformation (AVM; also known as *racemose hemangioma*) is an anomalous artery-to-vein anastomosis that can occur in the iris, near the

Table 17-1 Characteristics of Retinal Vascular Tumors

Tumor	Associations	Appearance	Leakage	Treatment
Retinal cavernous hemangioma	Intracranial vascular malformations caused by pathogenic variants in *CCM1*/*KRIT1*	"Cluster of grapes" with plasma-erythrocyte separation on FA	No	Required only in rare cases
Retinal AVM (racemose hemangioma)	Midbrain AVMs (Wyburn-Mason syndrome)	Tangle of large, tortuous vessels	No	Required only in rare cases
Retinal hemangioblastoma	VHL syndrome or sporadic	Red-orange lesion with large-caliber, tortuous afferent and efferent vessels	Yes	Anti-VEGF injections as adjunct, belzutifan, cryotherapy, brachytherapy, PDT, photocoagulation, proton beam radiotherapy, vitreoretinal surgery
Retinal vasoproliferative tumor (nodular retinal gliosis)	Idiopathic or associated with ocular disease (uveitis, inherited retinal disease, trauma)	Elevated pink-yellow mass in the peripheral retina	Yes	Anti-VEGF or steroid injections, brachytherapy, cryotherapy, laser photocoagulation, PDT, vitrectomy

AVM = arteriovenous malformation; FA = fluorescein angiography; PDT = photodynamic therapy; VEGF = vascular endothelial growth factor; VHL = von Hippel–Lindau.

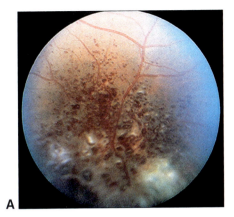 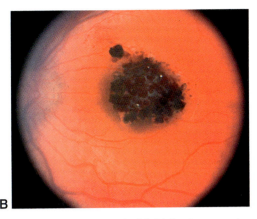

Figure 17-3 Retinal cavernous hemangioma, clinical photographs. **A,** Multiple tiny vascular saccules and associated white fibrotic tissue are visible in the retina. **B,** A smaller lesion consisting of a grapelike cluster of clumped vascular saccules is visible in the macula. *(Part B courtesy of Timothy G. Murray, MD.)*

ONH, or in the retinal periphery. Clinically, these malformations can range from a small, localized vascular communication to a prominent tangle of large, tortuous blood vessels throughout most of the fundus (Fig 17-4A, B). The term *racemose* refers to the clustered or bunched nature of the vessels. When associated with an AVM of the midbrain region, this condition is generally referred to as *Wyburn-Mason syndrome* (also known as *Bonnet-Dechaume-Blanc syndrome;* see BCSC Section 5, *Neuro-Ophthalmology,* and Section 6, *Pediatric Ophthalmology and Strabismus*). AVMs may also appear in the eyelid, orbit, and mandible.

An AVM of the retina is different from a congenital retinal macrovessel, which is a large aberrant retinal vessel that crosses the midline and, often, the macular area (Fig 17-4C, D). Retinal macrovessels occasionally show arteriovenous communications.

> Archer DB, Deutman A, Ernest JT, Krill AE. Arteriovenous communications of the retina. *Am J Ophthalmol.* 1973;75(2):224–241.
>
> Heimann H, Damato B. Congenital vascular malformations of the retina and choroid. *Eye (Lond).* 2010;24(3):459–467.

Postnatal Retinal Vascular Tumors: Leaking Lesions

Retinal hemangioblastoma

Retinal hemangioblastoma (RH; formerly known as *retinal capillary hemangioblastoma*) is a rare condition with a reported incidence of 1 in 40,000. It can be sporadic, occurring only in the retina, or it can be associated with a cerebellar and/or spinal hemangioblastoma, occurring as part of *von Hippel–Lindau (VHL) syndrome* (Fig 17-5). A variety of names are used for RH in the literature, including *angiomatosis retinae* and *retinal capillary hemangioma;* sporadic lesions have also been called *von Hippel lesions,* a term meant to differentiate the nonsyndromic retinal lesions from those seen in the systemic disorder (VHL syndrome). The term *retinal hemangioblastoma* most accurately reflects the pathogenesis of these lesions (see Chapter 10).

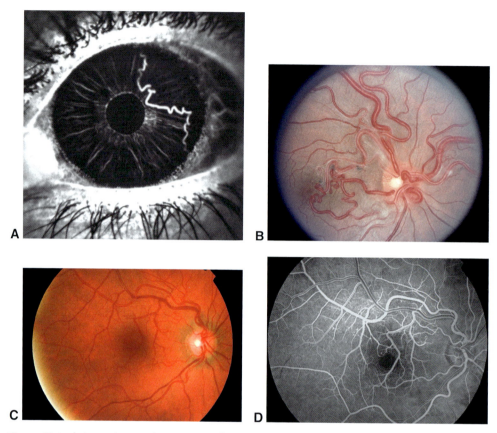

Figure 17-4 Intraocular arteriovenous malformations (AVMs) and retinal macrovessels, clinical photographs. Fluorescein angiography (FA) of arteriovenous malformation, or racemose hemangioma, in the iris **(A)** and color photograph of arteriovenous malformation of the retina **(B)** in 2 patients. **C,** Although it can occasionally have an arteriovenous communication, a retinal macrovessel is distinct from an AVM (racemose hemangioma). **D,** FA highlights the macrovessel, which crosses the macular area and the horizontal midline. Absence of leakage is characteristic of retinal AVMs. *(Part A courtesy of Cullen Barnett, MD, and Daniel Barajas, MD, USC Roski Eye Institute; part B courtesy of Robert H. Rosa Jr, MD; parts C and D courtesy of Tero Kivelä, MD.)*

Although RH may be present at birth in rare cases, these lesions typically are acquired and are usually diagnosed in the patient's second to third decades of life. RH may occur as a single lesion or as multiple lesions. The lesions appear as red-to-orange tumors that arise within the retina and have large-caliber, tortuous afferent and efferent retinal blood vessels (see Fig 17-5A, B, E, F; also see Chapter 10, Fig 10-5). Because the lesions occur postnatally, leakage and exudation are common. Associated yellow-white retinal and subretinal lipid exudates, often involving the fovea, and exudative retinal detachments may occur. Variations include tumors arising from the ONH (see Fig 17-5C) and in the retinal periphery, where vitreous traction may elevate the tumor from the surface of the retina (see Fig 17-5B). FA demonstrates rapid arteriovenous transit with immediate filling of the feeding arteriole, subsequent filling of the numerous fine blood vessels that constitute much of the tumor, and drainage by the dilated venule. Massive leakage of dye into the tumor and vitreous can occur.

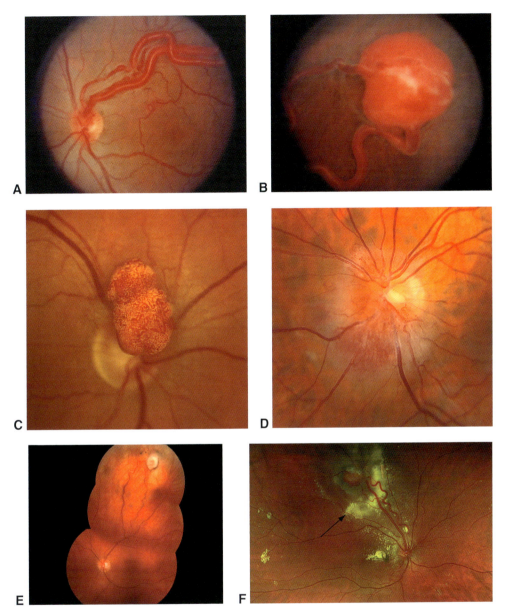

Figure 17-5 Retinal hemangioblastoma (RH), clinical photographs. Dilated, tortuous retinal feeder artery and draining vein emanate from the optic nerve head (ONH) **(A)**, leading to the red-to-orange peripheral retinal tumor **(B)**. **C**, Endophytic ONH RH extends into the vitreous cavity. **D**, Exophytic optic disc RH has a sessile appearance. **E**, Fundus photograph of a patient with a peripheral RH. **F**, Fundus photograph of a patient with an RH reveals extensive exudative response with lipid exudates *(arrow)*. *(Parts A and B courtesy of Robert H. Rosa Jr, MD; parts C, D, and F courtesy of Elaine M. Binkley, MD; part E courtesy of Mary Beth Aronow, MD.)*

Patients with RHs may wish to undergo genetic screening to determine whether they are at risk for developing systemic manifestations. RHs are often the first manifestation of VHL syndrome, and more than 60% of patients will have RHs. Pathogenic variants in *VHL*, which is located on chromosome 3, cause overproduction of VEGF and other hypoxia-inducible factors, leading to the development of highly vascular tumors. Several other types of tumors and cysts may develop in patients with this syndrome, the most serious of which are CNS hemangioblastomas, renal cell carcinoma, and pheochromocytoma. For more information on VHL syndrome, see BCSC Section 6, *Pediatric Ophthalmology and Strabismus*, and Section 12, *Retina and Vitreous*. Chapter 10 in this volume discusses the histologic features of RH.

In addition to appropriate genetic consultation, ongoing screening is critical for early identification of the ocular and systemic manifestations of the disease in patients with suspected VHL. By identifying the retinal lesions, the ophthalmologist is often the first medical specialist to diagnose VHL syndrome. Screening for systemic vascular anomalies (eg, CNS hemangioblastomas) and malignancies may reduce mortality, and aggressive screening for and early treatment of RHs may reduce complications and improve long-term visual outcomes.

Modalities for the treatment of RH include the following:

- *for small lesions:* photocoagulation
- *for larger lesions located in the peripheral retina:* cryotherapy or laser
- *for large lesions with more extensive retinal detachment:*
  - plaque brachytherapy
  - proton beam radiotherapy
  - pars plana vitrectomy with diathermy or endoresection of tumors, sometimes combined with scleral buckle
- *for selected cases (eg, some juxtapapillary tumors):* PDT

The use of VEGF inhibitors as monotherapy in the treatment of RH has been ineffective. However, these agents may have efficacy in reducing macular edema and exudation following PDT or brachytherapy. Although most ONH lesions are resistant to treatment, some have responded to treatment with PDT or and external beam radiation.

For patients with ONH or large retinal lesions, the visual prognosis remains guarded. Because additional tumors may develop over time in patients with VHL syndrome, careful serial examination of both eyes is important in order to identify and treat new tumors when they are small. Wide-field FA can be helpful in revealing small retinal hemangioblastomas in these patients. In 2021, the US Food and Drug Administration (FDA) approved belzutifan, a hypoxia-inducible factor (HIF)–2α inhibitor, for the treatment of renal cell carcinoma and CNS hemangioblastoma in patients with VHL; this medication may also have efficacy in controlling RH.

Jonasch E, Donskov F, Iliopoulos O, et al; MK-6482-004 Investigators. Belzutifan for renal cell carcinoma in von Hippel–Lindau disease. *N Engl J Med.* 2021;385(22):2036–2046.

Singh AD, Shields CL, Shields JA. von Hippel–Lindau disease. *Surv Ophthalmol.* 2001;46(2): 117–142.

Retinal vasoproliferative tumors

Retinal vasoproliferative tumors (VPTs; also called nodular retinal gliosis) are uncommon acquired retinal lesions. These lesions were initially called *presumed acquired retinal*

CHAPTER 17: Vascular Tumors • 351

hemangiomas to differentiate them from RH and have also been called by other names such as reactive retinal gliogliosis, reflecting the glial component of these tumors. VPTs may be idiopathic (74% of cases) or may develop in association with preexisting ocular disease (26% of cases), including inflammatory, traumatic, and degenerative ocular conditions (eg, retinitis pigmentosa). Primary VPTs manifest in the third or fourth decade of life, and both sexes are equally affected. Most patients present with a single solitary lesion; however, in secondary cases, multiple tumors may develop.

Clinically, VPTs appear as elevated pink and yellow vascular masses in the peripheral retina with associated subretinal exudation, which may be extensive. These lesions lack the prominent dilated feeder vessels typically seen in RHs (Fig 17-6). Macular fibrosis,

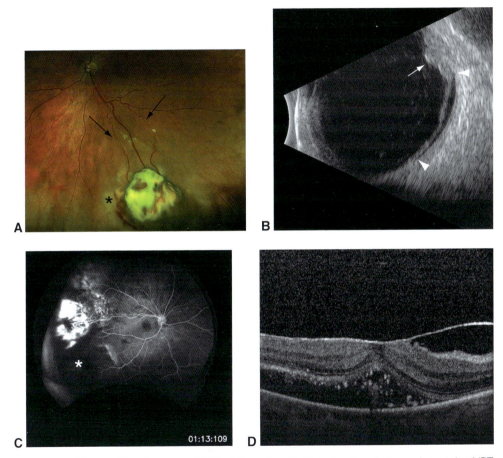

Figure 17-6 Vasoproliferative tumor (VPT) of the retina. **A,** Color fundus photograph reveals a VPT in the inferior periphery. Note the thin afferent and efferent vessels *(arrows)*, which contrast with the markedly dilated vessels seen in eyes with RH. The tumor appears as a yellow elevated mass with tortuous internal vasculature and associated exudation *(asterisk)*. **B,** B-scan ultrasonography demonstrates a heterogeneous, amorphous elevated mass *(arrow)*. There is an associated retinal detachment *(between arrowheads)*, which is not uncommon. **C,** FA highlights the internal vascular component, which demonstrates significant hyperfluorescent staining; late leakage is common. Loss of retinal vasculature is visible in the area of previous cryotherapy treatment *(asterisk)*. **D,** OCT reveals subretinal fluid tracking under the fovea, an epiretinal membrane, and significant foveal distortion. *(Part A courtesy of Elaine M. Binkley, MD; parts B–D courtesy of Jesse L. Berry, MD.)*

epiretinal membranes, CME, and subretinal fluid, which occur in association with VPTs, may lead to vision loss. Histologically, VPTs are composed of a mixture of glial cells and a network of fine capillaries with some larger dilated blood vessels.

Treatment of VPTs is notoriously difficult. Small peripheral VPTs that lack significant exudation or maculopathy may be managed with periodic observation. First-line treatment of symptomatic tumors generally involves triple freeze–thaw transconjunctival cryotherapy; repeated treatments are often required. Other treatment options include plaque brachytherapy, laser photocoagulation, and PDT. Anti-VEGF agents and intraocular steroids have also been used. Some cases may require vitrectomy with membrane peel.

> Shields CL, Shields JA, Barrett J, De Potter P. Vasoproliferative tumors of the ocular fundus. Classification and clinical manifestations in 103 patients. *Arch Ophthalmol.* 1995;113(5):615–623.

CHAPTER 18

Retinoblastoma

 This chapter includes related videos. Go to aao.org/bcscvideo_section04 or scan the QR codes in the text to access this content.

Highlights

- Retinoblastoma is a rare tumor, with an estimated incidence of 250–300 cases annually in the United States. Despite its infrequent occurrence overall, retinoblastoma is the most common primary intraocular cancer in children.
- In the United States, children with retinoblastoma most often present with leukocoria and/or strabismus.
- Retinoblastoma is typically caused by a pathogenic variation in *RB1,* a tumor suppressor gene. The *RB1* pathogenic variant may be inherited from a parent who carries it or can result from a new pathogenic germline (eg, heritable) or somatic variant. The type of variant—whether heritable or somatic—determines the patient's risk for secondary tumors and whether the patient's family should receive genetic counseling.
- Unlike with most tumors, including other intraocular tumors, biopsy is contraindicated in retinoblastoma, and diagnosis and classification are based solely on clinical features.
- In advanced unilateral cases, enucleation is traditionally performed. However, recent therapeutic improvements have led to more children undergoing eye-sparing treatment with intravenous or intra-arterial chemotherapy.

Introduction

Retinoblastoma is the most common primary intraocular malignant tumor of childhood and the second most common primary intraocular malignant tumor in all age groups (after uveal melanoma). Worldwide, the frequency of retinoblastoma ranges from 1 in 14,000 to 1 in 20,000 live births, with an estimated 7500–8000 new cases occurring each year. Both sexes and all races are affected equally, and the tumor occurs bilaterally in 30%–40% of patients. Approximately 90% of retinoblastoma cases are diagnosed in patients younger than 3 years. The age range or mean age at diagnosis depends on family history and disease laterality:

- patients with known family history of retinoblastoma: age range, 4–8 months
- patients with bilateral disease: mean age, 12 months
- patients with unilateral disease: mean age, 24 months

The retinoblastoma disease rate varies among countries by approximately 50-fold, mainly because of variances in birth rates. Disease registries indicate that the highest incidences of retinoblastoma occur in India, China, and some countries in Africa. In the Global Retinoblastoma Study, which included 4351 retinoblastoma cases from 153 countries, 85% of cases were from low- and middle-income countries.

> Abramson DH, Beaverson K, Sangani P, et al. Screening for retinoblastoma: presenting signs as prognosticators of patient and ocular survival. *Pediatrics.* 2003;112(6 Pt. 1):1248–1255.
>
> Global Retinoblastoma Study Group. Global retinoblastoma presentation and analysis by national income level. *JAMA Oncol.* 2020;6(5):685–695. Published correction appears in *JAMA Oncol.* 2020;6(11):1815.
>
> Orjuela M. Epidemiology. In: Rodriguez-Galindo C, Wilson MW, eds. *Retinoblastoma. Pediatric Oncology Series.* Springer; 2010:11–23.
>
> Wong JR, Tucker MA, Kleinerman RA, Devesa SS. Retinoblastoma incidence patterns in the US Surveillance, Epidemiology, and End Results program. *JAMA Ophthalmol.* 2014;132(4):478–483.

Diagnostic Evaluation

The diagnosis of retinoblastoma is made clinically. Obtaining a tumor specimen by fine-needle aspiration is contraindicated because of the risk of extraocular spread of the cancer. In rare diagnostic dilemmas in which there is visual potential, an expert ocular oncologist may perform a biopsy procedure through the clear cornea followed by cryotherapy. When visual potential is poor and retinoblastoma is part of the differential diagnosis, the safest option for the child is enucleation.

Clinical Examination

The presenting signs and symptoms of retinoblastoma correspond to the extent and location of the tumor. In the United States, the most common presenting signs in children are leukocoria (white pupillary reflex) and strabismus (Fig 18-1, Table 18-1). Other presenting features, such as iris heterochromia, spontaneous hyphema, and orbital inflammation, are

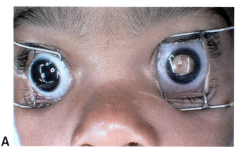
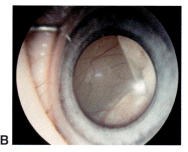

Figure 18-1 Retinoblastoma. **A,** Clinical photograph shows leukocoria associated with an advanced intraocular tumor. **B,** Higher-magnification view through the pupil. Note the large retrolental tumor and secondary total exudative retinal detachment. *(Courtesy of Timothy G. Murray, MD.)*

Table 18-1 **Presenting Signs and Symptoms of Retinoblastoma**

Leukocoria (most common)
Strabismus (~20%)
Ocular and/or orbital inflammation (~5%)
Pseudohypopyon
Hyphema
Iris heterochromia
Phthisis bulbi
Proptosis
Cataract
Glaucoma
Nystagmus
Tearing
Anisocoria

less common and are associated with more advanced tumors. A small tumor may be identified on routine examination, but this is rare and is generally limited to patients who receive screening evaluations because of a family history of the disease. Known vision problems at presentation are uncommon because most patients are very young children who cannot yet express the vision loss.

In all patients with suspected retinoblastoma, an examination under anesthesia (EUA) is indicated to completely assess the extent of ocular disease prior to treatment. During the EUA, intraocular pressures (IOPs) and corneal diameters of the eyes should be determined, and the iris should be evaluated carefully for neovascularization with a portable slit lamp. In addition, the locations of retinal tumors, the occurrence of subretinal fluid or exudative detachment, and the presence of either vitreous or subretinal tumor seeds should be ascertained for both eyes and clearly documented. Fundus photography and ultrasonography (echography) should also be performed to document findings and allow serial comparisons. Findings from the EUA are also used to classify each eye, as discussed in the Retinoblastoma Classification section. The group classification is useful in determining therapeutic options, visual prognosis, and potential for ocular salvage.

Retinoblastoma begins as a round, translucent, gray-to-white tumor in the retina (Figs 18-2, 18-3, 18-4). As the tumor enlarges, necrotic foci with calcification emerge, giving the tumor its characteristic chalky white appearance. Larger tumors also contain dilated, tortuous intratumoral vessels. In addition, retinoblastomas may exhibit exophytic and/or endophytic growth patterns. Exophytic tumors grow beneath the retina and often involve serous retinal detachment. As these tumors grow, the retinal detachment may become extensive, obscuring clear visualization of the tumor (Fig 18-5). In contrast, endophytic tumors grow on the retinal surface and into the vitreous cavity; therefore, blood vessels may be more difficult to discern in these tumors. Exophytic tumors cause subretinal seeding, whereas endophytic retinoblastomas are more likely to yield *vitreous seeds* (Fig 18-6; see also Fig 18-4); these cells, which are shed from the tumor, remain viable in the vitreous and may eventually implant in ocular tissue, resulting in new tumor foci within the eye. Vitreous seeds also may enter the anterior chamber; there, they may aggregate on the iris as nodules or settle inferiorly as a pseudohypopyon formed of tumor cells rather than inflammatory cells (Fig 18-7).

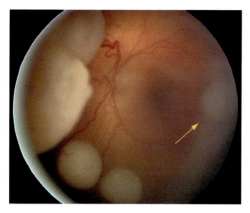

Figure 18-2 Retinoblastoma. Multiple tumor foci in an eye of a patient with International Intraocular Retinoblastoma Classification (IIRC) group D retinoblastoma (see Table 18-3). Note the diffuse vitreous seeds in the temporal periphery *(arrow)*. These clinical findings of multiple tumors denote a pathogenic germline *RB1* variant. *(Courtesy of Matthew W. Wilson, MD.)*

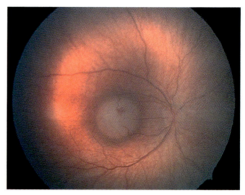

Figure 18-3 Retinoblastoma. Clinical photograph shows an IIRC group B tumor (tumor >3 mm). The discrete white macular tumor is supplied by dilated retinal blood vessels. *(Courtesy of Timothy G. Murray, MD.)*

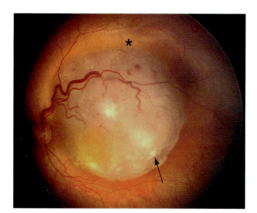

Figure 18-4 Endophytic retinoblastoma. Note the growth into the vitreous cavity, dilated retinal blood vessels, foci of calcification *(arrow)*, and cuff of subretinal fluid *(asterisk)*. Early seeding is visible, suggestive of IIRC group C retinoblastoma. *(Courtesy of Matthew W. Wilson, MD.)*

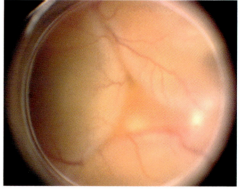

Figure 18-5 Exophytic retinoblastoma. Total exudative detachment due to tumor growth under the retina obscures visualization of the tumor. Note the normal-appearing retinal vessels, as opposed to those found in eyes with Coats disease. This is an IIRC group D tumor; however, anterior segment involvement and neovascular glaucoma need to be excluded to rule out a group E eye. *(Courtesy of Matthew W. Wilson, MD.)*

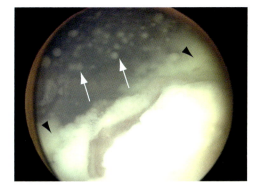

Figure 18-6 Retinoblastoma. Large endophytic tumor with extensive vitreous seeding (*arrows* indicate sphere-type seeding and *arrowheads* indicate cloud-type seeding). This presentation can be seen in either IIRC group D or IIRC group E retinoblastoma. *(Courtesy of Matthew W. Wilson, MD.)*

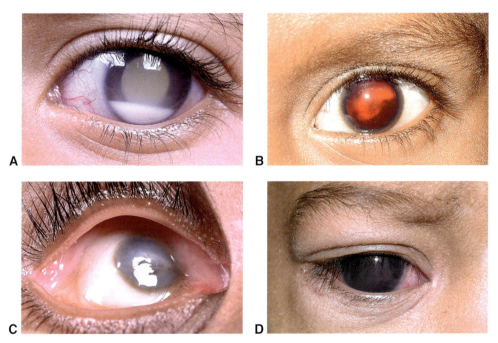

Figure 18-7 Clinical photographs show eyes with IIRC group E retinoblastoma. **A,** Pseudohypopyon resulting from migration of tumor cells into the anterior chamber. Note the clumped appearance of the cells, which is somewhat different from the appearance of inflammatory cells in a true hypopyon. **B,** Opaque media due to vitreous hemorrhage and neovascular glaucoma. **C,** Phthisis bulbi after an episode of aseptic orbital cellulitis. **D,** Aseptic orbital cellulitis with eyelid edema and conjunctival congestion. *(Courtesy of Swathi Kaliki, MD.)*

In approximately 50% of eyes with advanced disease, secondary glaucoma and rubeosis iridis occur. Most advanced tumors have mixed endophytic and exophytic growth.

Diffuse infiltrating retinoblastoma is a rare variant of retinoblastoma that is detected later in childhood (>5 years of age) and typically presents unilaterally. Diffuse infiltrating retinoblastoma presents a diagnostic challenge because dense vitreous cells impede visualization of the retina, and there is no isolated retinal mass. This variant is often mistaken for an intermediate or posterior uveitis of unknown etiology. A sign that supports a diagnosis of retinoblastoma is when the seeds are in clumps of various sizes, and some seeds may be spherical, which is atypical of vitritis.

Ancillary Imaging

In the initial EUA, patients with retinoblastoma may undergo imaging with fundus photography, fluorescein angiography (FA), handheld optical coherence tomography (OCT), and B-scan ultrasonography. Color fundus photographs help the clinician document the appearance and location of retinal tumors and the sites of vitreous and subretinal seeding; serial images over time are also helpful for determining treatment efficacy and disease recurrence. On FA, common findings of retinoblastoma include retinal vascular dilatation, capillary telangiectasia, intrinsic tumor vessel formation, and retinal venous leakage; subclinical iris neovascularization may also be seen.

In eyes with small tumors or a visible macula, OCT with a handheld device can be helpful in assessing macular anatomy and identifying and monitoring intraretinal tumors not otherwise visible clinically. Small tumors are smooth, round, homogeneous, and isodense on OCT. In addition, small tumors may involve the inner nuclear layer and the outer nuclear layer, whereas very small tumors have been described as limited to the outer nuclear layer, with draping of the overlying inner retinal layers beginning with the outer plexiform layer (Fig 18-8). So-called invisible tumors that are in very early stages may be detected on OCT before ophthalmoscopic visualization is possible. OCT also can be used to evaluate the extent and morphology of vitreous seeds (Fig 18-9). Use of ultrasonography may be critical for diagnosing retinoblastoma (its findings are a dome-shaped retinal lesion with scattered intratumoral calcifications), particularly when ophthalmoscopic visualization of the tumor is limited (Fig 18-10).

Imaging studies of the optic nerve, orbits, and brain are also essential for complete staging of retinoblastoma in children. For example, retinoblastoma may invade the optic nerve head (ONH) and spread through the lamina cribrosa into the central nervous system (CNS). In rare germline cases, retinoblastoma can be associated with a separate CNS tumor called a *pinealoblastoma* (a condition referred to as *trilateral retinoblastoma;* Fig 18-11). Magnetic resonance imaging (MRI) is the preferred diagnostic modality for evaluating these tumors. Soft-tissue resolution is better with MRI than with computed tomography (CT), and MRI does not expose the patient to potentially harmful radiation, which is especially important in children with a genetic cancer syndrome (see the Genetic Counseling section). Systemic metastatic evaluation with bone marrow biopsy and lumbar puncture is not indicated in children unless they have neurologic abnormalities or evidence of extraocular extension. When extension of the retinoblastoma into the retrobulbar optic nerve is suspected, lumbar puncture and bone marrow biopsy may be part of the workup, but they should not delay definitive enucleation or neoadjuvant chemotherapy.

In the United States, patients with retinoblastoma rarely present with metastases or intracranial extension at the time of diagnosis; in contrast, in resource-limited countries, advanced presentations are common. In children with retinoblastoma, the most frequent sites of metastatic involvement are the orbit, brain, distal bones, lymph nodes, skull bones, spinal cord, and abdominal viscera. Retinoblastoma cells may escape the eye by invading the optic nerve and extending into the cerebrospinal fluid. In addition, tumor cells may massively

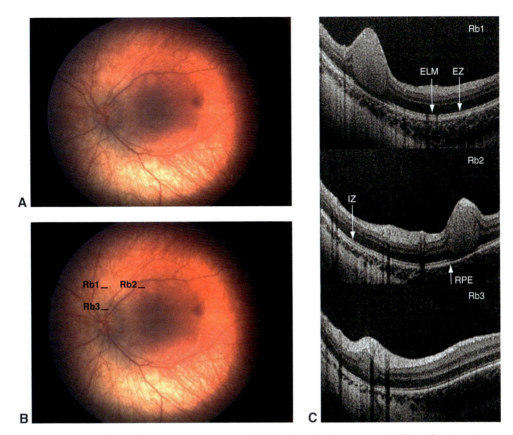

Figure 18-8 Optical coherence tomography (OCT) of retinoblastoma. **A,** Color fundus photograph of a left eye with 3 retinoblastoma tumors. Although these are small tumors, given their proximity to the optic nerve head (ONH), this is IIRC group B retinoblastoma. **B,** Color fundus photograph of the same eye with the 3 retinoblastomas labeled Rb1–3. The tumors are marked by lines through the body of the growths correlating with the OCT slice. The smallest one, barely visible on ophthalmoscopy, lies just superior to the optic nerve. **C,** Spectral-domain OCT of the 3 tumors shows homogeneous dome-shaped masses with overlying inner retinal draping. Tumor 3 is located in the outer retina, involving the outer nuclear layer and possibly the outer plexiform layer. The inner nuclear layer and inner plexiform layer drape over the tumor. There is also an outer retinal abnormality in all tumors affecting the external limiting membrane (ELM), ellipsoid zone (EZ), and interdigitation zone (IZ). There is shadowing on OCT from the retinal vessels overlying the tumor, which are also seen clinically. RPE = retinal pigment epithelium. *(Reproduced with permission from Berry JL, Cobrinik D, Kim JW. Detection and intraretinal localization of an 'invisible' retinoblastoma using optical coherence tomography.* Ocul Oncol Pathol. *2016;2[3]:149.)*

invade the choroid before traversing emissary canals, thereby spreading hematogenously or eroding through the sclera to enter the orbit. As the tumor grows in the orbit, extraocular extension may result in proptosis (Fig 18-12). In the anterior chamber, tumor cells may invade the trabecular meshwork, gaining access to the conjunctival lymphatics. Subsequently, palpable preauricular and cervical lymph nodes may develop.

> Kim JW, Ngai LK, Sadda S, Murakami Y, Lee DK, Murphree AL. Retcam fluorescein angiography findings in eyes with advanced retinoblastoma. *Br J Ophthalmol.* 2014;98(12):1666–1671.

360 • Ophthalmic Pathology and Intraocular Tumors

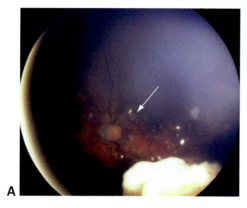
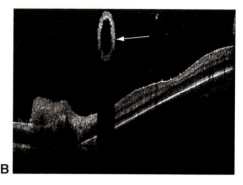

Figure 18-9 Vitreous seeds. **A,** Clinical photograph shows a large, spherical vitreous seed *(arrow)* in a retinoblastoma. **B,** OCT findings in a child with advanced (IIRC group D) retinoblastoma demonstrate an intact fovea, a dusting of small hyperreflective seeds on the retinal surface, and a hollow reflective cystic structure floating above the retina consistent with a spherical vitreous seed *(arrow)*. *(Reproduced from Berry JL, Anulao K, Kim JW. Optical coherence imaging of large spherical seed in retinoblastoma. Ophthalmology. 2017;124[8]:1208. With permission from Elsevier.)*

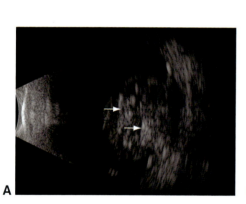
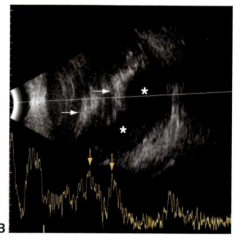

Figure 18-10 Ultrasonography of retinoblastoma. **A,** B-scan ultrasonographic findings demonstrate a dome-shaped retinal lesion with characteristic scattered calcifications within the tumor *(arrows)*. **B,** B-scan ultrasonographic findings demonstrate an irregular intraocular mass with characteristic calcifications within the tumor *(white arrows)* causing back shadowing *(asterisks)* with corresponding high internal echoes on A-scan ultrasonography *(yellow arrows)*. *(Part A courtesy of Jesse L. Berry, MD, and Jonathan W. Kim, MD; part B courtesy of Swathi Kaliki, MD.)*

Differential Diagnosis

In children, leukocoria can result from many types of lesions, some of which masquerade as retinoblastoma (Table 18-2). The most common conditions that simulate retinoblastoma are persistent fetal vasculature, Coats disease, and ocular toxocariasis. Most of these conditions can be differentiated from retinoblastoma on the basis of a comprehensive history, clinical examination, and ancillary testing.

CHAPTER 18: Retinoblastoma • 361

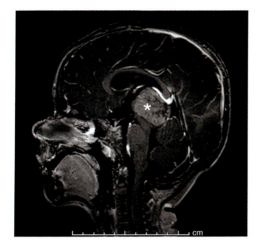

Figure 18-11 Contrast-enhanced sagittal T1-weighted magnetic resonance image (MRI) of the brain in a child with germline bilateral retinoblastoma demonstrates a large midline cerebral lesion *(asterisk)* involving the pineal region; this is consistent with a pinealoblastoma (primitive neuroectodermal tumor [PNET]). The presence of the bilateral retinoblastomas and the pineal tumor is diagnostic of a condition referred to as *trilateral retinoblastoma*. *(Courtesy of Jonathan W. Kim, MD.)*

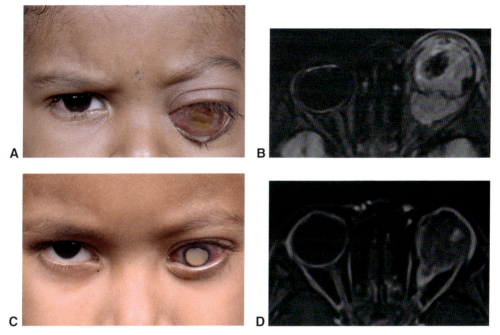

Figure 18-12 Advanced extraocular extension of retinoblastoma. **A,** Clinical photograph of a child with proptosis of the left eye and extraocular tumor extension. **B,** MRI of the orbits confirms extraocular extension of the tumor. **C,** Clinical photograph of a child with proptosis of the left eye with leukocoria and conjunctival congestion. **D,** MRI of the orbits confirms optic nerve tumor extension. This case also highlights the importance of orbital imaging to evaluate for orbital extension of the disease. *(Courtesy of Swathi Kaliki, MD.)*

Table 18-2 Differential Diagnosis of Retinoblastoma

Persistent fetal vasculature
Coats disease
Toxocariasis (larval granuloma)
Astrocytic hamartoma (retinal astrocytoma)
Organizing vitreous hemorrhage
Medulloepithelioma
Cataract
Retinal dysplasia
Retinopathy of prematurity
Coloboma of choroid or optic nerve head
Macular toxoplasmosis (scar)
Posterior uveitis

Persistent fetal vasculature

The most severe form of persistent fetal vasculature (PFV; formerly called *persistent hyperplastic primary vitreous*) is typically recognized within days or weeks of birth. The condition occurs unilaterally in 90% of cases and is associated with microphthalmia, a shallow or flat anterior chamber, a hypoplastic iris with prominent vessels, cataract with fibrovascular material adherent to the posterior capsule, and a retrolenticular fibrovascular mass that exerts traction on the ciliary body processes to draw them inward. On indirect ophthalmoscopy, a vascular stalk that extends from the ONH and attaches to the posterior lens capsule may be visible, or the remnants of a stalk at the capsule and optic nerve may be observed. Ultrasonographic findings that are diagnostic for PFV include a microphthalmic eye (eg, short axial length) with persistent hyaloid remnants arising from the ONH, usually in association with closed-funnel retinal detachment. Although PFV is not associated with retinal tumors, small foci of calcification may be present; if bilateral, Norrie disease should be considered. See also Chapter 9 in this volume and BCSC Section 6, *Pediatric Ophthalmology and Strabismus.*

Coats disease

Coats disease is clinically evident within the first decade of life and is more common in males. It is associated with unilateral retinal telangiectasia with characteristic lightbulb aneurysms and intraretinal yellow exudation without a distinct mass (Fig 18-13). The progressive leakage of fluid can result in extensive retinal detachment and neovascular glaucoma. On ultrasonography, retinal tumors are absent, and cholesterol accumulation is visible in the subretinal fluid. FA demonstrates the presence of telangiectatic vessels and areas of retinal ischemia. See Chapter 10 in this volume for discussion of the pathology of Coats disease; see also BCSC Section 6, *Pediatric Ophthalmology and Strabismus,* and Section 12, *Retina and Vitreous,* for additional discussion.

Ocular toxocariasis

Ocular toxocariasis is a parasitic infection caused by *Toxocara canis* or *Toxocara cati* that typically occurs in older children with a history of soil ingestion or exposure to puppies or kittens. Toxocariasis presents with posterior and peripheral granulomas and associated

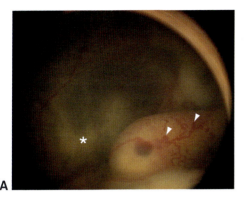 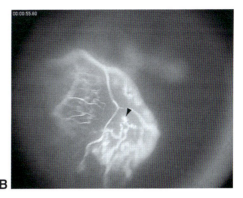

Figure 18-13 Coats disease. **A,** Clinical photograph demonstrates characteristic lightbulb aneurysms *(arrowheads)* and associated exudative retinal detachment with subretinal exudate *(asterisk)*. **B,** Fluorescein angiogram shows classic telangiectatic vessels *(arrowhead)*. This case highlights the way Coats disease can mimic a mass. *(Courtesy of Matthew W. Wilson, MD.)*

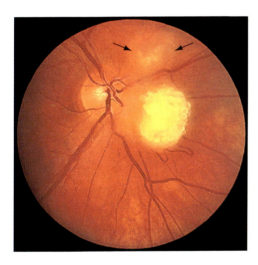

Figure 18-14 Clinical photograph of retinal astrocytic hamartomas reveals a more subtle opalescent lesion *(between arrows)* superonasal to the ONH and a larger "mulberry" lesion that is inferonasal to the ONH.

uveitis. The granulomas often have a slightly elevated, circumscribed appearance. Exudative retinal detachment, organized vitreoretinal traction, and cataracts may be present. Ultrasonographic findings include vitritis, retinal detachment, granulomas, retinal traction, and an absence of calcium. See BCSC Section 6, *Pediatric Ophthalmology and Strabismus,* and Section 9, *Uveitis and Ocular Inflammation,* for further discussion.

Astrocytoma

Retinal astrocytoma, or astrocytic hamartoma, generally appears as a small, smooth, white, glistening tumor located in the nerve fiber layer of the retina (Fig 18-14). Retinal astrocytoma may present as 1 or multiple lesions occurring unilaterally or bilaterally. In some cases, the lesion grows and calcifies, yielding a "mulberry" appearance. Astrocytomas occasionally arise from the ONH; such tumors often are referred to as *giant drusen.* Retinal astrocytomas commonly occur in patients with tuberous sclerosis and may be found in patients with neurofibromatosis; however, most cases are not associated with phakomatoses. Clinically, this lesion can masquerade as a small retinoblastoma, but handheld OCT imaging can demonstrate whether the tumor is confined to the nerve fiber layer. See BCSC Section 6, *Pediatric Ophthalmology and Strabismus,* for more information.

Medulloepithelioma

Medulloepithelioma typically appears as an off-white mass arising from the ciliary body (Fig 18-15A). In rare instances, this lesion has also been documented in the retina and optic nerve. Medulloepitheliomas may be benign or malignant, although the benign form is far more common. In most cases, this tumor becomes clinically evident in children aged 4–12 years, but it may also occur in adults. In 5% of patients, there may be an association between ciliary body medulloepithelioma and pleuropulmonary blastoma (*DICER1* syndrome). Smaller lesions may present with unexplained neovascular glaucoma accompanied by iris heterochromia. The tumor may erode through the iris root or grow along the lens zonular fibers, extending into the anterior chamber. Diagnostic imaging may reveal large cysts on the surface of the tumor or within the lesion (Fig 18-15B). See Chapter 10 for a discussion of the histologic features of medulloepithelioma.

Management of medulloepitheliomas includes cryotherapy for small tumors, plaque radiotherapy for eyes with tumors smaller than 4 clock-hours and normal IOP, and enucleation for eyes with larger tumors and secondary glaucoma. If malignant features are found on histopathology, systemic chemotherapy may be considered. For most medulloepitheliomas, local surgical resection is avoided because of the association with late complications and metastases. Fortunately, with appropriate management metastasis is rare, even when the tumor appears frankly malignant on histologic examination.

> Priest JR, Williams GM, Manera R, et al. Ciliary body medulloepithelioma: four cases associated with pleuropulmonary blastoma—a report from the International Pleuropulmonary Blastoma Registry. *Br J Ophthalmol.* 2011;95(7):1001–1005.

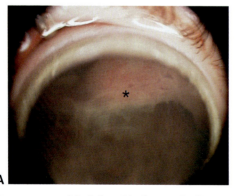 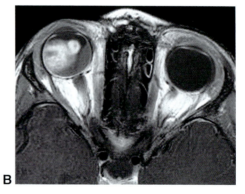

Figure 18-15 Medulloepithelioma. **A,** Pigmented lesion arising in the ciliary body, with an amelanotic apex *(asterisk).* The presence of melanin in these tumors is rare; most tumors are off-white to cream colored. **B,** T1-weighted MRI with gadolinium reveals diffuse enhancement and multiple cystic spaces. *(Courtesy of Matthew W. Wilson, MD.)*

Retinoblastoma Classification

The International Intraocular Retinoblastoma Classification

Various systems have been used to classify retinoblastoma. In 2005, the International Intraocular Retinoblastoma Classification (IIRC) (the first international classification system for intraocular retinoblastoma) was introduced; it is now the most commonly used system worldwide. The IIRC system was designed to predict ocular salvage in suitable cases with systemic chemotherapy combined with local consolidation therapy and to provide a uniform classification scheme for broad application across centers. In this system, tumors are grouped in terms of size, proximity to critical anatomical structures, presence of subretinal fluid, and extent of vitreous and subretinal seeding. Eyes are assigned a letter from A to E, indicating those most to least salvageable with chemotherapy. Eyes with anterior chamber involvement, neovascular glaucoma, vitreous hemorrhage, or necrosis are classified as group E and are generally considered unsalvageable. The grouping system and preferred treatments for the IIRC system are summarized in Table 18-3.

Other Retinoblastoma Classification Systems

Unfortunately, small inconsistencies in published grouping systems have undermined the uniform classification scheme offered by the IIRC. For example, the classification system used in the Children's Oncology Group (COG) clinical trials includes a small deviation from the IIRC system for staging of group B eyes in the allowed size of the fluid cuff. The International Classification of Retinoblastoma (ICRB), proposed in 2006, differs from the IIRC in that a tumor filling more than 50% of the globe is a criterion for group E disease. Thus, some eyes classified as group D in the IIRC would be staged as group E in the ICRB scheme. This has caused confusion in reporting of outcomes, particularly in eyes with advanced disease.

In 2017, the eighth edition of the American Joint Committee on Cancer TNM (tumor, node, metastasis) staging system introduced a comprehensive reclassification system for intraocular disease in eyes with retinoblastoma. This clinical classification is based on a retrospective multicenter study of 1728 eyes diagnosed with the disease between 2001 and 2011 that addressed the proportion of eyes salvaged without external beam radiotherapy (EBRT). The International Retinoblastoma Staging System, which can be used for both intraocular retinoblastoma and extraocular tumor extension, is summarized in Table 18-4.

> Chantada G, Doz F, Antoneli CBG, et al. A proposal for an international retinoblastoma staging system. *Pediatr Blood Cancer*. 2006;47(6):801–805.
>
> Mallipatna A, Gallie BL, Chévez-Barrios P, et al. Retinoblastoma. In: Amin MB, Edge SB, Greene FL, et al, eds. *AJCC Cancer Staging Manual*. 8th ed. Springer; 2017:819–831.
>
> Murphree AL. Intraocular retinoblastoma: the case for a new group classification. *Ophthalmol Clin North Am*. 2005;18(1):41–53.
>
> Reese AB. *Tumors of the Eye*. 3rd ed. Harper & Row; 1976.
>
> Shields CL, Shields JA. Basic understanding of current classification and management of retinoblastoma. *Curr Opin Ophthalmol*. 2006;17(3):228–234.

Table 18-3 International Intraocular Retinoblastoma Classification (IIRC)

Group	Image	Tumor Description	Helpful Mnemonic	Treatment
A		Tumor ≤3 mm in size, ≥3 mm to fovea, and ≥1.5 mm from optic nerve head	Small tumors **A**way from critical structures	For peripheral lesions: cryotherapy For equatorial lesions: transpupillary thermotherapy or laser photocoagulation
B		Tumor >3 mm in size, <3 mm to fovea, <1.5 mm from optic nerve head, or small cuff of subretinal fluid ≤5 mm from tumor margin	**B**igger tumors	Intravenous or intra-arterial chemotherapy
C		Tumor with localized subretinal or vitreous seeds or retinal detachment of ≤1 quadrant	Seeding is present **C**lose to the tumor	Intravenous or intra-arterial chemotherapy For subretinal seeds: adjunct cryotherapy or laser For vitreous seeds: intravitreal chemotherapy
D		Tumor with diffuse subretinal or vitreous seeds or retinal detachment of >1 quadrant	**D**istant and **D**iffuse seeds	Intravenous or intra-arterial chemotherapy For subretinal seeds: adjunct cryotherapy or laser For vitreous seeds: intravitreal chemotherapy

Group	Image	Tumor Description	Helpful Mnemonic	Treatment
E		Large tumor with 1 or more of the following features: • neovascular glaucoma • intraocular hemorrhage • aseptic orbital cellulitis • tumor touching the anterior vitreous face • tumor touching the lens • diffuse infiltrating tumor • necrosis • pseudohypopyon • phthisis or pre-phthisis bulbi	Tumor *E*verywhere	Enucleation is preferable

Adapted from Murphree AL. Intraocular retinoblastoma: the case for a new group classification. *Ophthalmol Clin North Am.* 2005;18(1):42. Also from Shields CL, Shields JA. Basic understanding of current classification and management of retinoblastoma. *Curr Opin Ophthalmol.* 2006;17(3):230, Table 1. Images courtesy of Swathi Kaliki, MD.

Table 18-4 **International Retinoblastoma Staging System**

Stage	Definition
0	Eye salvaged with conservative treatment
I	Eye enucleated, completely resected
II	Eye enucleated, microscopic residual tumor
III	Regional extension
	a. Overt orbital disease
	b. Regional lymph node extension
IV	Metastatic disease
	a. Hematogenous metastasis (without central nervous system involvement)
	1. Single lesion
	2. Multiple lesions
	b. Central nervous system involvement
	1. Prechiasmatic lesion
	2. Central nervous system mass
	3. Leptomeningeal and cerebrospinal fluid involvement

Adapted from Chantada G, Doz F, Antoneli CBG, et al. A proposal for an international retinoblastoma staging system. *Pediatr Blood Cancer.* 2006;47(6):801–805.

Treatment

Treatment of retinoblastoma has evolved dramatically in the last century: from enucleation as the only option, to attempts at globe salvage with primary radiotherapy in the 1940s, to the modern chemotherapy era. Intravenous chemotherapy was introduced for this purpose in the 1990s, intra-arterial chemotherapy in the 2000s, and intravitreal chemotherapy in the 2010s. Currently, when retinoblastoma is contained within the eye, the survival rate exceeds 95%. In cases with extraocular spread, the survival rate is substantially lower.

A multidisciplinary team consisting of an ocular oncologist, a pediatric ophthalmologist, a pediatric oncologist, an interventional radiologist, and a radiation oncologist is often needed to treat retinoblastoma. When determining the treatment strategy, the clinician's first goal must be preservation of life, then preservation of the eye, and finally preservation of vision. To that end, modern management of intraocular retinoblastoma involves a combination of treatment modalities, including enucleation, systemic and local chemotherapy, and local consolidation therapy such as laser therapy, cryotherapy, and plaque brachytherapy. EBRT is now performed only in rare cases. Metastatic disease is similarly managed with intensive combinations of chemotherapy, radiation, and bone marrow transplantation. For many of these therapeutic modalities, anesthesia is required for young patients. Because new tumors and recurrent tumors may develop in an eye, particularly in patients with a pathogenic germline variant, serial EUAs are also required for surveillance.

Attempts at globe-conserving therapy should be undertaken only by ophthalmologists well versed in the management of this rare childhood tumor and, as mentioned, in conjunction with similarly experienced pediatric oncologists. Failed attempts at eye salvage may place a child at risk of metastatic disease.

Enucleation

Enucleation remains a definitive treatment for retinoblastoma, enabling complete surgical resection of the disease in most cases. This intervention is often curative in patients with unilateral disease and is the typical treatment for unilateral eyes classified as group E in the IIRC system. Enucleation is also considered appropriate in the following situations:

- Optic nerve involvement is suspected, and the surgeon can enucleate with a clear optic nerve margin (ie, complete tumor resection).
- Anterior segment involvement is present.
- The patient has neovascular glaucoma.
- The eye has been otherwise anatomically or functionally destroyed by the tumor.
- The affected eye has limited visual potential.
- The tumor persists or recurs despite attempts at globe salvage.

Tumor enucleation is designed to minimize the potential for inadvertent globe penetration while obtaining the greatest possible length of resected optic nerve, typically at least 10 mm. Most surgeons place an implant postoperatively. The implants may be composed of nonporous silicone/acrylic or an integrated porous material such as hydroxyapatite or porous polyethylene.

Chemotherapy

For eyes classified in groups B, C, and D of the IIRC system, the foundation of any globe-sparing regimen is currently chemotherapy, either as a systemic intravenous (IV) treatment (Fig 18-16) or as a selective intra-arterial modality. Although no head-to-head clinical trials have compared the efficacy of systemic IV treatment with that of selective intra-arterial chemotherapy, both forms of chemotherapy are effective according to various retrospective studies. In addition, both forms of chemotherapy are available at many centers across the world.

Systemic IV chemotherapy typically includes 3–6 cycles of carboplatin, vincristine, and etoposide. Although tumor regression occurs initially (chemoreduction), adjunctive treatment

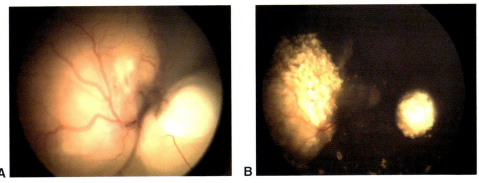

Figure 18-16 Retinoblastoma. **A,** Appearance before systemic chemotherapy. **B,** Reduced tumor volume after 6 cycles of systemic chemotherapy alone. *(Courtesy of Swathi Kaliki, MD.)*

with laser therapy, cryotherapy, and/or brachytherapy is necessary to completely treat the mass. For example, when combined with local therapies, systemic IV chemotherapy is highly successful in curing eyes classified according to the IIRC system as group B or C, although it has only a 50% success rate in group D eyes. Intravitreal injection of chemotherapy may also be needed to manage vitreous seeding.

Systemic chemotherapy is also frequently given to patients with bilateral disease with at least IIRC group B or AJCC group cT1b disease in the less affected eye. Although this treatment is generally well tolerated, even in very young children, complications can occur; these include pancytopenia, ototoxicity, and potentially secondary acute myelogenous leukemia. Thus, without serial ophthalmoscopic examinations and without the use of adjunctive local therapies, systemic chemotherapy is not sufficient for treatment of intraocular retinoblastoma and may lead to extraocular spread and metastases.

Selective intra-arterial chemotherapy has gained popularity in the last 2 decades because of its success in salvage for eyes in IIRC groups B, C, and D and minimal risk of systemic toxicity. Intra-arterial chemotherapy involves the selective infusion of chemotherapy agents into the ophthalmic artery via direct cannulation of the femoral artery (Fig 18-17). This modality usually involves administration of melphalan, topotecan, and/or carboplatin in 3 cycles. The effectiveness of intra-arterial chemotherapy is technique dependent and requires the expertise of an experienced interventional neuroradiologist. When this modality is used as a primary therapy, cure rates of more than 90% have been reported for advanced-stage group D eyes. When it is used after previous treatment failure and tumor recurrence, the cure rate is approximately 50%. Intra-arterial chemotherapy is typically reserved for patients older than 3 months (>6 months in many centers) and/or weighing at least 6 kg. At some centers, intra-arterial therapy is reserved for children with unilateral disease; at others, tandem therapy is given to patients with bilateral disease.

Complications of intra-arterial chemotherapy include periorbital edema and erythema, nasal eyelash loss, a 3% risk of ophthalmic vascular events per infusion (eg, retinal nonperfusion, vitreous hemorrhage, subretinal hemorrhage, branch retinal vein occlusion, choroidal ischemia), and stroke. There is extensive debate about whether the risk for metastatic disease is increased in children with advanced retinoblastoma treated with intra-arterial therapy because of the lack of systemic chemotherapy. When pathologic evaluation of the globe reveals high-risk features for metastasis in children, such as massive choroidal invasion or

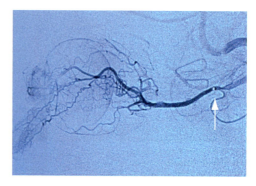

Figure 18-17 Angiogram of an eye with retinoblastoma under fluoroscopy during treatment with intra-arterial chemotherapy. *Arrow* demonstrates the location of the microcatheter injection into the ophthalmic vasculature. *(Courtesy of Dan S. Gombos, MD.)*

tumor infiltration into the retrolaminar optic nerve, most centers recommend adjuvant systemic chemotherapy after enucleation. A recent COG study found that the highest risk factor for metastatic disease is concomitant peripapillary choroidal invasion of more than 3 mm and postlaminar optic nerve invasion of 1.5 mm or more, thus supporting adjuvant chemotherapy in this cohort. When eyes with advanced disease (which are more likely to have high-risk pathologic features) are salvaged, histologic information is not available to the medical team to predict risk of systemic disease. For more information on the pathology of retinoblastoma, see Chapter 10.

> Berry JL, Jubran R, Kim JW, et al. Long-term outcomes of group D eyes in bilateral retinoblastoma patients treated with chemoreduction and low-dose IMRT salvage. *Pediatr Blood Cancer*. 2013;60(4):688–693.
>
> Chévez-Barrios P, Eagle RC Jr, Krailo M, et al. Study of unilateral retinoblastoma with and without histopathologic high-risk features and the role of adjuvant chemotherapy: a Children's Oncology Group study. *J Clin Oncol*. 2019;37(31):2883–2891.
>
> Dalvin LA, Ancona-Lezama D, Lucio-Alvarez JA, Masoomian B, Jabbour P, Shields CL. Ophthalmic vascular events after primary unilateral intra-arterial chemotherapy for retinoblastoma in early and recent eras. *Ophthalmology*. 2018;125(11):1803–1811.
>
> Francis JH, Levin AM, Zabor EC, Gobin YP, Abramson DH. Ten-year experience with ophthalmic artery chemosurgery: ocular and recurrence-free survival. *PLoS One*. 2018;13(5):e0197081. doi:10.1371/journal.pone.0197081

Local Consolidation Therapy

Laser photocoagulation

Various laser treatments have been used to manage retinoblastoma. Lasers can be a primary modality for treating group A/AJCC group cT1a eyes with small tumors or as adjuvant treatment after systemic or intra-arterial chemotherapy. Most practitioners use an 810-nm infrared or 532-nm green laser for these purposes. Laser techniques vary, but for all treatments, the laser is applied to the tumor surface, eliciting cytotoxic effects in tumor cells via photocoagulation or thermal injury. Multiple laser sessions are necessary for tumor control. Complications of this modality include iris atrophy, cataracts, tumor seeding into the vitreous, retinal traction, and fibrosis.

Cryotherapy

Cryotherapy is an effective primary or adjunctive treatment for peripheral tumors with an apical thickness of up to 3 mm. The clinician visualizes the tumor with an indirect ophthalmoscope and applies cryotherapy transsclerally using a triple freeze–thaw technique. Typically, laser photoablation is chosen for smaller, posteriorly located tumors, and cryoablation is performed in larger, anteriorly located tumors. Close monitoring is necessary so that tumor regrowth or treatment complications can be managed promptly. Complications, including retinal tear and retinal detachment, are more likely to occur in large, calcified tumors.

Plaque radiotherapy

When globe-conserving treatments have failed to destroy all of a viable tumor, radioactive plaque therapy (ie, brachytherapy) may be used as a salvage treatment; this technique can also serve as the primary treatment in eyes with small to medium tumors (ie, tumors less than 16 mm in basal diameter and less than 8 mm in apical thickness). The most commonly used isotopes for this procedure are iodine 125 and ruthenium 106. Ultrasound-assisted localization of the tumor intraoperatively enhances local tumor control. Compared with EBRT, plaque brachytherapy is associated with a greater likelihood of radiation optic neuropathy or retinopathy but a substantially lower risk of radiation-induced cancer.

Intravitreal chemotherapy

Intravitreal chemotherapy is now an accepted treatment modality for vitreous seeds, which were previously one of the most common reasons for treatment failure in retinoblastoma. Initially, use of intravitreal chemotherapy, which involves direct injections into the eye, was controversial because of concerns about possible spread of active cancer; however, these concerns have been ameliorated by the use of targeted safety measures. These measures include anterior ultrasonographic imaging to ensure that the injection is not inserted into a quadrant containing active tumor, reduction of IOP before the injection by means of anterior chamber paracentesis or ocular massage to prevent vitreous reflux, and cryotherapy during withdrawal of the injecting needle to kill any active tumor cells. The safety-enhanced technique is nearly 100% effective for prevention of vitreous seeding, and there have been no reports of extraocular tumor spread. Nevertheless, great care and attention to these safety precautions are imperative.

The number of injections needed for tumor control is based on the type of seeds and how they are classified (ie, as dust, spheres, or clouds). Melphalan, the most frequently used agent for this purpose, is known to induce chorioretinal toxicity; although this toxicity is not usually visually significant, it can be severe. Topotecan has also been used. Other adverse events associated with intravitreal injection include cataract, retinal detachment, and endophthalmitis. If any of these complications occur in a patient with retinoblastoma, enucleation may be required because intraocular surgery is rarely performed in these patients, given the risk of orbital seeding of the tumor. See Video 18-1 for a demonstration of intravitreal injection.

VIDEO 18-1 Intravitreal injection of melphalan for vitreous seeding in retinoblastoma.
Courtesy of Jesse L. Berry, MD.
Available at: aao.org/bcscvideo_section04

Berry JL, Bechtold M, Shah S, et al. Not all seeds are created equal: seed classification is predictive of outcomes in retinoblastoma. *Ophthalmology*. 2017;124(12):1817–1825.

Francis JH, Abramson DH, Ji X, et al. Risk of extraocular extension in eyes with retinoblastoma receiving intravitreous chemotherapy. *JAMA Ophthalmol*. 2017;135(12):1426–1429.

Munier FL, Gaillard M-C, Balmer A, et al. Intravitreal chemotherapy for vitreous disease in retinoblastoma revisited: from prohibition to conditional indications. *Br J Ophthalmol*. 2012;96(8):1078–1083.

Intracameral chemotherapy

Intracameral chemotherapy is a new modality for treatment of aqueous seeding, especially in cases with secondary seeding. Aqueous seeding may occur because of spillover of endophytic tumor cells into the aqueous after disruption of the anterior hyaloid membrane, from seeds at the vitreous base/ciliary body, or from contaminated aqueous production from the ciliary body. Although the seeds are apparent on the corneal endothelium, surface of the iris, and anterior chamber angle during clinical examination, they may also be hidden in the Petit and Hannover canals and in between ciliary processes, detectable only by ultrasound biomicroscopy.

In cases of aqueous seeding, injections of melphalan and topotecan via the clear corneal or limbal approach can achieve tumor control and globe salvage in 55% to 85% of eyes.

For injection of chemotherapeutic agent into the posterior and anterior chambers, the bicameral technique is recommended. When there are concomitant vitreous seeds, this technique should be combined with intravitreal chemotherapy. The chances of extraocular tumor extension are minimized by perioperative hypotony with antiglaucoma medications, paracentesis, triple freeze–thaw cryotherapy at the injection site, and a thorough wash of the eye with distilled water after the procedure. The patient may experience transient glaucoma and hyphema, but no serious anterior chamber complications have been reported yet. See Video 18-2 for a demonstration of intracameral injection for retinoblastoma.

 VIDEO 18-2 Intracameral chemotherapy for aqueous seeding in retinoblastoma.
Courtesy of Swathi Kaliki, MD.
Available at: aao.org/bcscvideo_section04

Kaliki S. Aqueous seeding in intraocular retinoblastoma: a review. *Clin Exp Ophthalmol.* 2021;49(6):606–614.

Munier FL, Moulin A, Gaillard M-C, et al. Intracameral chemotherapy for globe salvage in retinoblastoma with secondary anterior chamber invasion. *Ophthalmology.* 2018;125(4):615–617.

Stathopoulos C, Beck-Popovic M, Moulin AP, Munier FL. Ten-year experience with intracameral chemotherapy for aqueous seeding in retinoblastoma: long-term efficacy, safety and toxicity. *Br J Ophthalmol.* 2023;108(1):124–130.

External beam radiotherapy

In most centers, EBRT has largely been abandoned as a treatment for intraocular retinoblastoma, with use restricted to cases with extraocular tumor extension. Because retinoblastoma tumors are responsive to radiation, EBRT may be performed as a salvage technique; however, it is currently used only when chemotherapy has failed in the remaining eye. Two major concerns have limited use of EBRT:

- Pathogenic germline variants in *RB1* are associated with a lifelong increased risk of subsequent independent primary malignancies (eg, osteosarcoma); this risk is exacerbated by exposure to EBRT, especially in children younger than 12 months.
- Treatment with EBRT involves risks of radiation-related sequelae, such as orbital hypoplasia, midface hypoplasia, radiation-induced cataract, and radiation optic neuropathy and retinopathy.

Spontaneous Regression

Although the incidence of spontaneous regression is unknown, in rare cases, very large retinoblastoma tumors have undergone complete and spontaneous necrosis. The mechanism by which this occurs is also not well understood; however, tumor growth exceeding the vascular supply likely plays a role.

Children with spontaneous regression may present with vitreous hemorrhage, a dislocated crystalline lens, or phthisis. For this reason, retinoblastoma should be part of the differential diagnosis for young children who present with unilateral phthisis without a history of trauma. The presence of calcification on imaging is highly suggestive of retinoblastoma, and prompt enucleation should be considered. Certain histologic features of the enucleated globe can suggest or confirm the diagnosis:

- The vitreous cavity is filled with islands of calcified cells embedded in a mass of fibroconnective tissue.
- Close inspection of the peripheral portions of the calcified islands reveals ghosted contours of fossilized tumor cells.
- Exuberant proliferation of retinal pigment and ciliary epithelia is observed.

Genetic Counseling

Retinoblastoma is almost always caused by a pathogenic variation in both copies (ie, "2 hits") of the tumor suppressor gene *RB1*, located on the long arm of chromosome 13 at locus 14 (13q14); much less commonly, it is due to a deletion of part of this chromosomal arm. Retinal cells are not terminally differentiated at birth; therefore, pathogenic variants in *RB1* can still occur in retinal cells over the first few years of life as the retina matures, resulting in tumor formation.

When tumor DNA is analyzed, 1 or 2 pathogenic variants that cause loss of function of the retinoblastoma protein can be identified. Historically, this was done using tumor specimens from enucleated eyes. Now, with increased rates of globe salvage, aqueous humor or blood liquid biopsies are performed instead.

Retinoblastoma may be inherited (10% of cases) or sporadic, caused by a new pathogenic variant (90% of cases). Children with sporadic disease may have a solitary tumor related to a somatic event within a single retinal cell or may harbor a new spontaneous pathogenic germline variant, which can be inherited by their future children. Of patients with sporadic disease, two-thirds have nonhereditary pathogenic variants in which both *RB1* variants occurred as a somatic event in a single retinal cell. The remaining one-third of patients have a new germline variant that is present in all retinal cells or a variant that occurred during embryogenesis when the first *RB1* variant was present in many, but not all, retinal cells (ie, mosaicism). Thus, although these patients may have a family history of retinoblastoma (ie, 10% of them), it is more likely that the disease developed from a new sporadic variation in a parental germ cell or in the developing embryo. These patients therefore have a risk of passing a pathogenic variant copy of *RB1* to their offspring.

Retinoblastoma pathogenic variants are implicated in many different tumors in the body, thus predisposing affected patients with pathogenic germline *RB1* variants to multiple types of cancer. Patients with pathogenic germline variations in *RB1* often have bilateral or multifocal disease, with an earlier presentation than those with nongermline variants; however, approximately 15% of patients with unilateral disease also have a pathogenic germline variant. Clinical examination findings cannot distinguish patients with unilateral disease caused by germline versus nongermline variations unless there are multiple tumors in the affected eye. Thus, it is crucial for children with retinoblastoma to undergo molecular testing for a germline *RB1* variant.

Approximately 2% of unilateral retinoblastomas are caused by amplification of the N-myc proto-oncogene *(MYCN)* and not by a pathogenic variation in *RB1*. This occurs most commonly in children under 6 months of age. On clinical examination alone, it can be difficult to differentiate tumors driven by *MYCN* amplification from advanced unilateral disease caused by an *RB1* pathogenic variant. When *MYCN* is the suspected etiology, enucleation is recommended. With enucleation, distinct histologic features of *MYCN*-associated tumors can be observed, including undifferentiated cells with prominent nucleoli and little calcification. These cellular features are similar to those seen in other *MYCN*-amplified tumors such as neuroblastoma. Tumors driven by *MYCN* amplification appear to be nonheritable. The exact mechanism of the amplification remains under investigation.

Guidelines for Genetic and Family Counseling for Patients With Retinoblastoma
- The parents and siblings of the patient should be examined for evidence of untreated retinoblastoma or retinocytoma, which would represent a possible hereditary predisposition to the disease.
- Counseling with a genetic specialist is recommended for all families affected by retinoblastoma. Genetic testing of the child with retinoblastoma is recommended to determine the presence of a germline pathogenic variant. Genetic counseling in retinoblastoma includes the following important points:
  - A patient with bilateral retinoblastoma has a germline variant by definition.
  - A survivor of unilateral retinoblastoma has a 15% chance of having a germline pathogenic variant; thus, genetic testing is especially relevant in unilateral patients. If the germline status is unknown, there is a 7%–15% likelihood of having an affected child (based on the ~15% risk of having a germline alteration).
  - A survivor of retinoblastoma due to a pathogenic germline variant (regardless of whether the disease is unilateral or bilateral) has a 45% chance of having an affected child.
  - Unaffected parents of a child with bilateral retinoblastoma have a 5% risk of having another child with retinoblastoma. Thus, genetic testing should be offered to parents of a child with retinoblastoma.
  - If 2 or more siblings have retinoblastoma, there is a 45% chance that another child will be affected, as this represents hereditary disease.

Systematic screening for retinoblastoma by an ophthalmologist is recommended for all children in families with the disease. In 2018, the first national guidelines for retinoblastoma screening in the United States were published; these recommendations address practices and frequencies for screening of children at various risk levels. See also BCSC Section 6, *Pediatric Ophthalmology and Strabismus*.

- Abramson DH, Mendelsohn ME, Servodidio CA, Tretter T, Gombos DS. Familial retinoblastoma: where and when? *Acta Ophthalmol Scand*. 1998;76(3):334–338.
- Rushlow DE, Mol BM, Kennett JY, et al. Characterisation of retinoblastomas without *RB1* mutations: genomic, gene expression, and clinical studies. *Lancet Oncol*. 2013;14(4): 327–334.
- Skalet AH, Gombos DS, Gallie BL, et al. Screening children at risk for retinoblastoma: consensus report from the American Association of Ophthalmic Oncologists and Pathologists. *Ophthalmology*. 2018;125(3):453–458.
- Thériault BL, Dimaras H, Gallie BL, Corson TW. The genomic landscape of retinoblastoma: a review. *Clin Exp Ophthalmol*. 2014;42(1):33–52.

Associated Conditions

Retinocytoma

Retinocytoma is often clinically indistinguishable from retinoblastoma. See Chapter 10 for a summary of the histologic features that distinguish retinocytoma from retinoblastoma (also see Fig 10-43).

The developmental biology of retinocytoma is controversial. Some authorities assert that retinocytoma is a completely differentiated form of retinoblastoma—analogous to ganglioneuroma, the differentiated form of neuroblastoma. Others contend that retinocytoma is a benign counterpart of retinoblastoma in which biallelic *RB1* variants are present, but further genetic or genomic changes needed to promote tumorigenesis are absent. Although histologically benign, retinocytoma carries the same genetic implications as retinoblastoma. A child harboring a retinoblastoma in 1 eye and a retinocytoma in the other should be considered as having the same risk of transmitting an *RB1* variant to future offspring as children with bilateral retinoblastoma.

- Singh AD, Santos CM, Shields CL, Shields JA, Eagle RC Jr. Observations on 17 patients with retinocytoma. *Arch Ophthalmol*. 2000;118(2):199–205.

Primitive Neuroectodermal Tumor

Intracranial neoplasms known as *primitive neuroectodermal tumors (PNETs)* develop in some patients with germline retinoblastoma; PNETs represent the intracranial component of *trilateral retinoblastoma* (see Fig 18-11). The ectopic focus usually is located in the pineal gland or the parasellar region and traditionally is known as a *pinealoblastoma*. This tumor affects up to 5% of children with a germline *RB1* variation. In rare cases, the PNET arises prior to ocular involvement; more commonly, this independent malignant tumor presents months or years after treatment of intraocular retinoblastoma.

Several observations support the concept that an intracranial PNET constitutes a primary tumor, as opposed to intracranial spread of retinoblastoma. In some patients with terminal retinoblastoma, CT findings have shown that an intracranial tumor is anatomically separate from the ocular tumor(s). These intracranial tumors are not associated with metastatic disease elsewhere in the body and—unlike metastatic retinoblastoma—often have features of differentiation, such as *Flexner-Wintersteiner rosettes* (see Chapter 10, Fig 10-39B). Embryologic, immunologic, and phylogenic evidence of photoreceptor differentiation in the pineal gland further supports the concept of trilateral retinoblastoma.

It is recommended that all patients with retinoblastoma undergo baseline neuroimaging studies to exclude intracranial involvement. Experts disagree on the role of serial imaging in screening for PNETs. Studies have shown that the incidence of PNETs has decreased over time. It is unclear whether this is due to the prophylactic effect of systemic chemotherapy or a decrease in the use of radiation therapy.

> Friedman DN, Sklar CA, Oeffinger KC, et al. Long-term medical outcomes in survivors of extra-ocular retinoblastoma: the Memorial Sloan-Kettering Cancer Center (MSKCC) experience. *Pediatr Blood Cancer*. 2013;60(4):694–699.
>
> Jubran RF, Erdreich-Epstein A, Butturini A, Murphree AL, Villablanca JG. Approaches to treatment for extraocular retinoblastoma: Children's Hospital Los Angeles experience. *J Pediatr Hematol Oncol*. 2004;26(1):31–34.
>
> Moll AC, Imhof SM, Schouten-Van Meeteren AY, Kuik DJ, Hofman P, Boers M. Second primary tumors in hereditary retinoblastoma: a register-based study, 1945–1997: is there an age effect on radiation-related risk? *Ophthalmology*. 2001;108(6):1109–1114.

Prognosis

Ocular Prognosis

In patients with retinoblastoma, ocular prognosis is currently dictated by clinical staging and treatment modalities, with almost 100% ocular survival in IIRC group A, B, and C eyes and 30%–100% ocular survival in group D eyes. Molecular studies have shown that identification of chromosome 6p gain in cell-free DNA in the aqueous humor is associated with increased risk of treatment failure, thus serving as a potential prognostic biomarker. Additional studies have shown that the aggressiveness of the disease is defined by the *RB1* variant type, methylation status, and accompanying somatic chromosomal alterations.

Globe salvage rates have been very encouraging in high-income countries. However, there is a wide disparity in globe salvage rates in higher- versus lower-income countries. A meta-analysis revealed that the overall globe salvage rates for 2010–2020 were 70% for high-income countries versus 47% for upper middle–income countries, 34% for lower middle–income countries, and only 6% for low-income countries. This disparity is mainly attributed to poor socioeconomic status, lower educational level, and reduced availability and accessibility of health care facilities in lower-income countries.

> Berry JL, Xu L, Kooi I, et al. Genomic cfDNA analysis of aqueous humor in retinoblastoma predicts eye salvage: the surrogate tumor biopsy for retinoblastoma. *Mol Cancer Res*. 2018;16(11):1701–1712.

Bouchoucha Y, Matet A, Berger A, et al; European Retinoblastoma Group EuRbG. Retinoblastoma: from genes to patient care. *Eur J Med Genet*. 2023;66(1):104674. doi:10.1016/j.ejmg.2022.104674

Wong ES, Choy RW, Zhang Y, et al. Global retinoblastoma survival and globe preservation: a systematic review and meta-analysis of associations with socioeconomic and health-care factors. *Lancet Glob Health*. 2022;10(3):e380–e389. doi:10.1016/S2214-109X(21)00555-6

Life Prognosis

Similar to disparity in globe salvage rates, there is substantial variance in life salvage rates in individuals with retinoblastoma based on socioeconomic and health care factors. Survival rates for 2010–2020 were 98% for high-income countries versus 92% for upper middle–income countries, 83% for lower middle–income countries, and 57% for low-income countries. Early diagnosis may improve the outcomes in low-income countries. For more information on how social determinants of health affect prognoses, see Chapter 1 in BCSC Section 1, *Update on General Medicine*.

Children with intraocular retinoblastoma who have access to modern medical care have a very good prognosis (>95% survival rate in high-income countries). The main risk factor associated with death is extraocular extension of the tumor, either directly through the sclera or, more commonly, by invasion of the optic nerve, especially to the surgically resected margin (see Chapter 10, Fig 10-41). Massive choroidal invasion (≥3 mm of invasion), extrascleral extension, or postlaminar optic nerve disease increases the risk of metastatic disease. The risk is highest in patients with an active tumor at the cut end of the optic nerve; this clinical situation requires adjuvant chemotherapy and radiation therapy. Evidence also suggests that bilateral tumors may increase the risk of death because of the association with primary intracranial PNETs, due to germline disease.

Children with extraocular retinoblastoma historically had a very poor prognosis for survival. However, in a recent COG report, the authors demonstrated that intensive multimodal therapies—including high-dose chemotherapy, radiation, and bone marrow transplantation—have improved efficacy for curing regional extraocular retinoblastoma (87% event-free survival [EFS] at 36 months) and metastatic retinoblastoma not involving the CNS (79% EFS at 36 months), whereas rates for patients with CNS disease continue to be dismal (8% EFS at 36 months).

Recent molecular studies have shown that identification of higher *RB1* pathogenic variant allele frequencies from cell-free DNA in the blood may be associated with higher risk of metastatic disease. However, this finding needs to be validated in studies with larger cohorts.

Elam AR, Tseng VL, Rodriguez TM, Mike EV, Warren AK, Coleman AL; for the American Academy of Ophthalmology Taskforce on Disparities in Eye Care. Disparities in vision health and eye care. *Ophthalmology*. 2022;129(10):e89–e113. doi:10.1016/j.ophtha.2022.07.010

Kothari P, Marass F, Yang JL, et al. Cell-free DNA profiling in retinoblastoma patients with advanced intraocular disease: an MSKCC experience. *Cancer Med*. 2020;9(17):6093–6101.

Second Nonocular Tumors

Up to 20% of patients with bilateral retinoblastoma treated with chemotherapy will present with a second nonocular tumor within 20 years, and in up to 40% of those who were irradiated, a second or third nonocular tumor will develop. The 5-year survival rate in patients with sarcomas after retinoblastoma treatment is less than 50%. Patients with pathogenic germline *RB1* variants are advised to adhere to lifelong risk-modification practices, such as refraining from smoking, avoiding unnecessary radiation exposure (such as dental x-rays for screening), and applying sunscreen. An international consensus panel convened by the American Association for Cancer Research gave recommendations for second-primary tumor surveillance in germline retinoblastoma; these include an annual physical examination, with an assessment of the skin to identify second-primary skin cancers, as well as education regarding the signs and symptoms of bone and soft-tissue sarcomas. Although it may be feasible to conduct annual whole-body MRI procedures on patients with *RB1* germline variants beginning at age 8–10 years (when general anesthesia would no longer be required), there is no consensus on the use of whole-body imaging as a surveillance tool. Effective screening strategies for second-primary nonocular cancers in this population are an area of active research.

Second Nonocular Tumors in Retinoblastoma Survivors

- Children who survive germline retinoblastoma have an increased incidence of a second-primary nonocular malignancy later in life.
- A patient with a pathogenic germline *RB1* variant has an approximately 0.5%–1% risk of second-primary tumor development per year of life; thus, the risk exceeds 25% at 50 years of age. This risk is elevated further in patients who were treated with EBRT.
- The mean latency for development of a second tumor is approximately 9 years from management of the primary retinoblastoma.
- The most common type of second-primary cancer in these patients is osteosarcoma.
- Other relatively common second malignancies include soft-tissue sarcomas, cutaneous melanoma, PNETs, other brain tumors, and primitive unclassifiable tumors.

Dunkel IJ, Krailo MD, Chantada GL, et al. Intensive multi-modality therapy for extra-ocular retinoblastoma (RB): a Children's Oncology Group (COG) trial (ARET0321). *J Clin Oncol.* 2017;35(15 suppl):10506.

Kamihara J, Bourdeaut F, Foulkes WD, et al. Retinoblastoma and neuroblastoma predisposition and surveillance. *Clin Cancer Res.* 2017;23(13):e98–e106. doi:10.1158/1078-0432.CCR-17-0652

CHAPTER **19**

Ocular Involvement in Systemic Malignancies

Highlights

- The most common tumor occurring in the adult eye is a secondary metastatic tumor, disseminated from a carcinoma elsewhere in the body.
- The most common intraocular site for metastatic tumors is the posterior choroid, owing to its rich blood supply.
- Lymphoma can affect a single ocular tissue or multiple tissues, from the ocular adnexa to various parts of the eye; there may be systemic involvement.
- Ocular involvement is frequent in patients with leukemia; it most commonly manifests clinically as retinal hemorrhages and cotton-wool spots.

Secondary Tumors of the Eye

Metastatic Carcinoma

Since the first report in 1872 of a metastatic tumor in the eye of a patient with carcinoma, ocular metastases have been described as the most common intraocular tumor in adults. However, they may not be the lesions that are most commonly seen by ophthalmologists; many of the data regarding the incidence of these tumors are derived not from clinical studies but from evaluation of eyes at the time of autopsy.

Metastases to the eye are being diagnosed with increasing frequency for various reasons:

- increased incidence of certain tumor types that metastasize to the eye (eg, breast, lung)
- prolonged survival of patients with certain cancer types (eg, breast cancer)
- increased awareness among medical oncologists and ophthalmologists of the pattern of metastatic disease

As long-term survival rates for patients with primary systemic malignancies continue to improve and the incidence of intraocular and orbital metastatic disease increases, so will the need for prompt recognition and appropriate diagnostic and therapeutic management by the ophthalmologist.

> Shields CL, Kalafatis NE, Gad M, et al. Metastatic tumours to the eye. Review of metastasis to the iris, ciliary body, choroid, retina, optic disc, vitreous, and/or lens capsule. *Eye (Lond)*. 2023;37(5):809–814.

Mechanism of metastasis to the eye

The most common mechanism of intraocular metastasis is the hematogenous dissemination of tumor cells. The anatomy of the arterial blood supply to the eye dictates the location of tumor-cell deposits within the eye. The posterior choroid, with its rich vascular supply, is the most common site of intraocular metastasis; it is affected 10–20 times as frequently as the iris or ciliary body. The retina and optic nerve head, which are supplied by the single central retinal artery, are rarely the sole site of involvement. Bilateral ocular involvement has been reported in approximately 25% of cases of metastatic disease, and multifocal involvement is frequently seen within the eye. Many patients with ocular metastases also have concurrent central nervous system (CNS) (Fig 19-1) and other metastases. Ocular metastatic lesions are sometimes found before the primary tumor is detected; this happens most frequently in patients with lung adenocarcinoma.

Primary tumor sites

Ocular metastases represent a wide variety of primary tumor types. Most metastatic solid tumors to the eye are carcinomas from various organs. In a survey of 520 eyes with uveal metastases, the most common primary tumors to metastasize to the eye were breast (47%), lung (21%), and gastrointestinal tract (4%). In women, the breast is the most common primary tumor site; in men, the lung. Table 19-1 lists the most common primary tumors that metastasize to the choroid.

Clinical features and diagnosis

The clinical features of intraocular metastases depend on the location within the eye and are discussed in the following subsections. Metastatic tumors may be mistaken for other ocular

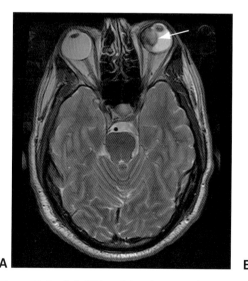 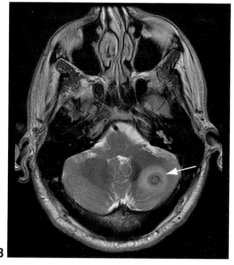

Figure 19-1 Axial T2-weighted magnetic resonance images of central nervous system (CNS) metastases. **A,** Metastatic intraocular tumor in the left eye *(arrow)*. **B,** Concurrent left cerebellar mass with surrounding edema *(arrow)*. *(Courtesy of Dan S. Gombos, MD.)*

Table 19-1 Primary Solid Tumors That Metastasize to the Uveal Tract (in Decreasing Order of Frequency)

Men	Women
Lung	Breast
Unknown	Lung
Gastrointestinal tract	Unknown
Kidney	Other
Prostate	Gastrointestinal tract
Skin	Skin
Other	Kidney
Breast	

Modified from Shields CL, Shields JA, Gross NE, Schwartz GP, Lally SE. Survey of 520 eyes with uveal metastases. *Ophthalmology.* 1997;104(8):1265–1276.

lesions, including primary tumors. See the sidebar for steps to take in order to make an accurate diagnosis.

> **Steps for Making an Accurate Diagnosis**
>
> - Take a thorough medical history.
> - Perform a careful ocular examination.
> - Use ancillary ophthalmic tests; the selection of these tests depends upon the location of the tumor(s).
> - Review patient medical records, including previous pathology reports, to determine the location of the primary tumor.
> - Take a biopsy of the lesion; this may be needed in a minority of cases to make the diagnosis of metastatic tumor (rather than primary intraocular tumor).
> - Refer the patient to an ocular oncologist; this should be considered when the ocular diagnosis is unclear, as this specialist has extensive experience in the diagnosis and management of ocular metastatic tumors.

Anterior segment: iris and ciliary body Metastases to the iris and ciliary body usually appear as gray-white to tan-pink gelatinous nodules (Figs 19-2, 19-3, 19-4). Metastases to the anterior uvea may include the following clinical features:

- iridocyclitis (sometimes before the tumor becomes clinically evident)
- secondary glaucoma

Figure 19-2 Metastatic tumor in the iris with associated hyphema *(arrow)*.

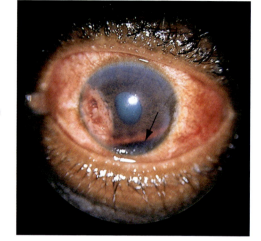

Figure 19-3 Metastasis from breast carcinoma to the iris. Note the 2 gray-white lesions on the iris surface. *(Courtesy of Timothy G. Murray, MD.)*

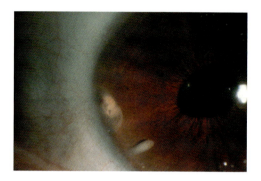

Figure 19-4 Metastatic cutaneous melanoma to the iris. Note the 2 peripheral amelanotic lesions.

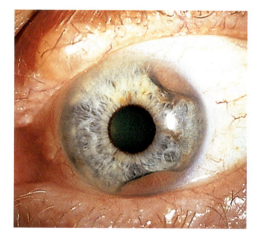

- iris neovascularization (rubeosis iridis)
- hyphema
- irregular pupil
- pseudohypopyon

Anterior segment tumors are best evaluated with slit-lamp biomicroscopy coupled with gonioscopy. High-frequency ultrasonography (eg, ultrasound biomicroscopy) may help quantify tumor size and anatomical relationships.

Posterior segment: choroid, retina, and optic nerve Patients with tumors in the posterior pole commonly report painless loss of vision. Indirect ophthalmoscopy may reveal an exudative retinal detachment associated with a placoid or "lumpy bumpy" tumor mass (Figs 19-5, 19-6, 19-7). These lesions are usually minimally elevated and ill defined, often amelanotic, gray, yellow, or off-white, with secondary alterations at the level of the retinal pigment epithelium (RPE) presenting as clumps of brown pigment ("leopard spots"; Fig 19-8).

The mushroom configuration present in eyes with primary choroidal melanoma from invasion through Bruch membrane is rarely present in uveal metastases. The retina overlying the metastasis may appear opaque and often detaches due to accumulation of subretinal fluid. Rapid tumor growth with necrosis and uveitis occasionally occur. Dilated epibulbar vessels may be visible in the quadrant overlying the metastasis. Table 19-2 presents a differential diagnosis of choroidal metastasis.

Although *fluorescein angiography* may be helpful in defining the margins of a metastatic tumor, it is typically less useful in differentiating a primary intraocular neoplasm from a metastasis. The double circulation pattern from an intrinsic intratumoral blood supply and

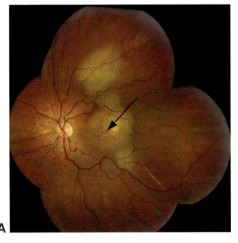
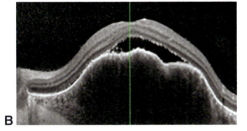

Figure 19-5 Metastases to the choroid from lung cancer. **A,** Note the multiple multifocal amelanotic lesions throughout the posterior pole and retinal pigmented changes over the lesion surface *(arrow).* **B,** Optical coherence tomography (OCT) image of 1 of the lesions reveals characteristic "lumpy bumpy" replacement of the choroid and overlying subretinal fluid. *(Courtesy of Elaine M. Binkley, MD.)*

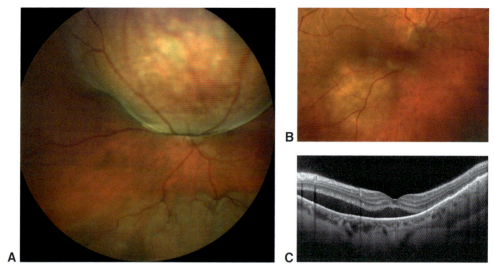

Figure 19-6 Metastases to the choroid from squamous cell carcinoma of the tonsil. **A,** Superior metastatic lesion to the choroid with inferior exudative retinal detachment. **B,** Metastatic lesion to the choroid that involves the inferior macula. **C,** OCT shows subretinal fluid from the lesion extending beneath the fovea. *(Courtesy of Elaine M. Binkley, MD.)*

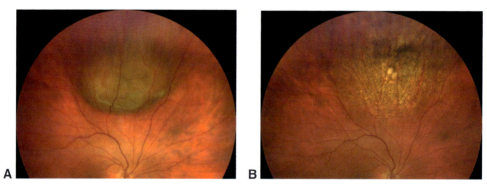

Figure 19-7 Metastases to the choroid from esophageal cancer. **A,** Fundus photograph shows an elevated, lightly pigmented choroidal lesion from esophageal cancer with overlying subretinal fluid. **B,** After the patient received treatment with systemic chemotherapy, the lesion regressed to a flat scar with overlying pigmentary changes. *(Courtesy of Elaine M. Binkley, MD.)*

the prominent early choroidal filling often associated with choroidal melanomas are found in metastatic tumors only in rare cases because of their rapid growth (ie, versus the slow growth of choroidal melanomas, which allows for the development of an intratumoral vascular supply).

Ultrasonography (echography) is diagnostically valuable in patients with choroidal lesions. In patients with a metastatic tumor, B-scan ultrasonography shows an echogenic choroidal mass with an ill-defined, sometimes lobulated or lumpy bumpy outline. Overlying

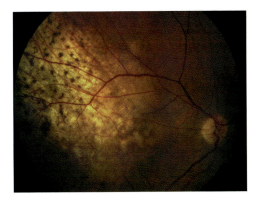

Figure 19-8 Clinical fundus photograph of metastatic breast carcinoma to the choroid. Note the amelanotic infiltrative choroidal mass with secondary overlying retinal pigment epithelial changes accounting for the characteristic leopard spots. *(Courtesy of Matthew W. Wilson, MD.)*

Table 19-2 Differential Diagnosis of Choroidal Metastasis

Amelanotic nevus	Extensive neovascular membranes
Amelanotic melanoma	Infectious/inflammatory lesions, granuloma
Central serous chorioretinopathy	Organized subretinal hemorrhage
Choroidal detachment	Posterior scleritis
Choroidal hemangioma	Rhegmatogenous retinal detachment
Choroidal osteoma	Vogt-Koyanagi-Harada syndrome

secondary exudative retinal detachment is commonly detected. A-scan ultrasonography demonstrates irregular and medium to high reflectivity.

Metastases to the optic nerve may produce edema of the optic nerve head, decreased vision, and visual field defects. Because metastases may involve the parenchyma or the optic nerve sheath, *magnetic resonance imaging (MRI)* and ultrasonography may be valuable in detecting the presence of additional lesions and identifying their location.

Enhanced depth imaging optical coherence tomography (EDI-OCT) may demonstrate a lumpy bumpy contour, choriocapillaris compression, and photoreceptor loss in the overlying retina. Metastases to the retina, which are quite rare, appear as white noncohesive lesions suggestive of cotton-wool spots, often distributed in a perivascular location (Fig 19-9). Because of secondary vitreous seeding of tumor cells, these metastases sometimes resemble retinitis rather than a tumor. Vitreous aspirates for cytologic studies may confirm the diagnosis (see Fig 19-9C).

Other diagnostic factors

One of the most important diagnostic factors in the evaluation of suspected ocular metastatic tumors is a history of systemic malignancy (see the section "Primary tumor sites" earlier in this chapter). When ocular metastasis is diagnosed, most patients have a known systemic malignancy, although the interval between the diagnosis of the primary tumor and that of the ocular metastasis may be many years. For example, in a study of 264 patients with uveal metastases from breast cancer, over 90% of patients had a history of systemic treatment before the development of ocular involvement. The ocular metastasis was the initial manifestation of

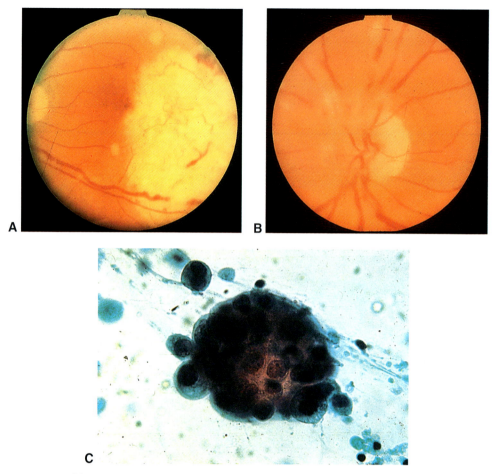

Figure 19-9 Metastases to the retina from lung carcinoma. **A,** Metastatic lung carcinoma involving the macula. Visual acuity was reduced to counting fingers. **B,** Fundus photograph of the same eye shows the characteristic perivascular distribution of metastases with obscuration of the retinal vessels by tumor infiltrates. **C,** Vitreous aspirate from the same eye demonstrates the characteristic tumor-cell clumping of carcinoma.

breast cancer in only 3% of patients, but the eye was the first site of metastatic disease in 16% of patients in this study, many of whom had been in remission for years.

For some patients, however, there is no history of systemic malignancy. Various studies have shown that in patients in whom an ocular metastatic lesion(s) was diagnosed, the ocular lesion was the first manifestation of cancer in about 30% of cases; that is, 30% of patients with an ocular metastatic lesion have an unknown primary tumor at the time of the ocular diagnosis. This is especially true of patients with ocular metastasis from lung cancer. A study of 194 patients with uveal metastases from lung carcinoma demonstrated that diagnosis of the uveal metastasis preceded the diagnosis of primary lung cancer in nearly half of the patients (44%). Thus, any patient with an amelanotic fundus mass suspected of representing metastases should be referred for a thorough systemic evaluation, including imaging of the breast, chest, abdomen, and pelvis. Suspicious lesions identified on systemic evaluation often require biopsy before further management can be determined.

Fine-needle aspiration biopsy (FNAB) of the choroidal lesion may be helpful in rare cases when the diagnosis cannot be established by noninvasive procedures. Although metastatic tumors may recapitulate the histology of the primary tumor, they are often less differentiated. For this reason, special histochemical and immunohistochemical stains facilitate the diagnosis of metastatic tumors. Although it may not be possible to narrow the differential to just 1 primary tumor type, FNAB with appropriate special studies may reduce the list to a few likely primary sites. In addition, FNAB may be helpful even when the primary cancer site is known. For example, breast cancer may demonstrate a change in receptor status during metastatic spread that warrants biopsy of new metastatic disease and often changes the therapeutic options for the patient. Communication between the patient's ophthalmologist and medical oncologist is paramount throughout the diagnostic workup.

> Demirci H, Shields CL, Chao AN, Shields JA. Uveal metastasis from breast cancer in 264 patients. *Am J Ophthalmol.* 2003;136(2):264–271.
> Shah SU, Mashayekhi A, Shields CL, et al. Uveal metastasis from lung cancer: clinical features, treatment, and outcome in 194 patients. *Ophthalmology.* 2014;121(1):352–357.

Prognosis

A diagnosis of an ocular metastasis is typically associated with a poor prognosis for survival because widespread dissemination of the primary tumor has typically already occurred. In 1 report, survival time after a diagnosis of metastasis to the uvea ranged from 1 to 67 months, depending on the primary cancer type. Overall, the average survival of patients with ocular metastases is less than 1 year. Although the overall survival rate for women with breast cancer has improved, patients with breast carcinoma metastatic to the uvea have historically survived an average of 9–13 months after the metastasis was detected. The 5-year survival rate in patients with metastatic ocular disease in patients with breast cancer is approximately 25% across studies. In patients with ocular metastases from lung carcinoma, survival time is typically shorter, with about half of patients deceased at 1 year.

Treatment

The goal in ophthalmologic management of ocular metastases is preservation or restoration of vision whenever possible and palliation of pain. Radical surgical procedures and treatments with risks that exceed the desired benefits should be carefully considered in the context of the patient's overall health status. All treatment should be coordinated with the patient's primary oncologist and should reflect the goals of the overall care plan.

Indications for ocular treatment include

- decreased vision
- pain
- diplopia
- severe ocular proptosis
- the patient's age and health status
- the condition of the fellow eye

Careful workup and systemic imaging help determine the treatment plan. In patients manifesting metastases in the eye alone, local therapeutic modalities may be sufficient, allowing conservation of visual function with minimal systemic morbidity. When ocular metastases are concurrent with widespread metastatic disease, systemic chemotherapy alone or in combination with local therapy is reasonable.

In patients with susceptible tumors, systemic chemotherapy or hormonal therapy may induce a prompt response in the ocular lesion as well. Choroidal metastatic lesions have been noted to respond well to targeted systemic chemotherapies in some cases. In such patients, no additional ocular treatment may be indicated. However, when vision is endangered by choroidal metastases despite the systemic therapy, additional forms of local therapy, such as external beam radiotherapy (EBRT), brachytherapy, photodynamic therapy, or transpupillary thermotherapy, may be indicated. Radiotherapy is frequently associated with rapid improvement of the patient's symptoms, along with resolution of exudative retinal detachment and often direct reduction in tumor size. Possible adverse effects of the radiation include cataract, radiation retinopathy, and radiation optic neuropathy. Ocular surface irritation and dry eye are expected and should be aggressively treated, because they can cause significant discomfort. In some cases, enucleation is performed because of severe, unrelenting pain.

Cohen VML. Ocular metastases. *Eye (Lond)*. 2013;27(2):137–141.

Jardel P, Sauerwein W, Olivier T, et al. Management of choroidal metastases. *Cancer Treat Rev*. 2014;40(10):1119–1128.

Direct Intraocular Extension

In contrast to intraocular metastases, direct extension of extraocular tumors into the eye is rare because the sclera is usually an effective barrier to such invasion. Intraocular extension occurs most commonly with conjunctival squamous cell carcinoma and less frequently with conjunctival melanoma and basal cell carcinoma of the eyelid. Only a small minority of carcinomas of the conjunctiva penetrate the globe, and these are often aggressive variants of squamous cell carcinoma: mucoepidermoid, adenoid, and spindle cell carcinoma. These neoplasms usually recur several times after local excision before they invade the eye. For more information on conjunctival tumors, see BCSC Section 8, *External Disease and Cornea*.

Lymphoid Tumors

Ocular lymphomas are typically a non-Hodgkin B-cell type; in rare cases, they are T-cell lymphomas. They may arise in different parts of the eye, expressing various clinical manifestations, and their nomenclature is as varied as the areas of anatomical involvement. Ocular lymphomas can be classified as *primary vitreoretinal lymphoma (PVRL)*, *primary uveal lymphoma*, *primary ocular adnexal lymphoma*, and *secondary lymphoma* from systemic disease. PVRL is often associated with primary central nervous system lymphoma (PCNSL); in fact, it is considered a variant of PCNSL with overlapping cytologic and clinical features.

Primary Vitreoretinal Lymphoma

See BCSC Section 12, *Retina and Vitreous*, for further discussion of PVRL.

Clinical evaluation

PVRL is a non-Hodgkin diffuse large B-cell lymphoma (DLBCL) and is the most aggressive ocular lymphoma. Ocular signs and symptoms may occur before, concurrently with, or subsequent to CNS disease. PVRL is considered a masquerade syndrome because it simulates many diagnoses, most commonly posterior uveitis, particularly when the eye is involved first. In patients older than 50 years with an onset of bilateral posterior uveitis, PVRL should be considered in the differential diagnosis. Although 30% of patients present with unilateral involvement, delayed involvement of the second eye occurs in approximately 85% of patients. Approximately 25% of patients with PCNSL will develop PVRL eventually, and at least 60% of patients who present with PVRL will develop CNS disease.

Patients with PVRL often report decreased vision and floaters. They present with diffuse vitreous cells and haze, which may be associated with deep subretinal and/or sub-RPE yellow-white infiltrates (Fig 19-10). Often, fine details of the retina are obscured by the density of the vitritis. Retinal vasculitis and/or vascular occlusion may be noted. The RPE may reveal characteristic clumping overlying the sub-RPE infiltrates (see Chapter 9, Fig 9-14). Anterior chamber reaction may be absent or minimal. See the discussion of cytologic findings of PVRL in Chapter 9.

Imaging

In patients with PVRL, fluorescein angiographic findings can vary; however, typically hypofluorescent spots are persistent from the early to late frames of the angiogram. The spots are thought to be secondary to tumor-cell aggregates between Bruch membrane and the RPE, which do not absorb fluorescein due to an intact overlying cell membrane. Hypofluorescent window defects may also be present because of damaged RPE. Indocyanine green (ICG) angiography is rarely indicated for PVRL but may show hypocyanescent spots. Ultrasonographic examination may reveal discrete nodular or placoid infiltration of the subretinal

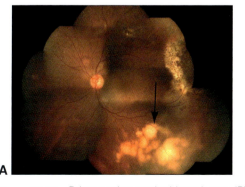
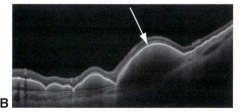

Figure 19-10 Primary vitreoretinal lymphoma (PVRL). **A,** Fundus photograph of a patient with PVRL shows extensive subretinal deposits *(arrow)*. **B,** OCT over the surface of the subretinal infiltrates *(arrow)*. *(Courtesy of Swathi Kaliki, MD.)*

space, associated retinal detachment, and vitreous syneresis with increased reflectivity. Although ocular coherence tomography (OCT) findings are not diagnostic, amorphous nodular lesions at the level of the RPE may be visible on OCT. If a diagnosis of PVRL is suspected, consultation with a neurologist and/or an oncologist should be considered, coupled with CNS imaging studies and lumbar puncture. Diagnostic vitrectomy is often performed to confirm PVRL even when the CNS imaging and/or cerebrospinal fluid analysis reveals lymphoma.

Pathologic studies

Diagnostic confirmation of ocular involvement requires sampling of the vitreous and, when appropriate, the subretinal space. Coordinated presurgical planning with the ophthalmic pathologist regarding sample handling is critical to clarify all the steps needed for obtaining a vitreous specimen and transporting it to the pathology laboratory; expedited transport to the laboratory is important to ensure cell viability. The staff at the pathology laboratory to which the vitreous sample is submitted must be skilled in the processing of small-volume cytologic specimens and experienced in the cytologic evaluation of vitreous samples. If the laboratory staff lacks the skills to process these samples, a second biopsy may be required after cells have reaccumulated in the vitreous. Even in cases in which the biopsy and laboratory evaluation are executed as planned, the diagnosis may be elusive. After consultation with the pathologist, diagnostic pars plana vitrectomy can be performed to obtain the vitreous specimen. When a subretinal nodule is accessible in a region of the retina that is unlikely to compromise visual function, subretinal aspiration of the lesion can be done.

The methodology for evaluation of the aqueous, vitreous, and subretinal specimens depends on the laboratory. Possible methods of pathologic analysis for lymphoma include

- cytopathology (see Chapter 9, Fig 9-14D), including immunohistochemical studies for characterization of the cells
- flow cytometry
- polymerase chain reaction for immunoglobulin H(IgH) gene rearrangements
- the ratio of interleukin 10 to interleukin 6
- *MYD88* variant studies

See Chapter 2 for a discussion of some of these methods. A diagnosis of large B-cell lymphoma is confirmed by specimens with atypical, large lymphoid cells (Fig 19-11) and characteristic cell surface markers.

Demerci H, Rao RC, Elner VM, et al. Aqueous humor–derived *MYD88* L265P mutation analysis in vitreoretinal lymphoma: a potential less invasive method for diagnosis and treatment response assessment. *Ophthalmol Retina*. 2023;7(2):189–195.

Treatment

In general, high-dose intravenous methotrexate is used to treat patients with PCNSL and may also be effective for treatment of PVRL. When there is only ocular involvement, intravitreal injections of methotrexate or rituximab or EBRT are usually employed. When there is minimal response of the ocular disease after systemic therapy for the CNS disease (the blood–ocular barrier may limit penetration of chemotherapeutic agents into the eye), these modalities may be used in addition to high-dose intravenous methotrexate.

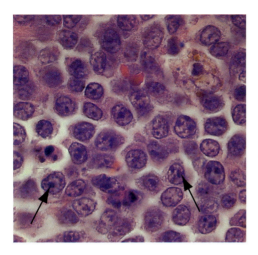

Figure 19-11 Histology image of large cell lymphoma reveals nuclear atypia with irregular nuclear contours and prominent nucleoli *(arrows)* of these neoplastic lymphoid cells, which were obtained by fine-needle aspiration biopsy.

There is no consensus as to whether irradiation of the affected eye using fractionated EBRT is more efficacious for the treatment of intraocular lymphoma than intravitreal injection of methotrexate or rituximab. Although radiotherapy may induce ocular remission, the tumor can recur, and further irradiation places the patient at risk for vision loss due to radiation retinopathy. Intravitreal injection of methotrexate or rituximab tends to produce very good local tumor response and low ocular recurrence rates; however, cystoid macular edema, keratopathy, and uveitis are potential adverse effects.

CNS or systemic lymphoma is treated by a medical oncologist in parallel with treatment for the intraocular disease.

Prognosis

Although the prognosis for patients with PVRL is poor, particularly in those with CNS involvement, advances in early diagnosis have produced a cohort of long-term survivors. Serial follow-up with the ophthalmologist and an experienced medical oncologist is critical in the management of this disease. Patients with PCNSL without ocular involvement should be observed longitudinally by an experienced ophthalmologist for possible ocular involvement, even after remission of the CNS disease.

> Habot-Wilner Z, Frenkel S, Pe'er J. Efficacy and safety of methotrexate for vitreo-retinal lymphoma—20 years of experience. *Br J Haematol.* 2021;194(1):92–100.
> Kim MM, Dabaja BS, Medeiros J, et al. Survival outcomes of primary intraocular lymphoma: a single-institution experience. *Am J Clin Oncol.* 2016;39(2):109–113.
> Soussain C, Malaise D, Cassoux N. Primary vitreoretinal lymphoma: a diagnostic and management challenge. *Blood.* 2021;138(17):1519–1534.

Primary Uveal Lymphoma

Many cases of uveal lymphoid infiltration, formerly known as *reactive lymphoid hyperplasia,* are now recognized as low-grade extranodal marginal zone B-cell lymphomas (EMZLs; formerly known as B-cell marginal zone mucosa-associated lymphoid tissue [MALT] lymphomas) of the uveal tract. Primary uveal lymphoma, though also a form of intraocular lymphoma, is distinct from PVRL (discussed in the previous section). These lesions, which typically present in patients in the sixth decade of life, can occur in any part of the uveal tract (Fig 19-12). There is an overlap between uveal lymphoma and similar lymphoid proliferations in the conjunctiva and orbit, termed *ocular adnexal lymphoma*. For information on the pathology of ocular adnexal lymphoma, see Chapter 4 (for conjunctival lymphoma) and Chapter 13 (for orbital lymphoma).

Clinical evaluation

Patients with uveal lymphoma typically report painless, progressive vision loss. Ophthalmoscopically, the presence of multifocal creamy-yellow amelanotic choroidal lesions tends to be most helpful in establishing the diagnosis (see Fig 19-12B). Although similar lesions may be visible in eyes with PVRL, those lesions are located between the RPE and Bruch membrane and *not* in the choroid. Associated subretinal fluid is present in some eyes, and diffuse uveal thickening is common. Secondary glaucoma may be present. Frequently, the delay between the onset of symptoms and diagnostic intervention is significant.

This rare disorder is characterized pathologically by localized or diffuse infiltration of the uveal tract by relatively mature lymphoid cells. Clinically, this condition can simulate posterior uveal melanoma, metastatic uveal carcinoma, sympathetic ophthalmia, Vogt-Koyanagi-Harada syndrome, and posterior scleritis. Proptosis of the affected eye may occur in a small proportion of patients who develop simultaneous episcleral orbital infiltration.

> Aronow ME, Portell CA, Sweetenham JW, Singh AD. Uveal lymphoma: clinical features, diagnostic studies, treatment selection, and outcomes. *Ophthalmology*. 2014;121(1): 334–341.

Imaging

In patients with uveal lymphoma involving the choroid, ICG angiography provides superior characterization than fluorescein angiography, which depicts variable findings. Classically, multiple scattered hypocyanescent lesions that correspond to the area of choroidal infiltration by the lymphoma are present. EDI-OCT reveals placoid or irregular lesions and thickening of the inner choroid (see Fig 19-12D), often associated with subretinal fluid. B-scan ultrasonography, the modality of choice for evaluation of choroidal lymphoma, typically reveals diffuse, homogeneous choroidal thickening with associated secondary retinal detachment. A pathognomonic feature of uveal lymphoma is crescent-shaped areas of acoustically hollow extrascleral extension (see Fig 19-12E).

Pathologic studies

Biopsy should be targeted to the most accessible tissue. When extraocular involvement is present, biopsy of the involved conjunctiva or orbit may be considered. For isolated uveal involvement, FNAB or pars plana vitrectomy with biopsy may be indicated. Histologic evaluation reveals dense lymphoid infiltrates. Coordination with the ophthalmic pathologist is crucial because appropriate specimen handling and cell marker studies increase the likelihood of establishing a diagnosis.

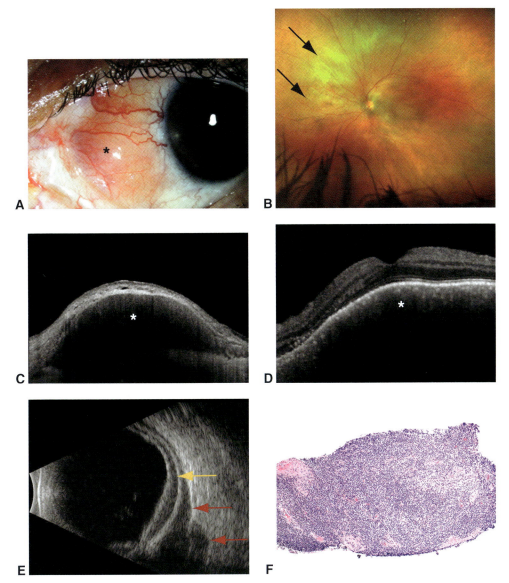

Figure 19-12 Uveal lymphoma, with concomitant ocular adnexal involvement. **A,** Slit-lamp photograph of a raised pink-orange "salmon patch" conjunctival lesion *(asterisk)* shows B-cell lymphoma. **B,** Multifocal creamy-yellow amelanotic choroidal lesions are visible ophthalmoscopically *(arrows)*. **C,** Anterior segment OCT of the conjunctival lesion demonstrates a homogeneous subepithelial mass *(asterisk)*. **D,** OCT through the macula reveals a diffusely thickened and irregular choroid *(asterisk)*. **E,** B-scan ultrasonography shows a diffusely thickened choroid *(yellow arrow)* and crescentic, extrascleral lucencies *(red arrows)* that are pathognomonic for uveal lymphoma and represent extraocular collections of lymphoid cells. **F,** Histologic examination of the conjunctival biopsy specimen demonstrates a monomorphic sheet of small lymphocytes consistent with extranodal marginal zone B-cell lymphoma, as determined with additional special pathologic studies. *(Courtesy of Jesse L. Berry, MD.)*

Treatment

Historically, eyes with uveal lymphoid infiltration were generally managed by enucleation. Current management strategies emphasize globe-conserving therapy aimed at vision preservation. Early intervention with low-dose ocular and orbital fractionated EBRT may definitively manage the disease.

Prognosis

The prognosis for survival is excellent for patients with uveal lymphomas; unlike PVRL, these are typically low-grade lymphomas. Early intervention appears to improve the chances of preservation of vision, which appears related to primary tumor location and secondary sequelae, including exudative retinal detachment or dysfunction from chronic tissue infiltration.

Secondary Involvement of Systemic Lymphoma

Ocular lymphoma may represent metastasis from systemic disease.

Clinical evaluation

The presentation of ocular involvement in systemic lymphoma can vary. Features may include uveitis; infiltration of any portion of the uveal tract; or a discrete mass of the conjunctiva, eyelid, or orbit. Diagnostic biopsy is performed on the most accessible region of the eye where a large amount of tissue can be obtained. Ideally, the pathologist is able to compare the results of the ocular biopsy with those of biopsies from other sites.

Treatment

The type of treatment is dictated by the type of lymphoma and extent of disease; when the site of tumor involvement is new, restaging of the lymphoma may be necessary. Treatment modalities may include systemic chemotherapy, orbital radiation, or bone marrow transplantation. Such cases are managed in collaboration with a medical oncologist.

Ocular Manifestations of Leukemia

Ocular manifestations of leukemia are common, occurring in as many as 80% of eyes from patients with the disease examined at autopsy. Clinical studies have documented ophthalmic findings in as many as 40% of patients when leukemia is diagnosed. Patients may be asymptomatic, or they may report blurred or decreased vision.

Clinically, the retina is the most commonly affected intraocular structure. Leukemic retinopathy is characterized by intraretinal and subhyaloid hemorrhages, hard exudates, cotton-wool spots, and white-centered retinal hemorrhages, also known as pseudo–Roth spots (Fig 19-13). (Classically, white-centered hemorrhages associated with endocarditis are termed *Roth spots;* they may be called *pseudo–Roth spots* when associated with other diseases.) In patients with leukemia, these findings are usually the result of associated anemia, hyperviscosity, and/or thrombocytopenia. True leukemic infiltrates are less common and appear as yellow-white deposits in the retina and the subretinal space. Perivascular leukemic infiltrates produce gray-white streaks in the retina. Vitreous involvement by leukemia is rare

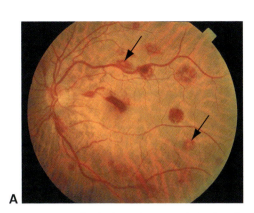 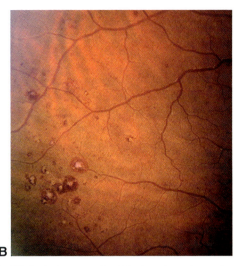

Figure 19-13 Retinal involvement in leukemia. **A,** Clinical photograph of leukemic retinopathy demonstrates scattered intraretinal hemorrhages, some of which have white centers *(arrows).* **B,** White-centered hemorrhages, also known as *pseudo–Roth spots. (Part A courtesy of Robert H. Rosa Jr, MD; part B courtesy of Jacob Pe'er, MD.)*

and most often results from direct extension via retinal hemorrhage. If necessary, a diagnostic vitrectomy can be performed to establish a diagnosis.

Although the retina is the most affected ocular structure clinically, histologic studies show that the uveal tract is more commonly affected by leukemia than is the retina. The uveal tract may serve as a "sanctuary site" for leukemic cells, making the eye more likely to be a site of recurrent disease. Choroidal infiltrates may be difficult to detect with indirect ophthalmoscopy; they may be better detected on ultrasonography as diffuse thickening of the choroid. Serous retinal detachments may overlie these infiltrates.

Leukemic involvement of the iris manifests as a diffuse thickening with loss of the iris crypts, and small nodules may be seen at the margin of the pupil in some cases. Leukemic cells may invade the anterior chamber, forming a pseudohypopyon. Infiltration of the angle by these cells can give rise to secondary glaucoma.

Patients with leukemic infiltration of the optic nerve (Fig 19-14) may present with severe vision loss and optic nerve edema. One or both eyes may be affected. This is an ophthalmic emergency that requires immediate treatment to preserve as much vision as possible. Systemic imaging, CNS assessment including lumbar puncture with cytology, and bone marrow evaluation are necessary to confirm the diagnosis. Urgent EBRT to the optic nerves is typically used to treat these patients, along with combined systemic and intrathecal chemotherapy.

Leukemic infiltrates may also involve the orbital soft tissue, with resultant proptosis. When these rare tumors occur, they have a predilection for the lateral and medial walls of the orbit. On direct visualization, the tumors appear to have a greenish hue. Because they are solid masses of granulocytic precursors, including myeloblasts and myelocytes from myelogenous leukemias, these tumors are sometimes referred to as *granulocytic sarcomas* or *chloromas.* However, the term *granulocytic sarcoma* is a misnomer, as this tumor is not a true sarcoma.

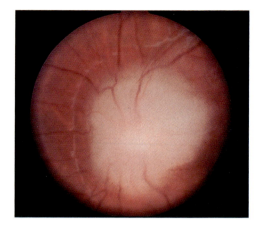

Figure 19-14 Leukemic infiltration of the optic nerve, which represents an ophthalmic emergency. *(Courtesy of Robert H. Rosa Jr, MD.)*

Ocular involvement in patients with leukemia may be found at initial diagnosis or relapse of leukemia; treatment typically consists of systemic chemotherapy. Depending on the ocular response to the systemic treatment, the patient may be treated with low-dose radiation to the eye; however, this should be undertaken with caution as it may limit future use of radiation therapy. The exception is patients with optic nerve infiltration with acute vision loss, for which radiotherapy is mandatory for treatment, as previously discussed. The prognosis for vision depends on the patient's particular subtype of leukemia and the extent of the ocular involvement.

Talcott KE, Garg RJ, Garg SJ. Ophthalmic manifestations of leukemia. *Curr Opin Ophthalmol.* 2016;27(6):545–551.

Additional Materials and Resources

Related Academy Materials

The American Academy of Ophthalmology is dedicated to providing a wealth of high-quality clinical education resources for ophthalmologists.

Print Publications and Electronic Products

For a complete listing of Academy clinical education products, including the BCSC Self-Assessment Program, visit our online store at aao.org/store. Or call Customer Service at 866.561.8558 (toll free, US only) or +1 415.561.8540, Monday through Friday, between 8:00 AM and 5:00 PM (PST).

Online Resources

Visit the Ocular Pathology and Oncology page on the **Ophthalmic News and Education (ONE®) Network** (aao.org/ocular-pathology-oncology) to find relevant videos, podcasts, webinars, online courses, journal articles, practice guidelines, self-assessment quizzes, images, and more. The ONE Network is a free Academy-member benefit.

The *Pathology Atlas* (aao.org/education/resident-course/pathology-atlas) is a comprehensive resource of microscopy images from the field contributed by ophthalmic pathologists, covering ocular anatomy and ophthalmic diseases and conditions. It also offers videos and interactive case studies.

The **Residents page** on the ONE Network (aao.org/residents) offers resident-specific content, including courses, videos, flashcards, and OKAP and Board Exam study tools.

The **Resident Knowledge Exchange** (resident-exchange.aao.org) provides peer-generated study materials, including flash cards, mnemonics, and presentations that offer unique perspectives on complex concepts.

Find comprehensive **resources for diversity, equity, inclusion, and accessibility** in ophthalmology on the ONE Network at aao.org/education/diversity-and-inclusion-education.

Access free, trusted articles and content with the Academy's collaborative online encyclopedia, **EyeWiki**, at aao.org/eyewiki.

Get mobile access to *The Wills Eye Manual* and *EyeWiki*, watch the latest 1-minute videos, listen to recent podcast episodes, challenge yourself with weekly Diagnose This activities, and set up alerts for clinical updates relevant to you with the free **AAO Ophthalmic Education app.** Download today: search for "AAO Ophthalmic Education" in the Apple app store or in Google Play.

Basic Texts and Additional Resources

American Academy of Ophthalmology. *Pathology Atlas*. aao.org/education/resident-course/pathology-atlas

Biscotti CV, Singh AD, eds. *FNA Cytology of Ophthalmic Tumors*. Karger; 2012. Monographs in Clinical Cytology; vol. 21.

Cummings TJ. *Ophthalmic Pathology: A Concise Guide*. Springer-Verlag; 2013.

Dutton JJ. *Atlas of Clinical and Surgical Orbital Anatomy*. 3rd ed. Elsevier; 2024.

Eagle RC Jr. *Eye Pathology: An Atlas and Text*. 3rd ed. Lippincott Williams & Wilkins; 2017.

Folberg R, Chévez-Barrios P, Lin AY, Milman T. *Tumors of the Eye and Ocular Adnexa*. American Registry of Pathology; 2021. *Atlases of Tumor and Non-Tumor Pathology*; series 5; vol. 3.

Grossniklaus HE, Bergstrom C, Baker Hubbard G, Wells JR, Singh AD, eds. *Pocket Guide to Ocular Oncology and Pathology*. Springer-Verlag; 2012.

Heegaard S, Grossniklaus HE, eds. *Eye Pathology: An Illustrated Guide*. Springer-Verlag; 2015.

Karcioglu ZA, ed. *Orbital Tumors: Diagnosis and Treatment*. 2nd ed. Springer-Verlag; 2015.

Naumann GOH, Holbach L, Kruse FE, eds. *Applied Pathology for Ophthalmic Microsurgeons*. Springer-Verlag; 2008.

Roberts F, Thum CK. *Lee's Ophthalmic Histopathology*. 4th ed. Springer; 2021.

Shields JA, Shields CL. *Eyelid, Conjunctival, and Orbital Tumors: An Atlas and Textbook*. 3rd ed. Wolters Kluwer; 2015.

Shields JA, Shields CL. *Intraocular Tumors: An Atlas and Textbook*. 3rd ed. Lippincott Williams & Wilkins; 2015.

Spencer WH, ed. *Ophthalmic Pathology: An Atlas and Textbook*. 4th ed. Elsevier/Saunders; 1996.

WHO Classification of Tumours Editorial Board. *WHO Classification of Tumours of the Eye*. 5th ed. International Agency for Research on Cancer; 2023. *WHO Classification of Tumours Series;* vol. 13. https://tumourclassification.iarc.who.int/chapters/7

Yanoff M, Sassani JW. *Ocular Pathology*. 8th ed. Elsevier; 2020.

Requesting Continuing Medical Education Credit

The American Academy of Ophthalmology is accredited by the Accreditation Council for Continuing Medical Education (ACCME) to provide continuing medical education for physicians.

The American Academy of Ophthalmology designates this enduring material for a maximum of 10 *AMA PRA Category 1 Credits*™. Physicians should claim only the credit commensurate with the extent of their participation in the activity.

To claim *AMA PRA Category 1 Credits*™ upon completion of this activity, learners must demonstrate appropriate knowledge and participation in the activity by taking the posttest for Section 4 and achieving a score of 80% or higher.

To take the posttest and request CME credit online:

1. Go to aao.org/education/cme-central and log in.
2. Click on "Claim CME Credit and View My CME Transcript" and then "Report AAO Credits."
3. Select the appropriate media type and then the Academy activity. You will be directed to the posttest.
4. Once you have passed the test with a score of 80% or higher, you will be directed to your transcript. *If you are not an Academy member, you will be able to print out a certificate of participation once you have passed the test.*

CME expiration date: June 1, 2027. *AMA PRA Category 1 Credits*™ may be claimed only once between June 1, 2024 (original release date), and the expiration date.

For assistance, contact the Academy's Customer Service department at 866.561.8558 (US only) or +1 415.561.8540 between 8:00 am and 5:00 pm (PST), Monday through Friday, or send an e-mail to customer_service@aao.org.

Study Questions

Please note that these questions are not part of your CME reporting process. They are provided here for your own educational use and for identification of any professional practice gaps. The required CME posttest is available online (see "Requesting Continuing Medical Education Credit"). Following the questions are answers with discussions. Although a concerted effort has been made to avoid ambiguity and redundancy in these questions, the authors recognize that differences of opinion may occur regarding the "best" answer. The discussions are provided to demonstrate the rationale used to derive the answer. They may also be helpful in confirming that your approach to the problem was correct or, if necessary, in fixing the principle in your memory. The Section 4 faculty thanks the Resident Self-Assessment Committee for developing these self-assessment questions and the discussions that follow.

1. What is the histologic description of a hamartoma?
    a. normal mature tissue at an abnormal location
    b. abnormal mature tissue at a normal location
    c. abnormal tissue derived from all 3 embryonic germ cell layers
    d. stereotypic, monotonous new growth of a specific tissue phenotype

2. What tissue is responsible for bone formation in phthisis bulbi?
    a. cataractous lens
    b. dystrophic calcification of Bowman layer
    c. gliotic and serously detached retina
    d. metaplasia of the retinal pigment epithelium (RPE)

3. What are the main features of the most used fixative?
    a. dyes tissues to allow visualization
    b. quickly penetrates tissues to preserve proteins and glycogen
    c. stabilizes proteins, lipids, and carbohydrates and prevents enzymatic destruction
    d. supports cell viability in biological samples

4. Which immunohistochemical stain is helpful in identifying lesions that arise from cells with a melanocytic origin?
    a. actin
    b. CD20
    c. Melan A
    d. pancytokeratin

5. Which layer of the cornea is not replaced when it is destroyed?

    a. Bowman layer

    b. Descemet membrane

    c. epithelium

    d. stroma

6. What type of cells in the retina proliferate in response to trauma?

    a. fibroblasts

    b. ganglion cells

    c. glial cells

    d. photoreceptors

7. Which is the most characteristic description of the histologic findings in a pterygium?

    a. acute inflammation

    b. elastotic degeneration

    c. eosinophilic deposits

    d. nuclear atypia

8. What are the histologic findings of complexion-associated melanosis?

    a. increased melanin production by melanocytes; no appreciable change in the number or morphology of melanocytes

    b. proliferation of melanocytes with cellular enlargement

    c. proliferation of melanocytes with hyperchromatic nucleoli

    d. proliferation of melanocytes arranged in nests

9. An ophthalmologist performs a slit-lamp examination of a male patient and notes aggregates of translucent, golden-brown spheroidal deposits in the interpalpebral superficial cornea in both eyes. A histologic stain for what material may be helpful in visualizing the deposits?

    a. amyloid

    b. calcium

    c. elastin

    d. glycosaminoglycan

10. On gonioscopy, which anatomical landmark marks the termination of Descemet membrane?

    a. iris root

    b. Schwalbe line

    c. scleral spur

    d. trabecular meshwork

11. Polymorphisms in what gene are associated with pseudoexfoliation syndrome?
    a. *FOXC1*
    b. *LOXL1*
    c. *PAX6*
    d. *PITX2*

12. Which histologic feature best explains the opaque appearance of the sclera?
    a. loose fibrovascular tissue
    b. presence of melanocytes
    c. sparse vascularization
    d. variable collagen orientation

13. Where in the lens are new cortical fibers produced?
    a. anterior capsule
    b. equator
    c. nucleus
    d. posterior capsule

14. Which histologic findings characterize the inflammation in eyes with phacoantigenic uveitis?
    a. central nidus of degenerating material surrounded by concentric layers of inflammatory cells
    b. deposition of abnormal protein on the lens zonular fibers
    c. protein-laden histiocytes clogging the trabecular meshwork
    d. sequestration of bacteria within the lens capsule

15. What degenerative lens change is caused by migration of lens epithelium followed by enlargement or swelling of those epithelial cells?
    a. cortical cataract
    b. duplication cataract
    c. nuclear sclerosis
    d. posterior subcapsular cataract

16. What type of developmental lens anomaly is associated with focal, internally directed excrescences of the lens capsule?
    a. congenital aphakia
    b. epicapsular star
    c. lens coloboma
    d. posterior lenticonus

17. What is the most prominent cell type that is found in eyes with vitritis associated with bacterial endophthalmitis?
    a. eosinophils
    b. epithelioid histiocytes
    c. neutrophils
    d. T and B lymphocytes

18. What is the composition of asteroid bodies in the vitreous?
    a. amyloid
    b. calcium
    c. cholesterol
    d. hyaline

19. Which primary cellular element is observed histologically in the periretinal membranes found in proliferative vitreoretinopathy?
    a. amacrine cells
    b. bipolar cells
    c. choroidal melanocytes
    d. RPE cells

20. What fundus finding is associated with Gardner syndrome?
    a. combined hamartoma of the retina and RPE
    b. congenital hypertrophy of the RPE
    c. hyperplasia of the RPE
    d. osseous metaplasia of the RPE

21. An area of peripheral retina demonstrates discontinuity of the internal limiting membrane, an overlying pocket of liquefied vitreous, focal sclerosis of retinal vessels, and condensation and adherence of vitreous at the margins of the lesion. What is the diagnosis?
    a. cystoid degeneration
    b. lattice degeneration
    c. paving-stone degeneration
    d. typical degenerative retinoschisis

22. What determines iris color?
    a. melanin granules in the anterior stromal melanocytes
    b. melanin granules in the posterior pigment epithelium
    c. thickness of the anterior stromal layer
    d. thickness of the posterior pigment epithelial layer

23. What is the predominant cell type found in Dalen-Fuchs nodules?
    a. eosinophils
    b. histiocytes
    c. neutrophils
    d. RPE cells

24. What is the most likely location for metastasis from uveal melanoma?
    a. bone
    b. brain
    c. liver
    d. lung

25. A 13-year-old patient presents with redness of the right eye; constant epiphora; and umbilicated, nodular, waxy lesions on the eyelid margin. Which kind of conjunctivitis does this patient most likely have?
    a. bacterial
    b. follicular
    c. giant papillary
    d. pseudomembranous

26. What is the most common form of basal cell carcinoma?
    a. morpheaform
    b. multicentric
    c. nodular
    d. pigmented

27. Keratoacanthoma is a variant of which other eyelid malignancy?
    a. basal cell carcinoma
    b. melanoma
    c. sebaceous carcinoma
    d. squamous cell carcinoma

28. A 70-year-old woman with a recurrent chalazion is referred to an ophthalmologist. She has an erythematous, nodular lesion on her upper eyelid. On closer examination, the ophthalmologist notes associated eyelash loss. What is the appropriate management of this lesion?
    a. Mohs micrographic surgery
    b. observation for change in size
    c. warm compresses and topical antibiotic ointment
    d. wide local excision with permanent margins

29. What is the typical mode of spread of adenoid cystic carcinoma of the lacrimal gland?
    a. hematologic metastasis
    b. local invasion
    c. lymphatic metastasis
    d. perineural invasion

30. What abnormality of embryologic development is responsible for the formation of optic nerve colobomas?
    a. failed induction of the surface ectoderm lens placode
    b. failure of neural crest differentiation
    c. incomplete closure of the embryonic fissure
    d. incomplete regression of the primary vitreous

31. What imaging modality is most helpful in assessing an iris melanoma that involves the angle?
    a. anterior segment optical coherence tomography (AS-OCT)
    b. computed tomography (CT) of the orbit
    c. fluorescein angiography of the iris
    d. high-frequency ultrasonography

32. What is the characteristic ultrasonography finding associated with circumscribed choroidal hemangiomas?
    a. acoustic hollowness
    b. choroidal excavation
    c. high internal reflectivity
    d. not visible on ultrasonography

33. Medulloepitheliomas are primary neuroepithelial tumors that most commonly arise in what part of the eye?
    a. choroid
    b. ciliary body
    c. optic nerve
    d. retina

34. What growth pattern of retinoblastoma is most likely to cause a serous retinal detachment?
    a. diffuse anterior
    b. diffuse infiltrative
    c. endophytic
    d. exophytic

35. What genetic alteration causes retinoblastoma (RB) to develop?
    a. complete loss of 1 copy of the *RB1* gene
    b. pathogenic variations in both copies of the *RB1* gene
    c. reciprocal rearrangement involving chromosome 13
    d. trisomy of the long arm of chromosome 13

36. Clinically, which intraocular structure is most commonly affected in patients with leukemia?
    a. iris
    b. optic nerve
    c. retina
    d. vitreous

Answers

1. **b.** Hamartomas are developmental anomalies that comprise both hypertrophy (abnormal size) and hyperplasia (abnormal amount) of mature tissue in a normal location. A choristoma consists of normal, mature tissue at an abnormal location and can contain 1 or 2 embryonic germ layers. A teratoma is a tumor that consists of a proliferation of tissue derived from all 3 embryonic germ cell layers. A neoplasm is a stereotypic, often monotonous new growth of a specific tissue phenotype.

2. **d.** Phthisis bulbi is defined as atrophy, shrinkage, and disorganization of the eye and intraocular contents. The globe becomes hypotonous and smaller, and it assumes a squared-off configuration as a result of the influence of the 4 rectus muscles. In the end stage of this process, osseous metaplasia of the retinal pigment epithelium (RPE) with bone formation may be a prominent feature. Over the course of this degenerative process, the lens becomes cataractous; extensive dystrophic calcification of Bowman layer, lens, retina, and drusen usually occurs; and the retina atrophies and becomes separated from the RPE due to serous fluid accumulation, but none of these cause bone formation.

3. **c.** Formalin is the most used fixative. It is a 10% neutral-buffered formalin solution that stabilizes proteins, lipids, and carbohydrates and prevents enzymatic destruction of the tissue by crosslinking proteins. Histochemical and immunohistochemical stains are used to stain tissue sections for visualization under the microscope. Glutaraldehyde fixative is used for electron microscopy; its fast penetration of tissues preserves proteins and glycogen and provides preservation of structures such as microtubules and smooth endoplasmic reticulum. Roswell Park Memorial Institute medium is a cell culture medium that supports cell viability in biological samples. It is not a fixative and is instead used when laboratory testing requires fresh specimens.

4. **c.** A given cell type can express specific antigens, a property that pathologists use to identify cell type or cell of origin, typically in tumors. Immunohistochemical staining is a common method used to detect specific antigens. The process typically involves using a primary antibody to bind to a specific antigen in or on the cell surface, and a secondary antibody linked to a chromogen that binds to the primary antibody. A specific antigen can be identified using this method, and depending on the antigen profile, the specific cell type can be ascertained. Melan A is used for diagnosis of tumors of melanocytic origin. Pancytokeratin is used for diagnosis of epithelial tumors. CD antigens are used for subtyping white blood cells, particularly lymphocytes. Actin is used for diagnosis of smooth muscle or skeletal muscle.

5. **a.** Bowman layer is not replaced when it is incised or destroyed. The wound healing response of the cornea is distinct due to its unique attributes. The corneal epithelium can regenerate itself rapidly. If a thin layer of anterior corneal stroma is lost with the abrasion, epithelial cells will fill the shallow crater, forming a facet. Corneal stromal healing occurs via the process of fibrosis. Stromal keratocytes (fibroblast-like cells) are activated and eventually migrate across the wound, laying down collagen and fibronectin. Activated corneal endothelial cells can deposit a new layer of Descemet membrane.

6. **c.** The retina is made of terminally differentiated cells that typically do not regenerate when injured. Because the retina is part of the central nervous system (CNS), glial cells (eg, Müller cells, astrocytes), rather than fibroblasts, proliferate in response to retinal

trauma. Ganglion cells and photoreceptors are not a part of the healing response of the retina.

7. **b.** Histologic examination of a pterygium typically reveals elastotic degeneration, fibrosis, and variable degrees of chronic inflammation, as well as prominent blood vessels that correlate with the vascularity seen clinically. The overlying epithelium may exhibit mild squamous metaplasia. Eosinophilic deposits are characteristic histologic findings of amyloid deposition. Nuclear atypia is a finding in conjunctival squamous intraepithelial neoplasia.

8. **a.** Complexion-associated melanosis (CAM) (also called benign epithelial melanosis, racial melanosis, and primary conjunctival melanosis) appears as bilateral flat patches of brown pigmentation with irregular margins, typically involving the bulbar conjunctiva in individuals with dark skin pigmentation. Streaks and whorls of melanotic pigmentation may extend onto the peripheral cornea, a condition called striate melanokeratosis. The caruncle and palpebral conjunctiva may also be involved. Histologically, pigmentation is limited to increased melanin in the epithelial cells while the epithelial melanocytes are normal in number or mildly increased in number and appear morphologically normal. Cellular enlargement, hyperchromatic nucleoli, and nesting are characteristics of melanocytes in primary acquired melanosis with atypia.

9. **c.** The clinical findings are characteristic of spheroidal degeneration (also known as actinic keratopathy, Labrador keratopathy, and climatic droplet keratopathy). This keratopathy is characterized by aggregates of translucent, golden-brown spheroidal deposits in the interpalpebral superficial cornea. The condition is generally bilateral and is more common in males. Smaller spheroidal deposits may mimic calcific band keratopathy; this phenomenon has been described as "actinic" band keratopathy. Histologic examination reveals irregular basophilic globules deep to the epithelium in the region of Bowman layer and the anterior stroma. Analogous to the actinic degeneration of collagen in pingueculae and pterygia, the deposits stain black with special stains for elastin, such as Verhoeff–van Gieson. Amyloid stains with Congo red stain; amyloid deposits are found in eyes with dystrophic and degenerative corneal disorders. Stains such as von Kossa and alizarin red are helpful in visualizing the calcium deposits present in calcific band keratopathy. Glycosaminoglycan deposits stain with Alcian blue or colloidal iron and are seen in eyes with macular corneal dystrophy.

10. **b.** The termination of Descemet membrane is manifested gonioscopically as the Schwalbe line. The iris root inserts into the anterior ciliary body posterior to the scleral spur. The scleral spur, a triangular extension of the sclera, appears gonioscopically as a white band and can be identified histologically by tracing the outermost longitudinal ciliary muscle fibers to its insertion. Anterior to the scleral spur in an internal indentation of the sclera are the trabecular meshwork and Schlemm canal.

11. **b.** Polymorphisms in the lysyl oxidase–like 1 gene *(LOXL1)* are associated with pseudoexfoliation syndrome. Lysyl oxidase is a pivotal enzyme in extracellular matrix formation; it catalyzes covalent crosslinking of collagen and elastin. Pathogenic variants in *FOXC1* and *PITX2* are associated with Axenfeld-Rieger syndrome. Pathogenic variants in *PAX6* are associated with various developmental abnormalities, such as aniridia and Peters anomaly.

12. **d.** In comparison to the collagen lamellae of the corneal stroma, scleral collagen fibers are thicker and more variable in thickness and orientation, resulting in the opaque appearance of the sclera. Loose fibrovascular tissue is present in the episcleral and lamina fusca

layers but does not contribute to the opacity of the sclera. Melanocytes are found in the lamina fusca, a delicate fibrovascular layer that binds the uveal tract to the sclera. The sparse vascularization of the scleral stroma also does not contribute to scleral opacity.

13. **b.** In the equatorial, or bow, region of the lens, the epithelial cells move centrally, elongate, produce crystalline proteins, lose organelles, and transform into lens fibers. As the lens epithelial cells differentiate, new fibers are continuously laid down over existing fibers, compacting them in a lamellar arrangement. Thus, the outermost fibers, derived from postnatally differentiated lens epithelial cells, are the most recently formed and make up the cortex of the lens, while older layers are located toward the center. The center of the lens contains the oldest fibers, the embryonic and fetal lens nucleus. Lens fibers are densely compacted in the nucleus. The anterior capsule is lined by a monolayer of lens epithelial cells. The posterior lens capsule is normally devoid of epithelial cells.

14. **a.** Phacoantigenic uveitis is a type of lens-induced intraocular inflammation. Histologically, an eye with phacoantigenic uveitis shows a central nidus of degenerating lens material surrounded by concentric layers of inflammatory cells. Deposition of abnormal protein on lens zonular fibers occurs in pseudoexfoliation syndrome. In phacolytic uveitis, lens proteins are engulfed by histiocytes; these histiocytes may clog the trabecular meshwork or induce an inflammatory response in the angle. In *Cutibacterium acnes* endophthalmitis, bacteria are sequestered within the lens capsule.

15. **d.** Posterior subcapsular cataract is a result of epithelial disarray at the lens equator, followed by posterior migration of the lens epithelial cells along the posterior capsule. As the cells migrate, they can enlarge significantly. These swollen cells are called Wedl, or bladder, cells. If these cells involve the center of the lens in the visual axis, they can cause a significant decrease in vision. The earliest sign of focal cortical degeneration is hydropic swelling of the lens fibers with decreased intensity of eosinophilic staining. Eosinophilic globules (morgagnian globules) accumulate in the slitlike spaces between the lens fibers. Ultimately, the entire cortex can become liquefied, allowing the nucleus to sink and the capsule to wrinkle. A duplication cataract occurs after injury to the lens epithelium. The lens epithelium undergoes metaplasia and forms anterior subcapsular fibrous plaques. After the resolution of the inciting stimulus, the lens epithelium may produce another capsule that surrounds the fibrous plaque. Nuclear cataracts take on a subtle homogeneous eosinophilic appearance and are thus difficult to assess histologically.

16. **d.** Histologically, the cataracts in eyes with posterior lenticonus display focal, internally directed excrescences of the lens capsule. Congenital aphakia results from failed lens induction from the surface ectoderm during embryogenesis. Primary lens coloboma is a wedge-shaped defect or indentation of the lens periphery that can be associated with faulty development of zonular fibers. An epicapsular star is a common remnant of tunica vasculosa lentis.

17. **c.** Because the vitreous is relatively acellular and completely avascular, it is not often a primary site of inflammation. However, it can become secondarily involved in inflammation of adjacent tissues. Vitritis refers to the presence of white blood cells, either benign or malignant, in the vitreous. In eyes with bacterial endophthalmitis, the vitritis consists predominantly of an infiltrate of neutrophils (polymorphonuclear leukocytes), which are acute inflammatory cells. Eosinophils are commonly associated with allergic reactions but may be present in some chronic inflammatory processes, such as sympathetic ophthalmia. Epithelioid histiocytes represent granulomatous inflammation. T and B lymphocytes

are chronic inflammatory cells. The vitreous infiltrate in noninfectious uveitis is typically composed of chronic inflammatory cells, including lymphocytes.

18. **b.** Histologically, asteroid bodies are rounded structures, typically attached to vitreous fibrils. The bodies are basophilic with hematoxylin and eosin stain and are usually positive with stains for calcium such as alizarin red and von Kossa. Occasionally, they will be surrounded by a foreign body giant cell reaction, but the condition is not generally associated with vitreous inflammation. Studies have shown that asteroid bodies are composed of complex lipids and also have a component with structural and elemental similarity to hydroxyapatite, a calcium phosphate complex. Asteroid bodies are not composed of amyloid or hyaline. Cholesterol deposits from chronic vitreous hemorrhage (synchysis scintillans) can clinically mimic asteroid hyalosis.

19. **d.** Proliferative vitreoretinopathy (PVR) membranes form as a result of the proliferation of RPE cells and other cellular elements, including glial cells (Müller cells, fibrous astrocytes), histiocytes, fibroblasts, and myofibroblasts. Amacrine and bipolar cells, which are found in the inner nuclear layer of the retina, are not a major constituent of PVR membranes. Unless there is rupture of Bruch membrane, choroidal melanocytes do not have access to the subretinal space or vitreous cavity and therefore are not typically observed in PVR membranes.

20. **c.** RPE lesions mimicking congenital hypertrophy of the RPE may be present in Gardner syndrome, a subtype of familial adenomatous polyposis. Histologic study of the RPE changes in Gardner syndrome reveals that these changes are more consistent with hyperplasia of the RPE than with hypertrophy. A combined hamartoma of the retina and RPE is characterized by disorganized glial tissue and vascular proliferation. RPE cells can undergo osseous metaplasia in an unrepaired or unresolved retinal detachment.

21. **b.** Histologically, the most important features of lattice degeneration are discontinuity of the internal limiting membrane of the retina, an overlying pocket of liquefied vitreous, focal sclerosis of retinal vessels, condensation and adherence of vitreous at the margins of the lesions, and variable degrees of atrophy of the inner layers of the retina. Cystoid degeneration involves the development of cystoid spaces in the outer plexiform layer of the retina. Paving-stone degeneration involves focal occlusion of the choriocapillaris and shows atrophy of the outer retinal layers and RPE with adhesion of the retina to Bruch membrane. Typical degenerative retinoschisis is caused by coalescence of cystoid spaces in the outer plexiform layer.

22. **a.** Iris color is determined by the number and size of melanin granules in the anterior stromal melanocytes. Melanin granules in the posterior pigment epithelium, the thickness of the anterior stromal layer, and the thickness of the posterior pigment epithelial layer do not determine iris color.

23. **b.** Dalen-Fuchs nodules are accumulations of epithelioid histiocytes and lymphocytes between the RPE and Bruch membrane (ie, sub-RPE granulomas) and may be seen in some cases of sympathetic ophthalmia. Eosinophils can be found in the uveal tract stroma in sympathetic ophthalmia. Neutrophils are not typical in sympathetic ophthalmia.

24. **c.** Metastases from choroidal melanoma almost invariably result from the hematogenous spread of melanoma to the liver; in more than 95% of tumor-related deaths there is liver involvement. In as many as one-third of tumor-related deaths, the liver is the sole site of metastasis. Other relatively frequent sites—generally after liver metastasis—include the lungs, bones, and skin. Among patients with metastases who were autopsied, liver

involvement was identified in 100%, whereas lung involvement was identified in 50%. Brain metastases from uveal melanoma are rare.

25. **b.** Molluscum contagiosum, which is caused by a member of the poxvirus family, is characterized by dome-shaped, waxy epidermal nodules with central umbilication. If present on the eyelid margin, these nodules may cause a secondary follicular conjunctivitis. Histologically, the lesions are distinctive in appearance with prominent Henderson-Patterson (molluscum) bodies, which are intracytoplasmic eosinophilic inclusions containing virus particles. Bacterial conjunctivitis, giant papillary conjunctivitis, and pseudomembranous conjunctivitis are generally not associated with molluscum lesions.

26. **c.** Basal cell carcinoma (BCC) is the most common malignant tumor of the eyelid, accounting for more than 90% of all malignant eyelid tumors. Nodular BCC (the most common type) is a slow-growing, slightly elevated lesion, often with ulceration and pearly, raised, rolled edges. Infiltrating BCC is the second most common type that frequently has a morpheaform, or sclerosing appearance. Only a small percentage of BCCs are pigmented or multicentric.

27. **d.** Keratoacanthoma is a rapidly growing dome-shaped nodular squamous epithelial proliferation with a keratin-filled crater that has the potential for spontaneous involution. Strong evidence supports the idea that keratoacanthomas are a variant of a well-differentiated squamous cell carcinoma. Histologically, keratoacanthomas show a cup-shaped invagination of well-differentiated squamous cells with parakeratin in the center. Basal cell carcinoma arises from epithelial cells of the epidermis or hair follicle stem cells and shows basaloid or hair follicle infundibular differentiation. Melanoma is a tumor of melanocytic lineage. Sebaceous carcinoma is a neoplasm of sebaceous gland lineage.

28. **d.** Eyelid erythema, loss of eyelashes, ulceration, and irregular eyelid thickening are clinical signs of sebaceous carcinoma. Sebaceous carcinoma can masquerade as an atypical chalazion that does not respond to warm compresses and topical antibiotic ointment and recurs following incision and drainage. When diagnosis of sebaceous carcinoma is suspected, observation for growth is not appropriate. Treatment of sebaceous carcinoma typically involves wide local excision of the tumor. Widespread conjunctival epithelial involvement or deeply invasive tumors may require exenteration. Because it can be difficult to identify pagetoid spread or sebaceous carcinoma in situ on frozen sections, permanent sections are generally considered more reliable for evaluation of surgical resection margins than frozen sections of margins or Mohs technique. Before definitive excision, staging of tumor extent via routine processing of multiple small "map" biopsies, typically of the conjunctiva, may afford a more accurate assessment of the extent of spread of the carcinoma, guiding management. Adjunctive therapies for sebaceous carcinoma include the use of topical chemotherapy, cryotherapy, radiotherapy, and systemic chemotherapy.

29. **d.** Although all of the modes of spread listed are possible, the typical mode is perineural invasion. Adenoid cystic carcinoma harbors a particular neurotropism for sensory nerves, traveling along the nerves to gain entry into the skull base.

30. **c.** Optic nerve coloboma results from defective closure of the posterior embryonic or choroidal fissure. It is often inferonasal and may be associated with colobomatous defects of the retina and choroid, ciliary body, and iris. Early in embryogenesis, the optic vesicle influences the specific region of head ectoderm to form the lens placode. The lens placode later invaginates to become the lens vesicle. Failure of induction of the lens placode

results in primary congenital aphakia. Failure of neural crest differentiation profoundly affects development of the ocular structures and results in cryptophthalmos (absence of the eyelids, conjunctiva, cornea, and lens). The primary vitreous consists of fibrillar material, mesenchymal cells, and vascular components. The tunica vasculosa lentis surrounds the developing lens, the vasa hyaloidea propria is a network of vessels posterior to the lens, and the hyaloid artery connects the vasa hyaloidea propria to the optic nerve. Failure of these vessels to regress results in persistent fetal vasculature and often microphthalmia.

31. **d.** Iris nevi are first evaluated with slit-lamp biomicroscopy coupled with gonioscopy. The clinician should pay specific attention to lesions involving the angle to rule out a ciliary body tumor, because the most important differential diagnosis is iris or ciliary body melanoma. When angle involvement is detected on clinical examination, high-frequency ultrasound biomicroscopy (UBM) is helpful in the evaluation of lesions that involve the angle as it can depict a ciliary body component. Investigations of the utility of anterior segment optical coherence tomography (AS-OCT) for iris lesions are ongoing, but this imaging modality has not replaced UBM. Iris fluorescein angiography may document intrinsic vascularity; however, this finding has limited value in confirming the diagnosis. Given the small size of these lesions, CT does not play a role in the evaluation of these lesions. CT or MRI may be performed to assist in planning for brachytherapy if an iris nevus has converted to a melanoma but is not needed for benign lesions.

32. **c.** Ancillary diagnostic studies are helpful in evaluating both circumscribed and diffuse choroidal hemangiomas. A-scan ultrasonography (echography) shows a high-amplitude initial echo and high-amplitude broad internal echoes (high internal reflectivity). B-scan ultrasonography reveals localized or diffuse choroidal thickening with prominent internal reflections but without choroidal excavation or acoustic shadowing. Choroidal melanomas exhibit low to medium internal reflectivity, acoustic hollowness, and choroidal excavation.

33. **b.** Medulloepithelioma usually appears as an off-white mass arising from the ciliary body. In rare instances, this lesion has also been documented in the retina and optic nerve. In most cases, this type of tumor becomes clinically evident in children aged 4–12 years, but it may also occur in adults. This lesion can mimic retinoblastoma and can cause glaucoma. Medulloepitheliomas do not arise from choroidal stroma.

34. **c.** Retinoblastoma begins as a round, translucent, gray to white tumor in the retina. As the tumor enlarges, necrotic foci with calcification emerge, giving the tumor its characteristic chalky white appearance. Larger tumors contain dilated, tortuous intratumoral vessels. Exophytic tumors grow beneath the retina and often involve serous retinal detachment. As these tumors grow, the retinal detachment may become extensive, obscuring clear visualization of the tumor. Endophytic tumors grow on the retinal surface and into the vitreous cavity; therefore, blood vessels may be more difficult to discern in these tumors. Exophytic tumors cause subretinal seeding, whereas endophytic retinoblastoma tumors are more likely to yield vitreous seeds; these cells shed from the tumor remain viable in the vitreous and may eventually become implanted in ocular tissue, resulting in new tumor foci within the eye. Diffuse infiltrative retinoblastoma is a rare subtype of retinoblastoma that infiltrates the retina with minimal tumefaction and generally does not cause retinal detachment. A diffuse anterior retinoblastoma is a variant of diffuse infiltrative retinoblastoma with high propensity for anterior segment and anterior chamber involvement.

35. **b.** Retinoblastoma (RB) is almost always caused by loss of a functional retinoblastoma tumor suppressor protein due to pathogenic alterations in both copies (ie, "2 hits") of the tumor suppressor gene *RB1*, located on the long arm of chromosome 13 at locus 14 (13q14). The *RB1* gene in retinoblastoma can be involved by a wide range of genetic alterations, including single nucleotide variations, small insertions and deletions, large deletions, and duplications. There can be 2 separate pathogenic alterations or loss of heterozygosity. Much less commonly, retinoblastoma occurs as a result of structural alterations in chromosome 13, such as deletion (but not a rearrangement) of the long arm of chromosome 13 that includes the *RB1* gene; the deletion causes a loss of an allele similar to the "first hit." Epigenetic events, including methylation and inactivation of the *RB1* promoter may also lead to retinoblastoma tumorigenesis. Fewer than 5% of retinoblastomas are caused by genetic alterations in other genes, such as *MYCN* protooncogene amplification.

36. **c.** Clinically, the retina is the most commonly affected intraocular structure. Leukemic retinopathy is characterized by intraretinal and subhyaloid hemorrhages, hard exudates, cotton-wool spots, and white-centered retinal hemorrhages, also known as pseudo–Roth spots. In leukemia, these findings are usually the result of associated anemia, hyperviscosity, and/or thrombocytopenia. True leukemic infiltrates are less common and appear as yellow-white deposits in the retina and the subretinal space. Perivascular leukemic infiltrates produce gray-white streaks in the retina. Vitreous involvement by leukemia is rare and most often results from direct extension via retinal hemorrhage. If necessary, a diagnostic vitrectomy can be performed to establish a diagnosis. Optic nerve involvement by leukemia is infrequent. Although the retina is the most commonly affected ocular structure clinically, histologic studies have shown that the uveal tract is more commonly affected by leukemia than is the retina. The optic nerve and uveal tract may serve as a "sanctuary site" for leukemic cells, making the eye more likely to be a site of recurrent disease.

Index

(*f* = figure; *t* = table)

A-scan ultrasonography, 322*f*, 323, 342*f*, 343, 360*f*, 387. *See also* Standardized ultrasonography
Abrasions, of cornea, 45, 192
Abscesses, 240, 271
Absolute ethanol or methanol, 23*t*
Abusive head trauma (AHT), 192–194, 193*f*, 194*f*
Acanthamoeba keratitis, 31*t*, 97–98, 98*f*
Acantholysis, 241, 249, 249*f*
Acanthosis, 241, 242, 248, 249*f*, 251*f*
Acanthosis nigricans, 250
ACC. *See* Adenoid cystic carcinoma
Accessory lacrimal glands of Krause, 240
Accessory lacrimal glands of Wolfring, 240
Acellular capillaries, 185, 187*f*, 189, 191
Actin, 39, 284, 284*f*
Actinic elastosis. *See* Solar (actinic) elastosis
Actinic keratitis, 101, 102, 103*f*
Actinic keratopathy. *See* Spheroidal degeneration
Actinic keratosis, 250, 251*f*
Actinomyces israelii, 273, 273*f*
Acute disseminated encephalomyelitis (ADEM), 293, 295
Acute retinal necrosis (ARN), 176, 177*f*
ADEM. *See* Acute disseminated encephalomyelitis
Adenoid cystic carcinoma (ACC), 17*f*, 274, 275*t*, 276–277, 277*f*
Adenomas and adenocarcinomas
 of ciliary body, 211, 212*f*, 213, 339–340
 classification, 17*t*
 of conjunctiva, 89, 89*f*
 of eyelids, 250*t*, 255–256, 256*f*
 of gastrointestinal system, 176, 250
 of lacrimal gland, 89, 89*f*, 274, 275*t*, 276–277, 276*f*, 277*f*
 of retina, 176, 213
 of retinal pigment epithelium, 339–340, 339*f*
Adenomatous polyposis coli gene *(APC)*, 176
Adenosquamous carcinoma, 72
Adenoviruses, 61
Adipocytic tumors, 286
Adipogenesis, 267
Adnexal appendages. *See* Hair follicles; Meibomian glands; Sebaceous glands; Sweat glands
Aflibercept, 186
Age-related calcific plaque, 136, 137*f*
Age-related macular degeneration (AMD)
 differential diagnosis, 181, 327, 328*f*
 overview, 194–199, 195*t*, 195*f*, 196*f*, 197*f*, 198*f*, 199*f*
 treatment, 344
AHT. *See* Abusive head trauma
AIDS/HIV infection, 72, 176
AJCC. *See* American Joint Committee on Cancer (AJCC) staging system
Albinism, 172, 173*f*
Alcian blue stain, 30*f*, 31*t*
ALH. *See* Atypical lymphoid hyperplasia
Alizarin red stain, 30*f*, 31*t*
Alkapton, 106

Alkaptonuria, 106
Allergic reactions, 9, 61
α-hemolytic strep, 99
Alport syndrome, 142–143
Alveolar rhabdomyosarcoma, 283–284
Amblyopia, 142, 172, 255
AMD. *See* Age-related macular degeneration
Amelanotic choroidal masses, 329, 329*t*, 342, 394, 395*f*
Amelanotic melanoma, 72, 238, 312*f*, 329*t*
Amelanotic nevus, 75–77
American Academy of Ophthalmology's Initiative in Vision Rehabilitation, 308
American Association of Cancer Research, 379
American Joint Committee on Cancer (AJCC) staging system
 about, 308
 for posterior uveal melanomas, 329, 331, 336
 for retinoblastoma, 308, 365
 on uveal melanoma, 232
Amiodarone, 106
Amyloidosis and amyloid deposits
 about, 160
 in conjunctiva, 68–69, 69*f*
 in cornea, 111, 113*f*, 115*f*, 116*t*
 in drusen, 196–197
 in eyelid, 246, 246*f*, 247*t*
 in orbit, 273
 in vitreous, 160–161, 162*f*
Angiofibroma, 282
Angioid streaks, 300
Angiomatosis, 343, 347
Angiomatosis retinae. *See* Retinal hemangioblastoma
Angiomatous tumors. *See* Vascular tumors
Angle-closure glaucoma, 123, 124*f*, 224, 319
Angle recession, traumatic, 50, 51*f*, 129
Aniridia, 218–219, 219*f*
Anisocoria, 355*t*
Anterior banded layer, 93
Anterior border layer, 216, 216*f*
Anterior chamber, 119–130
 degenerations, 122–129
  iridocorneal endothelial (ICE) syndrome, 122–123, 125*f*, 313*t*
  primary congenital glaucoma, 93
  secondary glaucoma, 124–129, 126*f*, 127*f*, 128*f*, 129*f*, 130*f*. *See also under* Glaucoma
 developmental anomalies, 120–122, 121*f*, 122*f*, 123*f*
 inflammation, 122, 124*f*, 176, 221
 neoplasia, 130, 130*f*, 230–231
 posterior uveal melanoma extension into, 319*f*, 320
 retinoblastoma and, 205–206, 205*f*, 359
 topography, 119–120, 120*f*, 216
 trauma, 127–129, 127*f*, 128*f*, 129*f*
Anterior chamber angle
 degenerations, 122–123, 125, 224
 developmental anomalies, 93, 94*f*, 121, 121*f*
 glaucoma and, 319
 inflammation, 122, 124*f*

419

iris melanoma extension into, 311, 313*f*
leukemia and, 397
neoplasia, 130, 130*f*
nevus extension of, 225
topography, 119, 120*f*
traumatic recession of, 50, 51*f*
Anterior lamella, of eyelids, 240
Anterior lens capsule
  degeneration, 124–126, 126*f*, 145–146, 146*f*
  depositions, 145
  developmental anomalies, 143
  topography, 140*f*, 141–142, 141*f*
  wound repair, 48
Anterior lenticonus, 142–143
Anterior lentiglobus, 142
Anterior optic nerve, 298
Anterior proliferative vitreoretinopathy (PVR), 53, 54*f*
Anterior segment dysgenesis, 93, 121–122, 122*f*, 123*f*
Anterior segment optical coherence tomography (AS-OCT), 73, 74*f*
Anterior subcapsular cataract, 48
Anterior subcapsular fibrous plaques, 146, 146*f*
Antibodies, for immunohistochemistry, 20, 33*f*, 36–39, 37*f*, 38*t*
Anti–vascular endothelial growth factor (VEGF), 186, 199, 334, 344, 350, 352
Antiviral drugs, 100
Antoni A and B patterns, 286, 287*f*
APC gene. *See* Adenomatous polyposis coli gene
Aphakia, 142, 157
Aphakia, congenital, 143
Apocrine glands (glands of Moll), 240, 241, 247, 266
Apocrine hidrocystoma, 247, 248*f*
Aqueous fluid samples, 23
Aqueous seeding, 372–373
Arachnoid sheath, 290, 290*f*, 291*f*, 303
Argyrosis, 145
ARM2/HTRA1 gene, 194
ARN. *See* Acute retinal necrosis
Array comparative genomic hybridization (CGH), 39
Arterial occlusions, 183, 183*f*, 185, 187–190, 188*f*, 190*f*. *See also* Ischemia, of retina
Arteriosclerosis, 190
Arteriovenous malformation (AVM), 345–347, 346*t*, 348*f*
Artifactitious clefts (laminations), 148, 149*f*
AS-OCT. *See* Anterior segment optical coherence tomography
Ascending optic atrophy, 298
Aspergillus spp, 97, 178, 272, 272*f*, 293
Asteroid bodies, 222, 223*f*
Asteroid hyalosis, 160
Astigmatism, 108, 320
Astrocytes
  macular holes and, 158, 159*f*
  optic atrophy and, 298
  of optic nerve, 290*t*, 291*f*
  of retina, 171
Astrocytic hamartoma, 363–364, 364*f*
Astrocytomas
  of optic nerve, 38*t*, 301–303, 303*f*
  of retina, 363–364, 363*f*
Atopy, 107

Atrophia bulbi, 15
Atypical lymphoid hyperplasia (ALH), 277–278
Avellino corneal dystrophy. *See* Granular corneal dystrophy type 2
AVM. *See* Arteriovenous malformation
Axenfeld anomaly, 123*f*
Axenfeld nerve loop, 132*f*
Axenfeld-Rieger syndrome, 121, 123*f*

B-cell lymphomas, 17*f*, 87–88, 88*f*, 162–164, 237, 279, 280*f*, 390–391, 393, 395*f*
B-cell marginal zone MALT lymphoma. *See* Extranodal marginal zone B-cell lymphoma
B cells, 10, 38*t*
B-scan ultrasonography. *See also* Standardized ultrasonography
  about, 323
  of lymphomas, 394, 395*f*
  of melanomas, 322*f*, 324*f*, 325
  of nevi, 321*f*
  for retinoblastoma, 358, 360*f*
  of secondary tumors, 386–387
  vascular tumors, 343
B&B stain. *See* Brown and Brenn (B&B) stain
B&H stain. *See* Brown and Hopps (B&H) stain
Bacterial infections. *See also specific bacteria*
  of conjunctiva, 61, 62*f*
  of cornea, 95, 95*f*, 99–100, 100*f*
  endophthalmitis, 143–144, 144*f*, 154, 155*f*, 372
  of eyelid, 242, 243*f*
  of lens, 143, 144*f*
  of optic nerve, 293
  of orbit and lacrimal drainage system, 271, 273, 273*f*
  of sclera, 134
  of vitreous, 154
Bacteroides spp, 271
"Bag of worms," 285, 285*f*
Balloon cells, 227, 228
Band keratopathy, 30*f*, 32*t*, 101–102, 102*f*
BAP1 (BRCA1-associated protein-1) gene, 39, 234, 234*t*, 316
Bartonella henselae, 64, 293
Bartonella quintana, 293
Basal cell carcinoma (BCC), of eyelid
  differential diagnosis, 256–258
  direct intraocular extension of, 390
  overview, 250–252, 250*t*, 251*f*, 252*f*
  specimen handling and processing, 34–35
Basal cell nevus syndrome, 250*t*
Basal laminar (cuticular) drusen, 195*t*
Basement membrane
  of anterior chamber. *See* Descemet membrane
  of conjunctiva, 57–58, 62, 62*f*, 72–73, 73*f*, 74*f*, 83*t*
  of cornea, 91, 92*f*, 104, 104*f*, 109, 110*f*, 192
  of lens, 139, 145
  of retinal pigment epithelium
    in age-related macular degeneration, 194
    diabetic intraocular changes, 192, 192*f*
    neoplasia, 181, 210–211, 212*f*
    topography, 172
  wound repair, 48
Basement membranes, staining of, 30*f*, 31*t*
Basophils, 9, 11*f*

BCC. *See* Basal cell carcinoma
BCOR gene, 209
Bear tracks, 326, 326*f*
"Beaten metal" appearance, of Descemet membrane, 113, 117*f*
Belzutifan, 350
Benign acquired melanosis. *See* Secondary acquired melanosis
Benign epithelial melanosis. *See* Complexion-associated melanosis
Benign intraepithelial dyskeratosis, 72
Benign lymphoid hyperplasia (reactive lymphoid hyperplasia), 86–88, 87*f*
Benign mixed tumor. *See* Pleomorphic adenoma
Benign neoplasia, classification of, 16–17, 17*f*
Berger space, 152*f*
Bergmeister papilla, 153, 154*f*, 291
Berlin edema. *See* Commotio retinae
β-blockers, 255, 344
β-pleated sheet, 160, 161*f*, 246
Bevacizumab, 186
Biopsies. *See* Specimen handling, processing, and testing
Bladder cells, 241, 242*f*
Blepharitis, 242
Blepharoconjunctivitis, 256, 257*f*
Blood staining, of cornea, 106, 106*f*
Blue cells, 258, 259*f*
Blue nevus, 77, 259
Blue tumor cells, 204, 204*f*, 211*f*. *See also* Retinoblastoma
Blunt trauma, to anterior chamber, 129
Boat-shaped hemorrhage, 186*f*
Bone marrow transplantation, 368, 396
Bones, metastases to, 330
Bonnet-Dechaume-Blanc syndrome. *See* Wyburn-Mason syndrome
Bony lesions of orbit, 286–288, 288*f*
Bony orbit. *See* Orbit and lacrimal drainage system
Bony tumors. *See* Osteomas
Borderline neoplastic proliferations, 16–17
Borrelia burgdorferi, 100, 293
"Bosselations," 276*f*
Botryoid variant, of rhabdomyosarcoma, 284
Bouin solution, 23*t*
Bowman layer
 degenerations, 18, 101*f*, 101–104, 102*f*, 103*f*, 105*f*
 diabetes and, 192
 dystrophies, 109–111, 111*f*, 112*f*
 ectatic disorders, 107*f*, 108
 inflammation, 95, 95*f*, 96*f*
 staining, 30*f*
 topography, 92, 92*f*
Bow region, of lens, 140*f*, 141
Brachytherapy
 for iris melanoma, 311
 for posterior uveal melanoma, 307, 333–336, 334*f*, 337
 for retinoblastoma, 371–372
 for secondary ocular tumors, 390
 for vascular tumors, 344, 350, 352
BRAF gene, 86
BRAO. *See* Branch retinal artery occlusion
Branch retinal artery occlusion (BRAO), 189

Branch retinal vein occlusion (BRVO), 189–190
BRCA1-associated protein-1 gene. *See* BAP1 (BRCA1-associated protein-1) gene
Breast, hamartomas of, 250*t*
Breast cancer
 metastases, 235, 250*t*, 288, 382, 383*t*, 384*f*, 387–389, 387*f*
 specimen handling and processing, 38*t*
Breslow thickness, 263
Brown and Brenn (B&B) stain, 31*t*
Brown and Hopps (B&H) stain, 31*t*
Bruch membrane
 choroidal melanoma and, 317*f*, 318–319
 degenerations, 181, 182*f*, 191, 191*f*, 194–199, 195*t*, 196*f*, 197*f*, 198*f*, 199*f*
 inflammation, 177*f*
 inflammation of uveal tract and, 221, 222*f*
 neoplasia of uveal tract and, 227, 230*f*, 233
 rupture of, 53–55
 staining, 31*t*
 topography, 168, 168*f*, 170*f*, 172, 218
 wound repair, 48–49
BRVO. *See* Branch retinal vein occlusion
Bulbar conjunctiva, 57, 58*f*, 66*f*
Bullae, 62*f*, 63, 104
Bullous hemorrhage, 186*f*
Bullous keratopathy, 103–105, 104*f*, 113, 117*f*
Busacca nodules, 222

Calcific band keratopathy, 101–102, 102*f*
Calcific drusen, 195*t*
Calcium deposits and calcification
 age-related, 136, 137*f*
 in astrocytomas, 363
 in lens, 148, 149*f*
 in optic nerve, 299–302, 300*f*, 304, 304*f*
 persistent fetal vasculature and, 362
 in retina, 204, 204*f*, 209, 355, 356*f*, 358, 360*f*, 374
 in vitreous, 160
Calcofluor white stain, 32*t*
Callender classification system (modified), 226, 229*t*, 231–232
CALT. *See* Conjunctiva-associated lymphoid tissue
CAM. *See* Complexion-associated melanosis
Canaliculitis, 272–273
Cancer Genome Atlas (TCGA) classification, 233–234, 234*t*
Candida albicans, 178
Candida spp, 97, 178
Candlewax drippings, of sarcoidosis, 222
Capillary hemangiomas. *See* Infantile hemangiomas
Capsule, of lens. *See* Lens capsule
Carbohydrate sulfotransferase 6 (*CHST6*) gene, 112, 116*t*
Carboplatin, 369–370
Carcinoma ex pleomorphic adenoma, 274
Carcinomas (general). *See also specific carcinomas*
 classification of, 17*f*, 17*t*, 381–390. *See also* Metastases
 specimen handling and processing, 30*f*, 32*t*, 34, 35*f*, 38*t*
Carney complex, 247*t*
Carotid occlusive disease, 183, 189
Caruncle, 58, 58*f*, 255, 256

Caseating granulomas, 12, 14*f,* 64, 293
Cataracts
    aniridia and, 219, 219*f*
    degenerations, 145–148, 145*f,* 146*f,* 147*f,* 148*f,* 149*f*
    developmental anomalies, 142–143
    diabetes and, 192
    glaucoma and, 125
    inflammation and, 144
    iris nevus and, 311
    of lens cortex, 147–148, 148*f,* 149*f*
    of lens epithelium, 145–147, 145*f,* 146*f,* 147*f*
    of lens nucleus, 148, 149*f*
    parasitic infections and, 363
    posterior uveal melanoma and, 320
    radiation and, 390
    retinoblastoma and, 355*t,* 362, 362*t*
    surgical complications, 103, 139
    trauma and, 48, 52–53
Cavernous hemangiomas, 8, 236, 275*t,* 281, 282*f,* 345, 346*t,* 347*f*
Cavernous optic atrophy, 31*t,* 298, 300*f*
Cavernous venous malformation, 275*t*
CCM1/KRIT1 gene, 345
CD3 markers, 279
CD20 markers, 279
CD antigens. *See* Cluster of differentiation (CD) antigens
cDNA (target), 41
Cellulitis, 242, 243*f,* 271, 283, 357*f*
Cemiplimab, 252
Central nervous system (CNS)
    cells of, 48, 290, 290*t,* 291*f*
    fungal infections spreading to, 272
    intraocular lymphoma extension to, 163, 163*f*
    leukemia and, 397
    lymphomas of, 390–391
    metastases, 382, 382*f*
    neoplasia of optic nerve and, 301
    neurosensory retina and, 48, 167
    retinoblastoma extension to, 358–359, 361*f,* 377
    tumors, 286
    vascular tumors of, 345, 350
Central retinal artery, 171, 189, 290*f*
Central retinal artery occlusion (CRAO), 185, 187–189, 188*f*
Central retinal vein, 290*f*
Central retinal vein occlusion (CRVO), 189–190, 190*f*
Cerebrospinal fluid, 291
CFH gene, 194
CGH. *See* Comparative genomic hybridization
Chalazion, 65–67, 244, 245*f,* 256, 257*f*
Chalcosis, 145
Chamber angle. *See* Anterior chamber angle
Chandler syndrome, 122
Charged-particle radiation, 333–335, 344
CHED. *See* Congenital hereditary endothelial dystrophy
Chemotherapy
    for leukemia, 398
    for lymphomas, 396
    for medulloepitheliomas, 364
    for posterior uveal melanoma, 335
    for retinoblastoma, 308, 368–373, 369*f,* 370*f*
    for sebaceous carcinoma, 258
    for secondary ocular tumors, 386*f,* 390
    for vitreous seeds, 370, 372–373
Cherry red spot, 187*f*
Children's Oncology Group (COG) clinical trials, 365, 371, 378
Chlamydia spp, 31*t,* 61, 62*f*
Chloromas, 397
Cholesterol crystals, 160
Cholesterol deposits, 53, 160, 173, 174*f,* 197, 362
Cholesterol emboli, 189
Choriocapillaris, 171–172, 181, 191, 191*f,* 197, 218, 218*f,* 221, 221*f,* 227
Chorioretinitis, 222, 223*f*. *See also* Toxoplasmic retinochoroiditis
Chorioretinitis sclopetaria, 55
Chorioretinopathy, 327, 328*f*
Choristomas
    of conjunctiva, 59, 60*f*
    of cornea, 93
    defined, 8, 59
    of lens, 241, 242*f*
Choroid. *See also* Choroidal neovascularization; Uveal tract
    blood supply, 171–172
    degenerations, 199, 200*f*
    detachment, 327
    developmental anomalies, 219–220, 291, 292*f,* 362*t*
    hemorrhage, 51, 52*f,* 53
    inflammation, 55, 55*f,* 178–179, 178*f,* 179*f,* 220, 221*f,* 222, 223*f*
    ischemia, 182, 183*f*
    neoplasia, 226–235
        amelanotic masses, 329, 329*t,* 342
        diabetes and, 191
        hemangiomas, 230, 230*f,* 233, 236, 236*f,* 319*f,* 320, 327, 341–345, 342*f,* 343*f*
        leukemia and, 397
        lymphomas and lymphoid proliferation, 164*f,* 165, 237, 237*f*
        melanocytomas, 326, 338
        melanomas, 228–234, 301, 314, 316, 317*f,* 318–320, 318*f*. *See also* Posterior uveal melanoma
        metastasis to, 234–235, 235*f*
        neural sheath tumors, 238, 238*f*
        nevus, 226–227, 228*f,* 314–316, 315*f,* 317*f,* 318, 324–325
        osteomas, 236–237, 237*f,* 288, 288*f,* 327, 328*f,* 342
        retinoblastoma extension, 206, 207*f,* 359, 371
        vascular tumors, 341–345, 342*f,* 343*f*
    rupture of, 53–55
    specimen handling and processing, 33*f*
    topography, 168*f,* 215, 216*f,* 217–218, 218*f*
    trauma to, 51, 52*f,* 53–55, 55*f*
    wound repair, 49
Choroidal neovascularization (CNV), 53–55, 186, 191, 195*f,* 197–199, 199*f,* 227, 314
    choroidal nevus and, 227, 314
    diabetes and, 191
    retinal degenerations, 186, 191, 195*f,* 197–199, 199*f*
    trauma-related, 53–55
Choroidal neovascular membranes (CNVMs), 198–199
Chromogens, 33*f,* 36–37, 37*f*

Chromogranin, 37f, 38t, 39, 258
CHRPE. *See* Congenital hypertrophy of the RPE
CHST6 gene. *See* Carbohydrate sulfotransferase 6 (*CHST6*) gene
Cilia. *See* Eyelashes
Ciliary arteries, 131, 132f
Ciliary body. *See also* Uveal tract
  degenerations, 224, 225f
  deposits and, 161
  developmental anomalies, 219–220
  diabetic changes, 192, 192f
  inflammation, 220
  neoplasia
    adenoma, 211, 212f, 213, 339–340
    leiomyoma, 238
    medulloepithelioma, 210, 364, 364f
    melanoma, 226, 228–234, 311, 314, 316, 319–320, 319f. *See also* Posterior uveal melanoma
    neurofibromas, 238
    nevus, 130, 130f, 314
    nodular hyperplasia, 211, 212f
  topography, 120f, 131, 140f, 157, 167–168, 215, 216f, 217, 217f
  trauma to, 50, 51f, 52f
  wound repair, 49
Ciliary epithelium
  diabetic changes, 192, 192f
  neoplasia, 209–211, 211f, 212f, 213, 339–340
  topography, 167–168, 217, 217f
Ciliary ganglion, 265
Ciliary muscle, 50, 119, 217, 217f
Ciliary nerves, 131, 132f
Ciliary pars plana, 140f
Ciliary pars plicata, 140f
Ciliochoroidal melanoma, 228
CIN. *See* Conjunctival intraepithelial neoplasia
Circular layer, of ciliary muscle, 217
Circulating tumor cells (CTCs), 19, 41–42
Circumferential perimacular folds, 192–193, 193f
Circumscribed choroidal hemangioma, 236, 236f, 341–345, 342f
Circumscribed iris nevus, 311
Climatic droplet keratopathy, 102, 103f
Cloquet canal. *See* Hyaloid canal
Clostridium spp, 271
Clouds (vitreous seed type), 206. *See also* Vitreous seeds
Cluster of differentiation (CD) antigens, 38t, 39
CME. *See* Cystoid macular edema
C-MIL. *See* Conjunctival melanocytic intraepithelial lesion (C-MIL) classification
C-MIN. *See* Conjunctival melanocytic intraepithelial neoplasia (C-MIN) scoring system
CMV. *See* Cytomegalovirus
CNS. *See* Central nervous system
CNV. *See* Choroidal neovascularization
CNVMs. *See* Choroidal neovascular membranes
Coats disease, 172–173, 174f, 356f, 360, 362, 363f
Coccidioidomycosis, 293
COG clinical trials. *See* Children's Oncology Group (COG) clinical trials
Cogan-Reese syndrome. *See* Iris nevus syndrome
COL4A3, *COL4A4*, and *COL4A5* genes, 142–143

Collaborative Ocular Melanoma Study (COMS), 307, 329–330, 330t, 333, 337–338
Collagen, orbital deposition of, 270
Collagen crosslinking (CXL), 108
Collagen genes, type IV, 142–143
Colloidal iron stain, 30f, 31t
Colobomas, 59, 133, 143, 219–220, 220f, 291, 292f, 362t
Combined hamartoma, 212–213, 212f, 339f, 340
Commotio retinae (Berlin edema), 53
Comparative genomic hybridization (CGH), 39
Complex choristomas, 59, 60f
Complexion-associated melanosis (CAM), 78, 79f, 80–81f, 82, 83t
Compound nevus, 76–77, 260, 260f
Computed tomography (CT)
  about, 323–324
  of posterior uveal melanoma, 323–324, 327, 330t, 334
  of retinoblastoma, 358
COMS. *See* Collaborative Ocular Melanoma Study
Congenital aphakia, 142
Congenital cataracts, 143
Congenital glaucoma, 93, 120–121, 121f, 136f
Congenital hereditary endothelial dystrophy (CHED), 114–115, 117f
Congenital hypertrophy of the RPE (CHRPE), 175–176, 175f, 213, 326–327, 326f
Congenital melanocytic nevus, 259
Congenital ocular melanocytosis, 313f, 313t, 314, 315f, 343
Congenital retinal arteriovenous malformation (AVM), 345–347, 346t, 348f
Congenital retinal macrovessel, 347, 348f
Congenital split nevus, 259, 260f
Congenital syphilis, 99–100, 100f
Congo red stain, 30f, 31t
Conjunctiva, 57–89
  about and overview, 57
  cysts, 266
  degenerations, 67–70, 68f, 69f, 70f
  developmental anomalies, 59, 60f, 76t
  hemorrhage, 69
  inflammation (conjunctivitis), 61–67, 63f, 64f, 78, 243, 244f
  lymphoma of, 394, 395f
  neoplasia, 70–89. *See also specific neoplasias*
    about and overview, 70
    carcinomas, 130
    differential diagnosis, 18
    glandular neoplasms, 89, 89f
    lymphoid lesions, 86–89, 87f, 88f
    melanocytic lesions and melanomas, 75–86, 76t, 77f, 78f, 79f, 80–81f, 83f, 85f, 86f, 263
    metastases to, 89
    other neoplasms, 89
    scleral involvement, 137
    squamous epithelial lesions, 67–68, 70–73, 71f, 73f, 74f
  retinoblastoma extension to, 359
  special testing and procedures, 23
  specimen handling and processing, 23, 26–28, 28f
  systemic malignancies and, 396
  topography, 57–59, 58f
  wound repair, 45

Conjunctiva-associated lymphoid tissue (CALT), 58
Conjunctival intraepithelial neoplasia (CIN), 72–73, 73*f*, 74*f*
Conjunctival melanocytic intraepithelial lesion (C-MIL) classification, 79*f*, 80–81*f*, 82, 83*t*
Conjunctival melanocytic intraepithelial neoplasia (C-MIN) scoring system, 79*f*, 80–81*f*, 82, 83*t*
Conjunctivitis, 61–67
  about and overview, 61
  acute *vs* chronic, 61
  follicular, 63, 63*f*, 64*f*
  granulomatous, 64–65, 65*f*, 66*f*
  infectious, 61, 62*f*, 64–65, 243, 244*f*
  noninfectious, 61–63, 62*f*
  papillary, 63, 63*f*, 64*f*
  pyogenic granuloma, 65–67, 66*f*
  secondary acquired melanosis and, 78
Conjunctivochalasis, 70
Constitutional melanosis. *See* Complexion-associated melanosis
Contact inhibition, 45
Contact lens wear, 97, 101
Copper deposits, 145
Corectopia, 121
Cornea
  about, 91
  abrasions, 45, 192
  degenerations, 100–105, 101*f*, 102*f*, 103*f*, 104*f*, 105*f*, 122–123
  depositions, 105–106, 106*f*
  deposits. *See* Cataracts
  developmental anomalies, 93–94, 94*f*
  dystrophies, 108–118
    classification system, 108–109
    Descemet membrane and endothelial, 113–118, 117*f*, 118*f*
    epithelial and subepithelial, 109, 110*f*
    epithelial–stromal *TGFB1*, 109–111, 111*f*, 112*f*, 113*f*, 114*f*, 115*f*
    stromal, 112–113, 116*f*, 116*t*
  ectatic disorders of, 106–108, 107*f*
  embryonic development, 93
  graft failure, 99, 104–105, 104*f*, 105*f*
  inflammation, 94–100, 95*f*, 96*f*, 98*f*, 99*f*, 100*f*. *See also* Keratitis
  neoplasia, 72, 118
  special testing and procedures, 23
  specimen handling and processing, 23
  staining, 30*f*, 31–32*t*
  topography, 91–93, 92*f*, 119, 120*f*
  ulcers, 45–46
  wound repair, 45–46, 46*f*, 47*f*, 48
Corneal button, 104*f*
Corneal deturgescence, 93
Corneal dystrophies, 30*f*, 31–32*t*
Corneal dystrophy of Bowman layer type I. *See* Reis-Bücklers corneal dystrophy
Corneal dystrophy of Bowman layer type II. *See* Thiel-Behnke corneal dystrophy
Corneal hydrops, 107*f*, 108
Corneal limbal stem cell deficiency, 219
Corneal macular dystrophy, 30*f*, 31*t*
Corneal melting, 100

Corneal pannus, 103, 103*f*, 104*f*, 104, 110–111, 112*f*
Cornea plana, 93, 94*f*
Cornea verticillata, 106
Cortex, of lens, 140*f*, 141, 147–148, 148*f*, 149*f*
Corticosteroid therapy, 97, 99, 271, 293, 297
Cotton-wool spots, 184, 189, 191, 387, 396
COVID-19, fungal infections and, 271
Cowden disease, 250*t*
CRAO. *See* Central retinal artery occlusion
Cribriform pattern of growth, 277, 277*f*
cRNA (target), 41
CRVO. *See* Central retinal vein occlusion
Cryotherapy
  for medulloepitheliomas, 364
  for retinoblastoma, 308, 354, 371
  sebaceous carcinoma treatment, 258
  for vascular tumors, 350, 352
Cryptococcosis, 293, 295*f*
Cryptophthalmos, 247*t*
Crystalline deposits, 148, 149*f*
Crystalline lens. *See* Lens (crystalline)
Crystalloid deposits, 110, 116*t*
CT. *See* Computed tomography
CTCs. *See* Circulating tumor cells
Cup-shaped lesion, 253, 254*f*
Curly collagen fibers, 111, 116*t*
Cutaneous melanoma, 262–263, 262*f*
Cutibacterium acnes endophthalmitis, 143, 144*f*
CXL. *See* Collagen crosslinking
Cyclodialysis, 50, 52*f*, 129
Cysticercosis, 272
Cystoid degeneration, 342
Cystoid macular edema (CME), 158, 159*f*, 171, 184, 185*f*, 190, 343–344, 352
Cystoid spaces
  corneal dystrophies, 110*f*
  optic atrophy, 298, 300*f*
  retinal degenerations, 179, 180*f*, 184, 184*f*, 185*f*, 190*f*
Cysts
  of conjunctiva, 266
  of cornea, 98*f*
  dermoid, 8, 93, 241, 266*f*, 267, 273
  of eyelid, 243, 247, 248*f*, 266
  of iris, 313*f*, 313*t*
  of orbit, 266–267, 266*f*, 272, 273
  with protozoal infection, 179, 179*f*
  retinal detachment sequelae, 181, 182*f*
  of sclera, 133
Cytoid bodies, 183, 184*f*
Cytokeratin 20 antibodies, 258, 259*f*
Cytokeratins, 38*t*, 39, 115
Cytokines, 335
Cytologic atypia, 80–81*f*, 82–84, 83*t*
Cytology fixatives, 19–20
Cytomegalovirus (CMV), 38*t*, 40, 176, 177*f*
Cytospin preparation, 33

Dacryoadenitis, 270
Dacryocystitis, 273, 288
Dacryolith, 273, 273*f*
Dacryops, 247
Dalen-Fuchs nodules, 221, 222*f*

DALK. *See* Deep anterior lamellar keratoplasty
Decapitation secretion, 240
Deep anterior lamellar keratoplasty (DALK), 92, 108, 115*f*
Degenerative pannus, 103, 103*f*
Degenerative retinoschisis, 179, 180*f*
"Delayed washout phenomenon," 342*f*, 343
DEM. *See* Diagnostic electron microscopy
Demodex folliculorum, 243
Demyelination of optic nerve, 293, 294*t*, 295, 295*f*
Dendrites, 95–97, 96*f*
Dendritic nevus cells (branching), 225
Dermal appendages. *See* Hair follicles; Meibomian glands; Sebaceous glands; Sweat glands
Dermal nevus, 260, 261*f*
Dermatomyositis, 247*t*
Dermis, of eyelids, 240, 240*f*
Dermoids (dermoid cysts)
 classification of, 8
 of cornea, 93
 of eyelid, 241
 of orbit, 266*f*, 267, 273
Dermolipomas, 59, 60*f*
Descemet membrane
 degenerations, 104, 105*f*
 developmental anomalies, 93, 94*f*, 121–122, 122*f*
 dystrophies, 112–118, 116*f*, 117*f*, 118*f*
 ectatic disorders, 107*f*, 108
 guttae and, 100, 112–114, 116*f*, 117*f*
 inflammation, 96*f*, 97, 98*f*, 100, 100*f*
 neoplasia, 207*f*
 rupture of, 50, 50*f*, 107*f*
 staining, 31*t*
 topography, 92*f*, 93, 119
 wound repair, 46, 47*f*, 50
Desmin, 38*t*, 39, 238, 284, 284*f*
Diabetes
 cornea and, 192
 fungal infections, 271
 optic nerve inflammation and, 293
 retinal ischemia and, 183, 185, 186*f*, 187*f*, 190–191, 191*f*
Diabetic choroidopathy, 191
Diabetic retinopathy, 186*f*, 187*f*, 190–191, 191*f*
Diagnostic electron microscopy (DEM), 42
DICER1 gene, 210
DICER1 syndrome, 364
Dichroism, 69
Differential diagnosis, 7*t*, 18
Diffuse choroidal hemangioma, 230, 230*f*, 233, 236, 319*f*, 320, 343–345, 343*f*
Diffuse choroidal melanoma, 230*f*, 233
Diffuse ciliary body melanoma. *See* Ring melanoma
Diffuse drusen, 195*f*, 197
Diffuse infiltrating retinoblastoma, 357–358
Diffuse iris nevus, 311, 313*f*, 313*t*, 315
Diffuse large B-cell lymphoma (DLBCL), 390–393
Diffuse photoreceptor dystrophies, 203, 203*f*
Diffuse scleritis, 133–134, 135*f*
Dilator muscle, 216, 216*f*, 224
Diode laser, 335
Direct immunofluorescence, 20, 23
Disciform keratitis, 96*f*, 97

Disease processes (general), 8–17. *See also specific eye structures*
 degenerations, 13–16
 developmental anomalies, 8
 dystrophies, 13
 inflammation, 7*t*, 8–13
 neoplasia, 16–17, 17*t*
Distichiasis, 241
DLBCL. *See* Diffuse large B-cell lymphoma
DNA, 39–41
DNA fragments (probes), 41
"Dot-and-blot" hemorrhage, 184, 186*f*
Down syndrome, 107
Drusen
 choroidal nevus and, 314, 315*f*, 321*f*, 324–325
 defined, 194–196
 degeneration and, 16
 macular degeneration and, 194–196
 neoplasia of choroid and, 227, 228*f*
 of optic nerve head, 299–301, 300*f*, 363
 types, 195*f*, 195*t*, 196*f*, 197*f*, 196–197
Dry (nonneovascular) age-related macular degeneration, 198, 198*f*
Dry eye, 101
Dua layer, 92
Ductal cysts, 247, 248*f*
Duplication cataract, 146, 146*f*
Dura, of optic nerve, 290, 290*f*, 291*f*, 295*f*, 301
Dust (vitreous seed type), 206. *See also* Vitreous seeds
Dutcher bodies, 280*f*
Dyscrasias, 246
Dyskeratosis, 72–73, 74*f*, 241, 250, 253
Dysplasia, of retina, 362*t*
Dysplastic nevus, 259
Dysplastic nevus syndrome, 316
Dystopia of globe, 265
Dystrophies. *See* Corneal dystrophies

EBM. *See* Epithelial basement membrane
EBMD. *See* Epithelial basement membrane dystrophy
EBRT. *See* External-beam radiotherapy
Eccrine hidrocystoma, 247
Echinococcus spp, 272
Echography. *See* Ultrasonography
Ectasias, 134, 136
Ectatic disorders, of cornea, 106–108, 107*f*
Ectropion uveae, 224, 224*f*, 310*f*, 311
"Eddies," 248, 249*f*
EDI-OCT. *See* Enhanced depth imaging optical coherence tomography
Ehlers-Danlos syndrome, 107
EK graft. *See* Endothelial keratoplasty (EK) graft
Electron microscopy, 42
Ellipsoid zone (EZ), of neurosensory retina, 169, 170*f*
ELM. *See* External limiting membrane
Elschnig pearls, 146, 147*f*
Embryonal rhabdomyosarcoma (botryoid variant), 283–284, 284*f*
Embryonic lens nucleus, 141
Emissary canals, 131, 132*f*, 215, 230, 231*f*, 319*f*
EMZL. *See* Extranodal marginal zone B-cell lymphoma
Encephalofacial angiomatosis (Sturge-Weber syndrome), 236, 343

Endophthalmitis, 143–144, 144f, 154, 155f, 178, 372
Endophytic retinoblastoma, 355, 356f, 357f
Endothelial keratoplasty (EK) graft, 104–105, 104f, 105f, 114
Endothelium
　of cornea
　　decomposition, 109, 110f
　　degenerations, 103–104
　　dystrophies, 103, 108–109, 110f, 112–115, 116f, 117f, 118f
　　graft failures and, 104–105, 104f
　　topography, 92f, 93
　　wound repair and, 46, 47f
Enhanced depth imaging optical coherence tomography (EDI-OCT), 321f, 323, 387, 394
Enterobacteriaceae, 95
Enucleation
　for choroidal melanoma, 307
　gross examination and dissection of, 24–25, 25f, 26f
　for lymphomas, 396
　for medulloepitheliomas, 364
　neovascularization and, 224
　outcome studies, 307
　for posterior uveal melanoma, 332–333
　processing and staining, 29f
　for retinoblastoma, 354, 368–369, 372, 374
　retinoblastoma management following, 208
　for uveal melanoma, 232, 236f
Eosinophils, 9, 11f
Epibulbar dermoids, 8, 59, 60f
Epidermal neoplasia, 248–253, 249f, 250t, 251f, 252f, 253f, 254f, 390. *See also* Squamous cell carcinoma
Epidermis, of eyelids, 240, 240f, 247
Epidermoid (inclusion) cysts, 247, 248f, 266, 273
Epiretinal membrane, 158, 159f
Episclera, 47, 131, 132f
Episcleral (Tenon) space, 59
Episcleral vessels. *See* Sentinel vessels
Episcleritis, 133
Epithelial basement membrane (EBM), 62f, 63, 72–73, 92f, 104, 104f, 192
Epithelial basement membrane dystrophy (EBMD), 109, 110f
Epithelial inclusion cysts, 69–70, 70f, 76, 77f
Epithelial ingrowth and downgrowth, 105, 105f
Epithelial–stromal *TGFB1* dystrophies, 108–111, 111f, 112f, 113f, 114f, 115f
Epithelial tumors, 17t
Epithelial whorling, 249
Epithelioid cells, 220–222, 221f, 222f, 223f, 225–226, 227f, 229t, 231–232
Epithelioid histiocytes, 12
Epithelioid melanoma, 231
Epithelium
　cataract formation and, 52–53
　of ciliary body, 217, 217f
　of conjunctiva, 57–58, 58f
　of cornea, 91, 92f, 108–111, 110f, 111f, 112f, 113, 113f, 117f
　of eyelid, 240, 244f
　of iris. *See* Iris pigment epithelium
　of lacrimal gland, 265
　of lens, 139, 140f, 141, 145f, 145–147, 146f, 147f, 241, 242f
　of retina. *See* Retinal pigment epithelium
　specimen handling and processing, 30f
　wound repair and, 43–46, 44f, 46f, 47f, 48–49
Epstein-Barr virus, 39, 100
Equilateral region. *See* Bow region, of lens
Erdheim-Chester disease, 245, 247t
Esophageal cancer, 386f
Essential iris atrophy, 122, 125f
Ethanol, 23t
Ethmoid bone, 265
Etoposide, 369–370
EUA. *See* Examination under anesthesia
Ewing sarcoma, 288
Examination under anesthesia (EUA), 355, 358, 368
Exciting (inciting) eye, 221
Exenteration, 335–336
Exfoliation syndrome, 124
Exogenous infections, 220
Exophthalmos. *See* Proptosis
Exophytic retinoblastoma, 355–357, 356f
Exposure keratitis, 267
Exposure keratopathy, 101
External-beam radiotherapy (EBRT)
　for leukemia, 397
　for lymphomas, 392–393, 396
　for posterior uveal melanoma, 335
　for retinoblastoma, 308, 372–373
　for secondary ocular tumors, 390
　for vascular tumors, 344, 350
External hordeolum, 242
External limiting membrane (ELM), 168f, 170f, 188f
Extranodal marginal zone B-cell lymphoma (EMZL), 88, 88f, 268, 275t, 279, 280f, 393–396, 395f
Extraocular muscles
　degenerations, 273
　inflammation, 267–268, 268f, 270, 270f
　thyroid eye disease and, 267
　wound repair, 49–50
Extravascular matrix patterns, 232, 233f
Exudative AMD. *See* Choroidal neovascularization
Exudative retinal detachment, 172–173
Eyelashes (cilia)
　extra row of, 241
　loss of, 251f, 253f, 254f, 257f, 370
　topography, 240–241
Eyelids, 239–263
　colobomas of, 59
　cysts, 243, 247, 248f, 266
　degenerations, 245–246, 245f
　deposits, 246, 246f, 247f
　developmental anomalies, 241, 242f, 254–255, 254f, 259
　inflammation, 242–244, 243f, 244f, 245f
　neoplasia, 248–263
　　basal cell, 34
　　dermal, 254–255, 255f
　　of dermal appendages, 255–258, 255f, 256f, 257f
　　epidermal, 30f, 32t, 248–253, 249f, 250t, 251f, 252f, 253f, 254f, 256–258, 257f
　　melanocytic, 259–263, 260f, 261f, 262f

neuroendocrine, 258–259, 259f
neurofibromas, 285, 285f
of sebaceous glands, 30f, 32t, 118, 255–258, 256f, 257f
squamous cell, 35
vascular tumors, 347
specimen handling and processing, 26–28, 28f, 34–35, 35f
systemic associations, 246, 247t, 250t, 396
topography, 239–241, 240f
wound repair, 49
EZ. *See* Ellipsoid zone

FA. *See* Fluorescein angiography
Facet, 45, 46f
FAF imaging. *See* Fundus autofluorescence (FAF) imaging
FAP. *See* Familial amyloid polyneuropathy
Familial adenomatous polyposis, 176, 326–327, 326f
Familial amyloid polyneuropathy (FAP), 160, 246
Familial amyloidosis, Finnish type, 246
Fascia bulbi, 58–59
Fat necrosis, 270, 271f
FECD. *See* Fuchs endothelial corneal dystrophy
Fetal lens nucleus, 141
Fiber-optic transillumination, 323
Fibrillin, 142
Fibroblasts, 43–45, 44f, 47, 49, 158
Fibrocytes, 267
Fibro-osseous dysplasia (juvenile ossifying fibroma), 287, 288f
Fibrosarcoma, 250t
Fibrosis, 270, 271
Fibrous and fibrovascular proliferation, 53
Fibrous differentiation tumors, 282–283, 283f
Fibrous dysplasia, 286–287, 288f
Fibrous hamartoma, 250t
Fibrous histiocytomas, 282
Fibrous ingrowth and downgrowth, 105, 105f
Fibrovascular plaques, 152, 153f
Filariasis, 272
Fine-needle aspiration biopsy (FNAB)
about and overview, 32–34, 33f
contradictions, 354
for gene expression profile testing, 307–308
handling and processing of, 23
indications, 325, 336–337
of metastases, 389
procedure, 336–337
Finnish type (familial) amyloidosis, 246
Fite-Faraco stain, 30f, 31t
5-fluorouracil, 48, 252
Fixatives, 22–24, 23t, 33
Flame-shaped intraretinal hemorrhage, 184, 186f
Flecks (retinal), 142, 200, 201f
Fleischer ring, 30f, 32t, 107–108, 107f
Fleurettes, 205–206, 205f, 209, 210f
Flexner-Wintersteiner rosettes, 205–206, 205f, 210, 211f, 377
Floaters, 391
Flow cytometry, 20, 23t, 32, 36
"Flower petal," 171

Fluid samples, 23
Fluorescein angiography (FA)
of choroidal nevus, 314
of iris melanoma, 311
of lymphomas, 391, 394
of posterior uveal melanoma, 323, 325, 327, 328f
of retinoblastoma, 358
of secondary tumors, 385–386
of vascular tumors, 343, 345, 348–350, 348f, 351f
FNAB. *See* Fine-needle aspiration biopsy
"Foamy" histiocytes, 173, 174f, 223f, 245f
"Foamy" stromal cells, 173, 175f
Focal choroidal extension, 179, 206
Focal cortical opacifications, 147
Focal posttraumatic choroidal granulomatous inflammation, 55, 55f
Follicular conjunctivitis, 63, 63f, 64f, 243, 244f
Follicular lymphoma, 279
Forceps injury, 50f
Foreign bodies
in choroid, 55
in conjunctiva, 65, 66f
dacryocystitis, 273
in iris, 313t
in lens, 147
in sclera, 47–48
Foreign body giant cells, 12, 15f
Forkhead box C1 *(FOXC1)* gene, 93, 284
Formalin fixative, 20, 22, 23t
Forniceal conjunctiva, 57, 58f
Fovea, 152f, 169f, 171, 219
Foveal pseudocyst, 158
Foveola, 170f, 171
FOXC1 (Forkhead box C1) gene, 93, 284
FOXE3 gene, 142
Fractionated stereotactic radiotherapy, 335
Fraser syndrome, 247t
Freckles (iris), 310, 310f, 313t
Fresh specimens, 23, 28
Frontal bone, 265
Frozen sections, 30f, 34–36, 35f
Fuchs adenoma. *See* Nodular hyperplasia
Fuchs endothelial corneal dystrophy (FECD), 100, 103, 113–114, 117f
Fundus autofluorescence (FAF) imaging, 320, 321f, 322f, 323
Fundus flavimaculatus, 200
Fundus photography, 320, 321f, 322f, 343f, 355, 358, 359f
Fungal infections
of choroid, 178, 178f
of cornea, 97, 98f, 99
of eyelids, 243–244
of optic nerve, 293, 295f
of orbit and lacrimal drainage system, 271–273, 272f
of retina, 178, 178f
staining, 30f, 31–32t
of uveal tract, 220
of vitreous, 154, 155f
Fungemia, 178
Fusarium keratitis, 97, 98f
Fusarium spp, 30f, 31t

Gamma knife radiosurgery, 335
Ganglion cells
  of optic nerve, 289, 290*f*, 295, 298
  of retina, 168–169*f*, 170*f*, 171, 183, 184*f*, 187, 189
Gardner syndrome, 176, 326–327, 326*f*
Gastrointestinal tract carcinoma, 38*t*, 250, 250*t*, 382, 383*t*
GCA. *See* Giant cell arteritis
GCD1. *See* Granular corneal dystrophy type 1
GCD2. *See* Granular corneal dystrophy type 2
Gelsolin amyloidosis, 246
Gene expression profile (GEP), 40–41, 233–234, 234*t*, 307–308
Genetic testing/counseling, 350, 374–376
Geographic atrophy, 181, 197–198, 198*f*, 201*f*
Geographic ulcer, 96*f*, 97
GEP. *See* Gene expression profile
GFAP. *See* Glial fibrillary acidic protein
Ghost cell glaucoma, 127, 128*f*, 160
Ghost cells, 160
Ghost vessels, 100, 100*f*
Giant cell angiofibromas, 282
Giant cell arteritis (GCA), 29, 295–297, 296*f*
Giant cells, 55*f*, 66*f*, 222*f*, 223*f*, 245*f*
Giant congenital melanocytic nevus, 259
Giant drusen, 363
Giemsa stain, 31*t*
Glands of Moll. *See* Apocrine glands
Glands of Zeis. *See* Sebaceous glands
Glandular neoplasms, of conjunctiva, 89, 89*f*
Glass slide preparations
  about and overview, 21
  communication with pathologist, 21–22
  gross examination and dissection, 24–29
  tissue handling and transfer, 22–24, 23*t*
  tissue processing and staining, 29–31
Glaucoma
  about, 126, 298
  degenerations and, 224, 298, 299*f*, 301
  developmental anomalies and, 93, 120–121, 121*f*, 143, 219
  inflammation and, 93, 144
  risk factors, 314
  secondary
    of anterior chamber, 123–129, 124*f*, 126*f*, 127*f*, 128*f*, 129*f*, 319
    iris and, 224, 311, 338, 383
    metastases and, 383
    retinoblastoma and, 355*t*, 357, 362, 364
    uveal tract and, 226, 231, 319, 334
    vascular tumors and, 343, 356*f*, 357*f*
    vitreous hemorrhage and, 160
  trauma and, 127–129, 127*f*, 128*f*, 129*f*
Glaucoma filtering surgeries, 48
Glaukomflecken, 147, 147*f*
Glial cells
  developmental anomalies, 220, 220*f*
  macular gliosis, 159
  macular holes and, 158–159, 159*f*
  neoplasia, 212–213, 212*f*
  of optic nerve, 289, 290*f*, 290*t*, 291*f*, 299*f*
  optic nerve gliosis, 203, 293, 298
  optic nerve neoplasia and, 301–303, 303*f*
  retinal developmental anomalies, 173
  retinal gliosis, 176, 178, 184, 189, 191
  vascular tumors and, 350–352, 351*f*
  wound repair, 48
Glial fibrillary acidic protein (GFAP), 159*f*
Glioblastoma multiforme, 302–303
Gliomas. *See* Astrocytomas
Globe. *See also* Enucleation
  degeneration, 14–16, 16*f*
  gross examination and dissection, 24–25, 25*f*, 26*f*
  protrusion (proptosis) and displacement (dystopia), 265. *See also* Proptosis
  specimen handling and orientation, 22–23
  topography, 265
  trauma to, 53–55, 55*f*
Glutaraldehyde fixative, 20, 23*t*
Glycogen staining, 31*t*
Glycosaminoglycans, 112, 116*f*, 116*t*, 137, 267
GMS stain. *See* Grocott methenamine silver (GMS) stain
GNA11 gene, 233
GNAQ gene, 233
Goblet cells, 31*t*, 57–58, 58*f*, 70*f*, 91
Goldenhar syndrome, 59
Golgi apparatus, 10, 13*f*
Gomori methenamine silver stain, 31*t*
Gonioscopy, 51*f*, 119, 120*f*, 310*f*, 311, 312*f*, 319*f*, 320, 385
Gorlin syndrome, 250*t*
Graft failure (corneal), 99, 104–105, 104*f*, 105*f*
Graft-vs-host disease, 100
Gram stain, 30*f*, 31*t*
Granular corneal dystrophies, 30*f*, 32*t*
Granular corneal dystrophy type 1 (GCD1), 110–111, 114*f*, 116*t*
Granular corneal dystrophy type 2 (GCD2), 110–111, 115*f*, 116*t*
Granulocytic chloromas, 397
Granulocytic sarcoma, 397
Granulomas
  about and overview, 12, 14*f*
  of choroid, 55, 55*f*, 342
  of conjunctiva, 64–67, 65*f*, 66*f*
  of optic nerve, 293, 297, 297*f*
  parasitic infections and, 362–363
Granulomatosis with polyangiitis, 247*t*
Granulomatous inflammation
  of choroid, 179
  cysts, 267
  of eyelid, 244, 245*f*
  of optic nerve, 295, 297, 297*f*
  of orbit, 271, 272*f*
  of retina, 177*f*, 178–179, 178*f*
  of sclera, 133–134, 135*f*
  of uveal tract, 220–222, 221*f*, 222*f*, 223*f*
  of vitreous, 154
Graves disease. *See* Thyroid eye disease
Grocott methenamine silver (GMS) stain, 30*f*, 31*t*
Grouped pigmentation of the retina (bear tracks), 326, 326*f*
Guide. *See* Quick-start guide
Guttae, 100, 112–114, 116*f*, 117*f*

H&E stain. *See* Hematoxylin and eosin (H&E) stain
Haemophilus influenzae, 271
Hair follicles, 247, 248*f*, 251*f*, 252, 262*f*, 266
Haller layer, 218
Hamartomas
    about, 8, 59
    conjunctival, 59, 75
    melanocytic, 313*f*, 313*t*
    of retina, 212–213, 212*f*, 363–364, 363*f*
    of retinal pigment epithelium, 176, 212*f*, 213, 326*f*, 338*t*, 339*f*, 340
    systemic malignancies and, 250*t*
Handling of specimens. *See* Specimen handling, processing, and testing
Hard drusen, 16, 195*t*, 196*f*
Hard exudates, in retina, 177*f*, 184, 185*f*, 190
Head trauma, 192–194, 193*f*, 194*f*. *See also* Trauma
"Healed arteritis," 297
Healing wounds. *See* Wound healing and repair
Hedgehog signaling pathway, 250
Hedgehog signaling pathway inhibitors, 252
Heinz bodies, 128*f*
Hemangioblastoma, 172–173, 175*f*, 346*t*, 347–350, 349*f*
Hemangiomas
    choroid, 230, 230*f*, 233, 236, 236*f*, 319*f*, 320, 327, 341–345, 342*f*, 343*f*
    of eyelid, 254–255, 254*f*
    of orbit, 8, 275*t*, 281, 282*f*
    of retina, 345–347, 346*t*, 347*f*, 348*f*
Hemangiopericytomas, 282
Hematoxylin and eosin (H&E) stain, 29–31, 29*f*, 30*f*, 31*t*, 37*f*
Hemoglobin, 128
Hemolytic glaucoma, 126–129, 128*f*
Hemosiderin, 106, 106*f*, 126, 127*f*, 128–129, 128*f*
Hemosiderosis bulbi, 53, 127, 129, 147
Henderson-Patterson bodies. *See* Molluscum bodies
Henle fiber layer, 169*f*, 171, 184, 185*f*, 197*f*
Herpes simplex virus (HSV)
    IHC stains for, 38*t*
    keratitis, 95–97, 96*f*
    molecular pathology, 39, 40
    optic nerve and, 293
    retinal infections, 176
Herpes zoster virus, 38*t*, 39
Heterochromia, of iris, 314, 354–355, 355*t*
Hidrocystomas, 247, 248*f*
HIF-2α inhibitor. *See* Hypoxia-inducible factor (HIF)–2α inhibitor
Histiocytes (macrophages)
    Coats disease and, 173, 174*f*
    neoplasia of uveal tract and, 231
    overview of, 10–12, 14*f*
    uveal tract inflammation, 220–222, 221*f*, 222*f*, 223*f*
    wound repair and, 43, 47
Histiocytomas, 282
Histochemical stains, 20, 29–31, 29*f*, 30*f*, 31–32*t*
HIV infection/AIDS, 72, 176
HMB-45 immunohistochemical stain, 33*f*, 38*t*, 39
Hodgkin lymphoma, 87
Hollenhorst plaques, 189
Homer Wright rosettes, 205–206, 205*f*, 210

Hordeolum (stye), 242, 244
Hormonal therapy, for secondary ocular tumors, 390
HPV. *See* Human papillomavirus
HSV. *See* Herpes simplex virus
Human papillomavirus (HPV), 71–72, 242–243, 243*f*
Hyaline deposits, 111, 114*f*, 115*f*, 116*t*
Hyalinization, of ciliary body, 224, 225*f*
Hyalocytes, 151
Hyaloid artery, 152, 153*f*
Hyaloid canal (Cloquet canal), 151, 152*f*
Hyaloideocapsular ligament (Wieger ligament), 151, 152*f*
Hyaluronic acid (hyaluronan), 267
Hydatid cyst, 272
Hydrops (corneal), 107*f*, 108
Hydroxyapatite, 160
Hypercalcemia, 102
Hyperchromic heterochromia, 311
Hyperkeratosis, 241, 242, 248, 250
Hyperlipoproteinemias, 245, 247*t*
Hypertension, 190
Hyphema, 106, 127, 127*f*, 222, 223*f*, 225, 354–355, 355*t*, 384*f*, 385
Hypoplasia, of optic nerve, 291
Hypopyon, 98*f*, 124*f*
Hypotony, 50, 53
Hypoxia-inducible factor (HIF)–2α inhibitor, 350

ICE (iridocorneal endothelial) syndrome, 122–123, 125*f*, 313*t*
ICG. *See* Indocyanine green (ICG) angiography
ICK. *See* Infectious crystalline keratopathy
ICRB. *See* International Classification of Retinoblastoma
IC3D. *See* International Committee for Classification of Corneal Dystrophies
IgG4-RD. *See* Immunoglobulin G4–related disease
IHC. *See* Immunohistochemistry
IIRC. *See* International Intraocular Retinoblastoma Classification (IIRC) system
IK. *See* Interstitial keratitis
ILM. *See* Internal limiting membrane
Imiquimod, 252
Immunocompromised patients
    fungal infections and, 178, 272
    infectious crystalline keratopathy and, 99
    keratoacanthoma and, 253
    optic nerve inflammation and, 293, 295*f*
    protozoal infection and, 178–179
    squamous lesion risk factor, 72
    viral infections, 176
Immunoglobulin G4–related disease (IgG4-RD), 246, 268, 269*f*, 270
Immunohistochemistry (IHC), 20, 33*f*, 36–39, 37*f*, 38*t*, 42
Immunomodulatory therapy, 221
Immunophenotyping, 20
Immunotherapy, 335
Inclusion cysts. *See* Epidermoid (inclusion) cysts
Indeterminate neoplastic proliferations, 16–17
Index features, for differential diagnosis, 18
Indirect immunohistochemistry (IHC), 20, 33*f*, 36–39, 37*f*, 38*t*, 42
Indirect ophthalmoscopic examination, 320

Indocyanine green (ICG) angiography, 323, 342*f*, 343, 391, 394
Infantile glaucoma. *See* Congenital glaucoma
Infantile hemangiomas, 59, 236, 254–255, 254*f*, 281
Infections. *See* Bacterial infections; Fungal infections; Parasitic infections; Viral infections; *specific organisms*
Infectious crystalline keratopathy (ICK), 99, 99*f*
Infectious endophthalmitis, 154, 155*f*
Inferior rectus muscle, 267
Inflamed juvenile conjunctival nevus, 77
Inflammation (general). *See also specific eye structures*
　about, 7*t*, 8–12
　acute *vs* chronic, 9–12, 9*f*
　of anterior chamber, 122, 124*f*
　cells of, 9–12, 9*f*, 10*f*, 11*f*, 12*f*, 13*f*, 14*f*
　classification, 8
Inflammatory pannus, 103
INL. *See* Inner nuclear layer
Inner ischemic retinal atrophy, 182, 183*f*, 191
Inner nuclear layer (INL)
　degenerations, 182, 183*f*, 184, 186*f*, 189
　topography, 168*f*, 170*f*, 171–172
Inner plexiform layer (IPL), 168*f*, 170*f*, 171, 183*f*, 184, 189
In situ hybridization (ISH), 20, 39
Intercellular bridges, 241, 252. *See also* Acantholysis
Interdigitation zone (IZ), 169, 170*f*
Internal hordeolum, 242
Internal limiting membrane (ILM)
　degenerations, 180, 181*f*, 185, 186*f*, 187*f*
　posterior vitreous detachment and, 156–157
　topography, 168*f*
　wound repair, 48
Internal ulcer of von Hippel, 93, 94*f*
International Classification of Retinoblastoma (ICRB), 365, 368*t*
International Committee for Classification of Corneal Dystrophies (IC3D), 108
International Intraocular Retinoblastoma Classification (IIRC) system, 356*f*, 365, 366–367*t*
Interstitial keratitis (IK), 96*f*, 97, 99–101, 100*f*
Intracameral chemotherapy, 372–373
Intradermal nevus, 260, 261*f*
Intraepithelial dyskeratosis, 72
Intraepithelial melanocytic proliferation without atypia, 78
Intraepithelial melanosis, 77–84, 79*f*, 80–81*f*, 83*t*
Intraepithelial nonproliferative melanocytic pigmentation, 77–78
Intraepithelial sebaceous carcinoma, 258
Intraocular lymphoma, 162–165, 163*f*, 164*f*
Intraocular pressure, 48, 122, 147
Intraocular silicone oil, 102
Intraretinal microvascular abnormalities (IRMAs), 185, 185*f*, 186*f*, 187*f*, 191
Intravitreal chemotherapy, 372
Inverted follicular keratosis. *See* Irritated seborrheic keratosis
Iodine 125, 337, 372
IPL. *See* Inner plexiform layer
Iridocorneal endothelial syndrome. *See* ICE (iridocorneal endothelial) syndrome

Iridodialysis, 50, 51*f*, 129
Iridoschisis, 121
Iridotomies, 49
Iris. *See also* Uveal tract
　color, 217
　cysts, 313*f*, 313*t*
　degenerations, 122–123, 125*f*, 126*f*, 129, 129*f*, 224, 224*f*
　developmental anomalies, 93, 94*f*, 121, 121*f*, 123*f*, 173, 173*f*, 219–220, 219*f*
　glaucoma, 129
　inflammation, 220, 222
　leukemia and, 397
　neoplasia
　　differential diagnosis, 313*t*
　　extension of iris due to, 230–231
　　medulloepithelioma extension of, 364
　　melanoma, clinical aspects of, 311–314, 312*f*, 313*f*, 313*t*
　　melanoma pathology, 130, 130*f*, 225–226, 227*f*, 230*f*
　　neurofibroma, 238, 238*f*
　　nevus, clinical aspects of, 310–311, 310*f*, 313*f*, 313*t*
　　nevus pathology, 130, 225–226, 226*f*
　　retinoblastoma and, 207*f*
　　vascular tumor, 345–347, 348*f*
　neovascularization, 192*f*, 205, 205*f*, 319
　secondary glaucoma, 129
　specimen handling and processing, 32
　topography, 120*f*, 140*f*, 215–216, 216*f*. *See also* Iris pigment epithelium
　trauma to, 50, 51*f*
　wound repair, 49
Iris freckles, 310, 310*f*, 313*t*
Iris nevus syndrome, 122–123, 125*f*, 313*t*. *See also* ICE (iridocorneal endothelial) syndrome
Iris pigment epithelium
　degenerations, 192, 192*f*, 224
　developmental anomalies, 173
　glaucoma and, 125, 126*f*, 129
　topography, 216*f*, 217
Iris root, 120*f*, 121, 121*f*, 230*f*
Iris sphincter, 50
Iris strands, 93, 94*f*, 121, 123*f*
IRMAs. *See* Intraretinal microvascular abnormalities
Iron deposits, 106–108, 106*f*, 107*f*, 128–129, 160, 301
Iron foreign bodies, 147
Irregular astigmatism, 108
Irritated seborrheic keratosis, 249–250, 249*f*
Ischemia, of lens, 146
Ischemia, of retina, 182–192
　about, 182–183, 183*f*
　cellular responses to, 183–184, 184*f*
　specific disorders, 187–190, 188*f*, 190*f*, 191*f*, 192*f*
　vascular responses to, 184–187, 185*f*, 186*f*, 187*f*
ISH. *See* In situ hybridization
IZ. *See* Interdigitation zone

Junctional nevus, 76, 260, 260*f*
Juvenile ossifying fibroma. *See* Fibro-osseous dysplasia
Juvenile xanthogranuloma, 222, 223*f*, 313*t*

Keratectomy, 109, 110f
Keratin
    cysts and, 247, 248f
    epidermal neoplasms and, 248–249, 249f
Keratin whorls, 73
Keratitis
    infectious
        bacterial, 95, 95f, 99–100, 100f
        crystalline, 99, 99f
        fungal, 97, 98f, 99
        protozoal, 97–98, 98f
        viral, 95–97, 96f, 100
    noninfectious, 100, 101, 267
Keratoacanthoma, 250t, 253, 254f
Keratoconjunctivitis, 101
Keratoconus, 30f, 50, 50f, 106–108, 107f
Keratocytes, 45–46, 47f
Keratoectasias, 106–108, 107f
Keratoepithelin, 109
Keratopathy, 30f, 32t, 96f, 97, 99, 99f, 101–105, 102f, 103f, 104f, 113, 117f
Ki-67 (proliferation marker), 67
Kidney, metastases from, 383t
Kissing nevus, 259, 260f
Klebsiella spp, 271
Koeppe nodules, 222
KOH with calcofluor white stain, 32t
Koilocytosis, 243, 243f
KRIT1 gene, 345
Krukenberg spindle, 129

Labrador keratopathy, 102, 103f
Lacrimal bone, 265
Lacrimal drainage system. *See* Orbit and lacrimal drainage system
Lacrimal gland
    cysts of, 247
    inflammation, 268, 269f, 270, 270f
    neoplasia, 17f, 274–277, 275f, 276f, 277f
    topography, 240, 265
Lacrimal sac, 273, 288
Lacy vacuolation, 31t, 192, 192f
Lamellar bone, 236–237, 237f
Lamina cribrosa
    degenerations, 298, 299f
    developmental anomalies, 292
    retinoblastoma and, 207f
    topography, 131, 289–290, 290f
    vein occlusions and, 189
Lamina fusca, 131, 132f, 218, 218f
Langerhans cells, 240
Langhans cells, 12, 15f
Large B-cell lymphoma (LBCL), 17f, 279, 391–393, 393f
Large cell (primary intraocular) lymphoma, 162–165, 163f, 164f
Larval granuloma. *See* Toxocariasis
Laser-assisted in situ keratomileusis (LASIK) flap, 46
Laser photocoagulation, 181, 191, 191f, 350, 352, 368, 371
Laser therapy, for retinoblastoma, 308
LASIK flap. *See* Laser-assisted in situ keratomileusis (LASIK) flap
Lattice corneal dystrophy, 30f, 31–32t, 111, 113f, 116t

Lattice degeneration, 157, 180, 181f
LBCL. *See* Large B-cell lymphoma
Leaking tumors. *See* Postnatal vascular (leaking) tumors
Leiomyoma, 238
Lens (crystalline), 139–149
    degenerations, 15–16, 16f, 124–126, 126f, 127f, 145–148, 145f, 146f, 147f, 148f, 149f. *See also* Cataracts
    developmental anomalies, 93, 94f, 142–143, 143f, 152–153, 153f
    dislocation, 374
    inflammation, 143–144, 144f, 145f, 313
    ischemia and, 146
    neoplasia, 149
    staining, 30f, 31t
    topography, 139–142, 140f, 141f, 216
    trauma to, 52–53, 143, 146
    wound repair, 48
Lens capsule
    degenerations, 145–146, 145f, 146f, 147f
    developmental anomalies, 241
    inflammation, 143, 145f
    pigment dispersion syndrome, 129, 129f
    staining, 30f, 30t
    topography, 139, 140f, 141f
Lens-induced granulomatous endophthalmitis, 143–144, 145f
Lenticonus, 142–143, 142f
Lentiglobus, 142–143
Lentigo maligna melanoma, 262f, 263
"Leopard spots," 385, 387f
Leptomeningeal carcinomatosis, 301
Leser-Trélat sign, 250
Leukemia, 17f, 17t, 273, 301, 396–398, 397f, 398f
Leukocoria (white pupillary reflex), 174f, 354, 354f, 355t, 360
Leukocyte common antigen, 39
Leukocytes, 9
Lightbulb aneurysms, 362, 363f
Limbal dermoid, 60f
Limbal stem cell deficiency, 219
Linear nevus sebaceous syndrome, 59
Lipid degenerations, 245, 245f
Lipid dropout spaces, 245f
Lipid exudates, 184, 185f, 190
Lipids, in asteroid bodies, 160
Lipoblasts, 286
Lipofuscin
    choroidal melanoma and, 317f, 318, 318f, 320, 322f, 324
    choroidal nevus and, 314, 315f, 324–325
    retinal degenerations, 198f
    retinal dystrophies, 200, 201f, 203
    in retinal pigment epithelium, 172
Lipomas, 286
Liposarcoma, 286
Lisch nodules, 313f, 313t
Liver, 234, 330
Loa loa, 272
Loiasis, 272
Longitudinal layer, of ciliary muscle, 217
Low-dose radiation. *See* Brachytherapy; External-beam radiotherapy
Lowe syndrome, 143
LOXL1 gene. *See* Lysyl oxidase–like 1 *(LOXL1)* gene

Luetic keratitis, 99–100
"Lumpy bumpy" tumor mass, 385, 385f, 387
Lungs
  infections, 293
  metastases from, 235, 235f, 313f, 382, 383t, 385f, 388, 388f
  metastases to, 330
  specimen handling and processing, 38t
Lymphadenopathy, 64
Lymphangiomas. *See* Lymphatic-venous malformations
Lymphatic-venous malformations, 280–281, 281f
Lymphocytes, 9f, 10, 12f, 38t, 58, 58f
Lymphoid hyperplasia, 86–88, 87f, 277–278, 279f
Lymphoid lesions, of conjunctiva, 86–89, 87f, 88f
Lymphoid proliferation, 237, 237f
Lymphoid tumors. *See specific tumors*
Lymphomas
  B-cell lymphomas, 237, 279, 280f
  classification of, 17f, 17t
  of conjunctiva, 68, 87
  differential diagnosis, 270
  non-Hodgkin lymphomas, 87, 279, 390–393
  of orbit and lacrimal drainage system, 275t, 277–280, 394, 395f
  overview, 390–396, 391f, 393f, 395f
  primary intraocular lymphoma, 162–165, 163f, 164f
  specimen handling and processing, 33, 36, 38t
  T-cell lymphomas, 279
  of uveal tract, 237, 237f
Lymphoplasmacytic lymphoma, 275t
Lymphoproliferative lesions, 275t, 277–280, 279f, 280f
Lynch syndrome, 256
Lysyl oxidase–like 1 *(LOXL1)* gene, 124

Macrophages (monocytes), 10, 14f. *See also* Histiocytes
Macrovessels, 347, 348f
Macula
  degenerations, 158–159, 159f, 171, 184, 185f, 186, 194–199, 195t. *See also* Age-related macular degeneration
  dystrophies, 30f, 31t, 112, 116f, 116t, 200–203, 201f, 202f, 203f
  edema
    cystoid macular edema, 158, 159f, 171, 184, 185f, 190, 292f, 293, 343–344, 352
    macular holes and, 158, 159f
    morphological features of, 171, 292f, 293
    vascular responses and, 184, 185f, 186, 189
    vascular tumors and, 343–344
  inflammation (toxoplasmosis), 362t
  metastases and, 388f
  topography, 168–169f, 170f, 171–172. *See also* Cystoid spaces
Macula lutea, 171
Macular corneal dystrophy (MCD), 30f, 31t, 112, 116f, 116t
Macular holes, 158–159, 159f
Macular star formation, 184, 185f, 293
Madarosis, 251f, 253f, 254f, 257f, 370
Magnetic resonance imaging (MRI)
  about, 323–324
  of optic nerve, 387
  of posterior uveal melanoma, 323–324, 331, 334
  RB1 germline whole-body scans, 379
  of retinoblastoma, 358, 361f, 364f
  of secondary tumors, 387
Magnocellular nevus. *See* Melanocytomas
MALT. *See* Mucosa-associated lymphoid tissue
MALT lymphoma. *See* Extranodal marginal zone B-cell lymphoma
"Maltese-cross" birefringence, 161f
Mandible, 347
Mandibulofacial dysostosis, 247t
Mantle cell lymphoma, 275t, 279
Map-dot-fingerprint dystrophy, 109, 110f
Masquerade syndrome, 256, 391
Massive choroidal extension, 206–208, 207f
Masson trichrome stain, 30f, 32t
Mast cells, 9
Maxillary bone, 265
MCC. *See* Merkel cell carcinoma
MCD. *See* Macular corneal dystrophy
MDM2 gene, 286
Measles virus, 176
Medial canthus, 250–251
Medial rectus muscle, 267
Medulloblastoma, 250t
Medulloepithelioma, 209–210, 211f, 364f
Meibomian gland dysfunction (MGD), 101
Meibomian glands, 64f, 240–242, 244, 255–256, 256f
Melan-A, 38t, 39
Melanin, 106, 126, 130, 130f, 172, 217, 228
Melanocytes
  of conjunctiva, 58, 58f
  of eyelids, 240
  of iris, 225, 226f
  of uveal tract, 236, 238, 238f
Melanocytic neoplasia, 309–340. *See also specific lesions and tumors*
  about, 309
  of anterior chamber, 126, 130, 130f
  classification of, 16–17, 17f, 17t
  of conjunctiva, 75–86
    about and overview, 75, 76t
    differential diagnosis, 85, 86, 86f
    intraepithelial melanosis, 77–84, 79f, 80–81f, 83t
    invasive melanoma, 83t, 85
    melanocytic nevi, 75–77, 77f, 78f
    melanoma in situ, 79f, 80–81f, 82, 83t, 84–85
    melanomas, 72, 79f, 80–81f, 83t, 84–86, 85f, 86f
    metastatic, 84–85
  of cornea, 118
  differential diagnosis, 18, 238, 250
  direct intraocular extension of, 390
  of eyelids, 250, 259–263, 260f, 261f, 262f
  of optic nerve, 301, 302f
  of retina, 301, 302f
  specimen handling and processing, 33, 33f, 37, 38t
  of uveal tract. *See also* Posterior uveal melanoma
    clinical aspects of, 301, 307–308, 311–338
    pathology of, 85, 130, 176, 225–234
Melanocytomas
  classification of, 17t
  differential diagnosis, 326, 338, 338t

malignant changes, 338
of optic nerve, 301, 302*f*, 326
of uveal tract, 227–228, 313*t*, 326, 338
Melanoma-associated spongiform scleropathy, 136–137
Melanomalytic glaucoma, 126, 129, 130*f*, 231
Melanosomes, 129, 129*f*, 172
Melphalan, 370, 372–373
Meningiomas, 38*t*, 286, 303–304, 304*f*
Meningitis, 294*t*
Meningothelial meningioma, 303, 304*f*
Meretoja syndrome, 246
Merkel cell carcinoma (MCC), 258–259, 259*f*
Merkel cell polyomavirus, 258, 259*f*
Mesectodermal leiomyoma, 238
Mesenchymal chondrosarcoma, 288
Mesenchyme neoplasia, 17*t*
Metaherpetic ulcer, 96*f*, 97
Metamorphopsia, 313
Metastases
 general
  about, 17*f*, 17*t*, 381–382, 382*f*, 383*t*
  clinical features and diagnosis, 38*t*, 382–383, 387–389
  direct intraocular extension, 390
  mechanism, 382, 382*f*
  prognosis, 389
  treatment, 389–390
 primary ocular tumor sites
  conjunctiva, 390
  eyelids, 250, 252, 258–259, 263, 390
  iris, 311
  posterior uvea, 232–234, 233*f*, 234*f*, 329–332, 329*t*, 330*t*
  retina, 358–359, 361*f*, 378
 secondary ocular tumors, 381–390
  of anterior segment, 382–385, 384*f*
  of conjunctiva, 89
  differential diagnosis, 387*t*
  of optic nerve, 382, 387
  of orbit, 288
  of posterior segment, 342, 382, 383*t*, 385–387, 385*f*, 386*f*, 387*f*, 387*t*, 388*f*, 390
  primary tumor sites (overview), 382, 383*t*, 387–389
  of uveal tract, 234–235, 235*f*, 313*f*, 313*t*, 382, 383*t*
 systemic malignancies and, 396
Methanol, 23*t*
Methotrexate, 392–393
MGD. *See* Meibomian gland dysfunction
Michel transport medium, 23*t*
Microaneurysms, 185, 187*f*, 189, 191
Microarrays, 40–41
Microcornea, 143
Microcystic adnexal carcinoma, 255
Microcysts, 104
Microglial cells, 183, 290*t*, 291*f*
Microphthalmia, 133, 142–143, 152, 362
MicroRNA microarrays, 41
Middle limiting membrane (MLM), 168
Mitomycin C, 48
Mittendorf dot, 153
Mixed-cell type melanoma, 231, 233
MLM. *See* Middle limiting membrane
MMP. *See* Mucous membrane pemphigoid

Modified Callender classification system, 226, 229*t*, 231–232
Mohs micrographic surgery, 35, 35*f*
Molecular diagnosis and prognosis, 307–308
Molecular pathology
 circulating tumor cells, 19, 41–42
 diagnostic electron microscopy, 42
 microarrays, 20, 40–41
 polymerase chain reaction, 20, 39–41
Molluscum bodies, 243, 244*f*
Molluscum contagiosum, 243, 244*f*
Monoclonal immunoglobulin, 68
Monocytes (macrophages), 10, 14*f*. *See also* Histiocytes
Monosomy 3, 233–234, 234*t*
Morgagnian cataract, 144, 148, 149*f*
Morgagnian globules, 148, 149*f*
Morning glory disc anomaly, 291
Morpheaform basal cell carcinoma, 251–252, 252*f*
"Moth-eaten" appearance, 180*f*
MRI. *See* Magnetic resonance imaging
Mucin staining, 31*t*
Mucoceles, 266
Mucoepidermoid carcinoma. *See* Adenosquamous carcinoma
Mucormycosis, 271–272, 274*f*, 293
Mucor spp, 271–272, 272*f*
Mucosa-associated lymphoid tissue (MALT), 58, 86, 88, 88*f*, 268, 393
Mucous membrane pemphigoid (MMP; ocular cicatricial pemphigoid), 23, 61–63, 62*f*
Muir-Torre syndrome, 250*t*, 256, 256*f*
"Mulberry" lesion, 363, 363*f*
Müller cells, 158, 159*f*, 181
Multinucleated giant cells, 12, 15*f*, 222, 223*f*, 295, 296*f*
Multiple recurrent serosanguineous RPE detachments. *See* Polypoidal choroidal vasculopathy
Multiple sclerosis, 295, 295*f*
Muscle differentiation tumors, 283–285, 284*f*
Mutton-fat keratic precipitates, 221
MYCN oncogene, 208, 209*f*, 375
Mycobacterium leprae, 30*f*, 31*t*, 100
Mycobacterium tuberculosis, 31*t*, 40, 100, 293
Mycosis. *See* Fungal infections
MYD88 gene, 164
Myelinated nerve fiber developmental anomalies, 172
Myeloma, 68, 246*f*
Myogenin, 284
Myoglobin, 38*t*, 39
Myoid zone (MZ), 169, 170*f*
Myopia, 157, 172
Myositis, 270, 270*f*
Myxoma, 247*t*
MZ. *See* Myoid zone

Nanophthalmos, 132–133
National Comprehensive Cancer Network (NCCN) clinical practice guidelines, 331
Natural killer (NK) cell lymphoma, 87
NBF. *See* Neutral-buffered formalin
NCCN. *See* National Comprehensive Cancer Network (NCCN) clinical practice guidelines
Necrobiosis, 134*f*

Necrobiotic granuloma, 245
Necrosis, 163, 163f, 271–272
Necrotic melanoma, 231–232
Necrotizing granulomas, 12, 14f, 64, 293
Necrotizing retinitis, 176, 177f, 178–179
Necrotizing scleritis, 133–134, 134f, 135f
Necrotizing ulcerative keratitis, 95f
Neoplasia (general). *See also specific tumors and eye structures*
   about and overview, 16–17
   classification of, 17f, 17t
   specimen handling and processing, 70
Neovascular age-related macular degeneration. *See* Choroidal neovascularization
Neovascular glaucoma (NVG), 224, 334, 356f, 357f, 362, 364, 369
Neovascularization
   age-related macular degeneration and, 198–199, 199f, 327
   choroidal, 53–55, 186, 191, 195f, 197–199, 199f, 227, 314
   of iris, 189, 192f, 205, 205f, 224, 224f, 319, 385
   of retina, 185–186, 187f, 189–190
   of vitreous, 185–186
Nerve fiber layer (NFL)
   degenerations, 180f, 182, 183f, 184, 186f, 187, 189
   developmental anomalies, 172
   topography of, 168, 168f, 170f, 171
Neural cysts, 266
Neural sheath tumors, 238, 238f
Neurilemoma. *See* Schwannoma
Neuroblastoma, 38t, 273, 288
Neuroendocrine tumors, 38t, 258–259, 259f
Neuroepithelial tumors, 206, 209–210
Neurofibromas, 238, 238f, 247t, 285–286, 285f
Neurofibromatosis, 247t, 285, 286, 301, 303, 313f, 340, 364
Neuroretinitis, 293, 294t
Neurosensory retina, topography of, 167–172, 168–169f. *See also* Retina
Neutral-buffered formalin (NBF), 20, 22, 23t, 27
Neutrophils, 9, 9f, 43, 44f, 45, 47f
Nevus cells, 261, 261f
NFL. *See* Nerve fiber layer
NHLs. *See* Non-Hodgkin lymphomas
NK cell lymphoma. *See* Natural killer (NK) cell lymphoma
Nodular basal cell carcinoma, 251, 251f
Nodular drusen. *See* Hard drusen
Nodular episcleritis, 134
Nodular hyperplasia, 211, 212f
Nodular melanoma, 262f, 263
Nodular retinal gliosis. *See* Retinal vasoproliferative tumor
Nodular scleritis, 133–134, 134f
Noncaseating granulomas, 12, 14f, 297, 297f
Non-Hodgkin lymphomas (NHLs), 87, 279, 390–393
Nonleaking tumors. *See* Prenatal vascular (nonleaking) tumors
Nonnecrotizing granulomas, 222, 223f
Nonnecrotizing scleritis, 133–134
Nonneovascular age-related macular degeneration, 198, 198f
Nonspecific orbital inflammation (NSOI), 270, 270f, 271f

Nonsteroidal anti-inflammatory drugs. *See* NSAIDs
Nonsulfated glycosaminoglycan, 112, 116f, 116t
Norrie disease, 362
NSAIDs (nonsteroidal anti-inflammatory drugs), 100
NSOI. *See* Nonspecific orbital inflammation
Nuclear cataracts, 148, 149f
Nucleus, of lens, 140f, 141, 148, 149f
NVG. *See* Neovascular glaucoma
Nystagmus, 172, 355t

OAL. *See* Ocular adnexal lymphoma
Observation, of posterior uveal melanoma, 332
OCRL gene, 143
OCP. *See* Ocular cicatricial pemphigoid
OCT. *See* Optical coherence tomography
Ocular adnexal lymphoma (OAL), 275t, 277–280, 394, 395f
Ocular albinism, 172
Ocular cicatricial pemphigoid (OCP; mucous membrane pemphigoid), 23, 61–63, 62f
Ocular melanocytosis, 77, 78f
Ocular surface squamous neoplasia (OSSN), 72–73, 73f, 74f, 118
Ocular toxocariasis, 360, 362–363
Ocular toxoplasmosis. *See* Toxoplasmic retinochoroiditis
Ocular trauma. *See* Foreign bodies; Trauma
Oculoauriculovertebral dysgenesis, 59
Oculocerebrorenal syndrome (Lowe syndrome), 143
Oculocutaneous albinism, 172
Oculodermal melanocytosis, 77
"Oil droplet," 142
Oil red O stain, 30f, 31, 32t
Oligodendrocytes, 290, 290t, 291f, 298
Oligonucleotides, 41
Onchocerca volvulus, 100
Oncocytoma (oxyphilic adenoma), 89, 89f
ONE Network online resource, 308
ONH. *See* Optic nerve head
ONL. *See* Outer nuclear layer
Open-angle glaucoma, 124–130, 126f, 127f, 128f, 129f
Operculum, 159f
Ophthalmic artery, 291
Ophthalmic pathology (general)
   about, 5
   organizational framework and pathological concepts, 6–18
      differential diagnosis, 18
      disease process, 8–17
      overview, 6, 7t
      topography, 6–8
   specimens, 19–42. *See also* Specimen handling, processing, and testing
   wound repair, 43–55. *See also* Wound healing and repair
Ophthalmoplegia, 42, 273
OPL. *See* Outer plexiform layer
Optical coherence tomography (OCT)
   of astrocytomas, 364
   of choroid nevus, 316, 321f, 323, 325
   of conjunctiva, 73, 74f
   of iris nevus, 310f
   of lymphomas, 392, 394, 395f

posterior uveal melanoma differential diagnosis, 321*f,* 323, 325, 327
of retinal layers, 169, 170*f*
for retinoblastoma, 358, 359*f*
of secondary tumors, 385*f*
of vascular tumors, 342*f,* 343
Optic atrophy, 298–299, 298*f,* 299*f,* 300*f,* 301
Optic disc. *See* Optic nerve head
Optic nerve, 289–304
 atrophy, 203, 203*f*
 blood supply, 290*f,* 291
 compression of, 286
 degenerations, 298–301, 298*f,* 299*f,* 300*f*
 developmental anomalies, 152–153, 153*f,* 154*f,* 171–172, 220, 291–292, 292*f,* 362*t*
 edema, 189
 glioma, 38*t*
 gliosis, 203
 inflammation, 222, 267, 270, 292–297, 294*t,* 295*f,* 296*f,* 297*f*
 leukemia and, 397–398, 398*f*
 neoplasia
  hemangioblastomas, 173
  intraocular lymphoma and, 164–165
  medulloepithelioma, 209–210, 364
  melanocytoma, 326
  overview, 301–304, 302*f,* 303*f,* 304*f*
  retinoblastoma extension, 206, 207*f,* 361*f*
  specimen handling and processing, 38*t*
 specimen handling and processing, 33, 38*t*
 topography, 131, 168, 171, 215, 289–290, 290*f,* 290*t,* 291*f,* 298
 trauma, 193, 194*f*
 wound repair, 49
Optic nerve head (ONH)
 blood supply, 291
 degenerations, 298–301, 298*f,* 300*f*
 deposits, 299–301, 300*f*
 developmental anomalies, 292*f*
 edema, 298, 298*f,* 387
 neoplasia
  hamartomas, 363, 363*f*
  overview, 301–303, 302*f,* 303*f*
  retinoblastoma extension of, 358, 359*f,* 360*f*
  vascular tumors, 345, 347–350, 349*f*
 persistent fetal vasculature and, 362
 topography, 289
Optic nerve hypoplasia, 291
Optic nerve pits, 292, 292*f*
Optic neuritis, 222, 267, 270, 292–297, 294*t,* 295*f,* 296*f,* 297*f*
Optic neuropathy, 292–293, 294*t,* 300, 390
Optic perineuritis, 293, 294*t*
Ora serrata, 53, 53*f,* 157, 171, 182*f,* 193*f,* 218
Orbicularis oculi muscle, 49, 239–240, 240*f*
Orbital cavernous venous malformation, 8, 281, 282*f*
Orbital lymphatic malformations, 280–281, 281*f*
Orbital myositis, 270, 270*f*
Orbital pseudotumor (idiopathic) orbital inflammatory syndrome. *See* Nonspecific orbital inflammation
Orbit and lacrimal drainage system, 265–288. *See also* Lacrimal gland
 cysts, 266–267, 266*f,* 272–273
 degenerations, 273
 deposits, 270, 273
 developmental anomalies, 266–267, 266*f*
 inflammation
  infectious, 271–273, 271*f,* 272*f,* 273*f*
  noninfectious, 267–270, 268*f,* 269*f,* 270*f,* 271*f,* 354–355, 355*t,* 357*f*
 neoplasia, 273–288, 275*t*
  bony lesions, 286–288, 288*f*
  central nervous system tumors, 286
  with fibrous differentiation, 282–283, 283*f*
  lacrimal gland neoplasia, 274–277, 275*t,* 276*f,* 277*f*
  lacrimal sac, 288
  lymphoproliferative lesions, 275*t,* 277–280, 279*f,* 280*f*
  with muscle differentiation, 283–285, 284*f*
  overview, 273–274
  peripheral sheath tumors, 275*t,* 285–286, 285*f,* 287*f*
  secondary tumors, 273, 288
  soft-tissue tumors, 280, 282
  vascular tumors, 275*t,* 280–281, 281*f,* 282*f,* 347
 retinoblastoma extension of, 359, 361*f*
 systemic malignancies and, 394, 396–397
 topography, 265–266
 wound repair, 49–50
Osseous tumors of orbit, 286–288, 288*f*
OSSN. *See* Ocular surface squamous neoplasia
Osteoblastoma, 288
Osteomas, 236–237, 237*f,* 288, 288*f,* 327, 328*f,* 342
Osteosarcoma, 288
Outer ischemic retinal atrophy, 182, 183*f*
Outer nuclear layer (ONL), 168*f,* 170*f,* 172, 183*f,* 188*f*
Outer plexiform layer (OPL), 168–169*f,* 170*f,* 171–172, 179, 180*f,* 183, 186*f,* 188*f*
"Owl's eye" inclusions, 177*f*
Oxidative stress, 194

p53 gene, 67, 72
p63 gene, 67
Pagetoid spread, 84, 257*f,* 258, 262*f,* 263
Paired box protein 6, 93
Paired-like homeodomain transcription factor 2 (*PITX2*) gene, 93
Palatine bone, 265
Palisaded Antoni A pattern, 286, 287*f*
Palisades of Vogt, 91
Palpebral conjunctiva, 57, 64*f,* 239–240, 240*f*
PAM. *See* Primary acquired melanosis
Pannus
 of conjunctiva, 67
 of cornea, 103–104, 103*f,* 104*f,* 110–111, 112*f*
 differential diagnosis, 72
Panuveitis, 179, 221
Papillary conjunctivitis, 63, 63*f,* 64*f*
Papillitis, 300
Papillomas, 17*t,* 72, 242–243, 243*f,* 288
Papillomatosis, 248
Papules, 246, 247*t,* 248, 249*f,* 250
Paraffin block (cell block), 33, 33*f*
Paraffin tissue sections, 20, 29–31, 29*f,* 30*f,* 31*t*
Parakeratosis, 241, 242, 250, 251*f*
Paranasal sinus, 242

Parasitic infections
  of eyelid, 243
  of orbit, 266, 272
  retinoblastoma differential diagnosis, 360, 362–363, 362t
Parinaud oculoglandular syndrome, 64
Pars plana, 53, 53f, 157, 217, 217f
Pars plana vitrectomy, 350
Pars plicata, 212f, 217, 217f
PAS. *See* Peripheral anterior synechiae
PAS stain. *See* Periodic acid–Schiff (PAS) stain
Pathology. *See* Ophthalmic pathology
Pattern dystrophies, 202–203, 202f
Paving-stone (cobblestone) degeneration, 181, 182f
PAX3-FOXO1 gene, 284
PAX6 gene, 93, 219
PAX7-FOX1 gene, 284
PCG. *See* Primary congenital glaucoma
PCNSL. *See* Primary central nervous system lymphoma
PCR. *See* Polymerase chain reaction
PD-1 inhibitors, 252
PDT. *See* Photodynamic therapy
Pedunculated papillomas, 70–71, 71f
PEHCR. *See* Peripheral exudative hemorrhagic chorioretinopathy
Pellucid marginal degeneration (PMCD), 108
Penetrating keratoplasty (PK) graft, 99, 104–105, 104f, 105f, 108, 114, 117f
Perifoveal outer plexiform layer. *See* Henle fiber layer
Perifoveal vitreous detachment, 158
Perimacular circumferential retinal folds, 192–193, 193f
Periodic acid–Schiff (PAS) stain, 29–31, 30f, 31t
Peripapillary choroidal nevus, 318f
Peripapillary retina, 152
Peripheral anterior synechiae (PAS), 123, 124f, 125f, 127, 192f, 219, 224
Peripheral corneal vascularization, 101
Peripheral cystoid degeneration, 179, 180f
Peripheral exudative hemorrhagic chorioretinopathy (PEHCR), 327, 328f
Peripheral nerve sheath tumors, 285–286, 285f, 287f
Peripherin 2 gene. *See PRPH2* (peripherin 2) gene
Periphlebitis, 222
Perls Prussian blue stain, 30f, 32t
Permanent sections, 31, 34
Persistent fetal vasculature (PFV; formerly persistent hyperplastic primary vitreous), 133, 143, 152, 153f, 360, 362
"Petaloid" cystoid macular edema (CME), 184, 185f
Peters anomaly, 93, 94f, 121
PFV. *See* Persistent fetal vasculature
Phacoantigenic uveitis. *See* Lens-induced granulomatous endophthalmitis
Phacolytic glaucoma, 125–126, 127f, 144
Phacolytic uveitis, 144
Phakomatous choristoma, 241, 242f
Pheochromocytoma, 350
Phlyctenular keratitis, 101
Photocoagulation, 350, 352
Photodynamic therapy (PDT), 252, 335, 343–344, 350, 352, 390
Photoreceptors
  atrophy of, 197–198
  degenerations, 181–183, 181f, 183f
  developmental anomalies, 175–176, 175f
  dystrophies, 201f, 202–203, 203f
  topography, 168–169f, 171–172
Phthisis, 374
Phthisis bulbi, 14–16, 16f, 53, 355t, 357f
Pial sheath, 290, 290f, 291f, 298, 299f, 302
Pial vessels, 291
Pigmentary glaucoma, 311
Pigment deposits (corneal), 106, 106f
Pigment dispersion syndrome, 129, 129f
Pigment epithelial cyst, 313f, 313t
Pilocytic astrocytoma, 301
Pilosebaceous units, 240–241
Pinealoblastoma (primitive neuroectodermal tumor), 358, 361f, 376–377
Pinguecula, 67–68, 68f, 72
Pink necrosis, 204, 204f
PIOL. *See* Primary intraocular lymphoma
PITX2 (paired-like homeodomain transcription factor 2) gene, 93
PK graft. *See* Penetrating keratoplasty (PK) graft
Plaque radiotherapy. *See* Brachytherapy
Plaques
  calcific, 136, 137f, 189
  cholesterol, 189
  on eyelids, 245, 245f
  of lens, 146, 146f
Plasma cell myeloma, 68, 246f
Plasma cells, 9f, 10, 13f
Plasmacytoma, 68
Platelet-fibrin emboli, 189
Pleomorphic adenoma, 274, 275t, 276, 276f
Pleomorphic rhabdomyosarcoma, 284
Pleuropulmonary blastoma, 364
Plexiform neurofibromas, 247t, 285–286, 285f
Plica semilunaris, 58, 58f
Plump fusiform dendritic nevus cells, 227, 228f
Plump polyhedral nevus cells, 226
PMCD. *See* Pellucid marginal degeneration
PMNs. *See* Polymorphonuclear leukocytes
PNET. *See* Primitive neuroectodermal tumor
PO section. *See* Pupil–optic nerve (PO) section
Polyarteritis nodosa, 247t
Polychondritis, 247t
Polymerase chain reaction (PCR), 39–41
Polymorphonuclear leukocytes (PMNs), 9, 10f
Polypoidal choroidal vasculopathy, 199, 200f
Posterior banded layer, 93
Posterior capsule opacification, 146
Posterior ciliary arteries, 171, 231f, 291, 297
Posterior embryotoxon, 121–122, 122f, 123f
Posterior keratoconus, 121
Posterior lamella, 240
Posterior lens capsule
  degenerations, 145, 145f
  developmental anomalies, 152
  inflammation, 143
  topography, 139, 140f, 141–142, 141f
Posterior lenticonus, 142–143, 142f
Posterior lentiglobus, 142–143
Posterior polymorphous corneal dystrophy (PPCD), 115, 118, 118f
Posterior subcapsular cataract, 145, 145f, 146f

Posterior synechiae, 48
Posterior uveal bleeding syndrome. *See* Polypoidal choroidal vasculopathy
Posterior uveal melanoma
    clinical aspects of, 316–338
        about, 311, 316–317
        characteristics, 316, 317*f*, 318–320, 318*f*, 319*f*
        classification, 329, 330*t*
        diagnostic evaluation, 318*f*, 320–324, 321*f*, 322*f*, 324*f*
        differential diagnosis, 85, 86*f*, 311, 321*f*, 324–329, 326*f*, 328*f*, 329*t*, 338*t*, 340
        metastatic evaluation, 329–332, 330*t*
        prognosis and prognostic factors, 336–337
        risk factors, 314, 316, 324–325
        treatment, 332–336, 334*f*
    differential diagnosis, 394
    pathology, 228–234
        about, 228
        cell types associated with, 228, 229*t*, 232
        growth patterns, 228–231, 230*f*, 231*f*, 232*f*
        histological prognostic factors, 229*t*, 231–233, 233*f*
        molecular genetics of, 233–234, 234*t*
Posterior uveitis, 362*t*, 391
Posterior vitreous detachment (PVD), 156–159, 156*f*, 160
Postherpetic neurotrophic keratopathy, 96*f*, 97
Postnatal vascular (leaking) tumors, 347–352, 348*f*, 349*f*, 351*f*
PPCD. *See* Posterior polymorphous corneal dystrophy
PRAME gene, 234
Prenatal vascular (nonleaking) tumors, 345–347, 347*f*
Prepapillary vascular loops, 153
Preretinal membrane, 152, 158*f*, 212
Presbyopia, 224
Preseptal cellulitis, 242, 243*f*
Presumed acquired retinal hemangioma. *See* Retinal vasoproliferative tumor
Primary acquired melanosis (PAM)
    with atypia, 77, 79*f*, 80–81*f*, 82–84, 83*t*, 85*f*
    of conjunctiva, 77–78, 79*f*, 80–81*f*, 82–84, 83*t*, 85*f*
Primary aphakia, 142
Primary central nervous system lymphoma (PCNSL), 390–393
Primary choroidal lymphomas, 237
Primary congenital glaucoma (PCG), 93, 120–121, 121*f*
Primary conjunctival lymphoma, 68
Primary conjunctival melanosis. *See* Complexion-associated melanosis
Primary intraocular lymphoma (PIOL), 162–165, 163*f*, 164*f*. *See also* Large B-cell lymphoma
Primary uveal lymphoma, 38*t*, 278, 279*f*, 393–396, 395*f*
Primary vitreoretinal lymphoma (PVRL), 33, 40, 162–165, 163*f*, 164*f*, 390–393, 391*f*, 393*f*
Primary vitreous, 151, 152
Primitive neuroectodermal tumor (PNET; pinealoblastoma), 358, 361*f*, 376–377
Procedures. *See* Specimen handling, processing, and testing
Progressive iris atrophy. *See* Essential iris atrophy
Proliferative vitreoretinopathy (PVR), 53, 54*f*, 157, 158*f*

Proptosis
    defined, 265
    inflammation and, 272–273
    leukemia and, 397
    lymphomas and, 394
    metastases and, 389
    neoplasia and, 274, 276*f*, 278, 279*f*, 280*f*, 281–283, 283*f*, 284*f*
    thyroid disease and, 267, 268*f*
    tumors causing, 355*t*, 359, 361*f*
Prostate cancer, 38*t*, 288, 383*t*
Protein microarrays, 41
Proteus spp, 271
Proton beam therapy, 311, 350
Protozoal infections, 178–179, 179*f*, 220
PRPH2 (peripherin 2) gene, 202
Prussian blue iron stain, 30*f*, 32*t*
Psammoma bodies, 303–304, 304*f*
Psammomatous meningioma, 287, 288*f*
Pseudocoloboma, 247*t*
Pseudocysts, 109, 158
Pseudoexfoliation syndrome, 124–125, 126*f*, 148
Pseudoglands of Henle, 58*f*
Pseudohorn cysts, 248–249, 249*f*
Pseudohypopyon, 355, 355*t*, 357*f*, 385, 397
Pseudomonas aeruginosa, 95
Pseudophakia, 157
Pseudopolycoria, 121, 123*f*
Pseudorosettes, 204, 204*f*
Pseudo–Roth spots, 396, 397*f*
Pterygium, 67–68, 68*f*, 72, 101
Ptosis, 247*t*, 273
Pulmonary conditions. *See* Lungs
Punctum, 65–67
Pupil, 216, 313*f*
Pupil–optic nerve (PO) section, 24–25, 27*f*
Purple calcification, 204, 204*f*
PVD. *See* Posterior vitreous detachment
PVRL. *See* Primary vitreoretinal lymphoma
Pyogenic granuloma, 65–67, 66*f*

Quick-start guide, 19–42. *See also* Specimen handling, processing, and testing

Racemose hemangioma. *See* Congenital retinal arteriovenous malformation
Racial melanosis. *See* Complexion-associated melanosis
Radial layer, of ciliary muscle, 217
Radial perivascular lattice degeneration, 180, 181*f*
Radiation retinopathy, 183, 390
Radiation therapy
    for leukemia, 398
    for lymphomas, 396
    for posterior uveal melanoma, 333–335, 334*f*
    for retinoblastoma, 368
    for vascular tumors, 344
Radiotherapy. *See also* External-beam radiotherapy
    basal cell carcinoma treatment, 252
    for choroid and ciliary body melanomas, 333–335, 334*f*
    for lymphomas, 392–393
    for medulloepitheliomas, 364
    for retinoblastoma, 368, 371–373

sebaceous carcinoma treatment, 258
for secondary ocular tumors, 390
for vascular tumors, 344, 350, 352
"Railroad track"–like lesions, of Descemet membrane, 115, 118*f*
Ranibizumab, 186
Rapid processing of specimens, 29
RB1 (retinoblastoma) gene, 208–209, 308, 356*f*, 373–379
RBCD. *See* Reis-Bücklers corneal dystrophy
Reactive lymphoid hyperplasia (RLH). *See* Primary uveal lymphoma
Reactive melanosis. *See* Secondary acquired melanosis
Rectus muscles, 267
Recurrent pterygium, 67
Red chromogen, 33*f*, 37*f*
Red reflex, 142
Reis-Bücklers corneal dystrophy (RBCD), 109, 111*f*, 116*t*
Relapsing polychondritis, 247*t*
Renal cell carcinoma, 350
Repair, defined. *See* Wound healing and repair
Respiratory infections, 281
Reticular degenerative retinoschisis, 179
Reticular peripheral cystoid degeneration (RPCD), 179, 180*f*
Reticular pseudodrusen (RPD), 195*t*, 196–197, 197*f*
Retina, 167–213. *See also* Subretinal fluid
   blood supply, 171, 183, 187–190. *See also* Ischemia, of retina
   degenerations, 15–16, 16*f*, 179–199, 179*f*, 180*f*, 181*f*, 182*f*, 183*f*, 184*f*, 185*f*, 186*f*, 187*f*, 188*f*, 190*f*, 191*f*, 195*t*, 200*f*
   deposits, 161
   detachments
      choroidal nevus and, 314
      Coats disease and, 362, 363*f*
      developmental anomalies, 172–173, 174*f*
      hemangiomas and, 327, 342–343
      macular holes and, 158
      neoplasia and, 230–231, 230*f*
      optic nerve pits and, 292
      parasitic infections, 363
      persistent fetal vasculature and, 362
      posterior uveal melanoma and, 317*f*, 318–320
      radiation complication, 334, 390
      retinal degenerations and, 180–181, 181*f*
      retinoblastoma and, 354*f*, 355, 356*f*
      secondary tumors and, 386*f*, 387
      sequelae, 181, 182*f*
      trauma-related, 53–55
   developmental anomalies, 152–153, 153*f*, 172–176, 173*f*, 174*f*, 175*f*, 220, 220*f*, 291–292, 292*f*, 353–379. *See also* Retinoblastoma
   dystrophies, 200–203, 201*f*, 202*f*, 203*f*
   hemorrhage
      abusive head trauma and, 192–193, 193*f*
      choroidal vasculopathy, 200*f*
      ischemia and, 184–185, 186*f*, 187*f*, 189–190, 190*f*
      subretinal, 53, 193, 317*f*, 319, 323–325, 328*f*, 387
   inflammation (retinitis)
      chorioretinitis, 222, 223*f*
      infectious etiologies, 38*t*, 176–179, 177*f*, 178*f*, 179*f*
      noninfectious etiologies, 179
      specimen handling and processing, 38*t*
   neoplasia, 204–213
      adenoma and adenocarcinoma, 176, 213
      of ciliary body epithelium, 212*f*
      developmental anomalies, 173, 174*f*
      differential diagnosis, 18
      hamartoma, 212–213, 212*f*, 339*f*, 340, 363–364, 363*f*
      lymphomas, 164–165, 164*f*
      medulloepithelioma, 209–210, 211*f*, 364, 364*f*
      nodular hyperplasia, 211, 212*f*
      posterior uveal melanoma extension into, 317*f*, 318–320
      retinoblastoma, 204–209, 204*f*, 205*f*, 207*f*, 209*f*, 353–379. *See also* Retinoblastoma
      retinocytoma, 209, 210*f*
      uveal tract melanomas, 227, 230, 230*f*, 232*f*
      vascular tumors, 345–352, 346*t*
   neovascularization, 185–186, 187*f*, 189–190
   opacification of, 53
   staining, 30*f*
   systemic malignancies and, 396–397, 397*f*
   tears (breaks), 53, 157–158, 157*f*, 158*f*
   topography, 167–172. *See also* Retinal pigment epithelium
      neurosensory retina, 168–172, 168*f*, 169*f*, 170*f*
      overview, 167–168
   trauma to, 53–55, 53*f*, 54*f*
   vitreous detachment and, 156–158, 156*f*
   wound repair, 48–49
Retinal arteriovenous malformation (AVM), 345–347, 346*t*, 348*f*
Retinal artery and vein occlusions, 183, 183*f*, 185, 187–190, 188*f*, 190*f*
Retinal capillary hemangioblastoma. *See* Retinal hemangioblastoma
Retinal capillary hemangioma. *See* Retinal hemangioblastoma
Retinal cavernous hemangioma, 345, 346*t*, 347*f*
Retinal dialysis, 53, 53*f*
Retinal flecks, 142, 200, 201*f*
Retinal ganglion cells (RGCs), 289, 290*f*, 298
Retinal hemangioblastoma (RH), 346*t*, 347–350, 349*f*
Retinal pigment epithelium (RPE)
   blood supply, 218, 218*f*
   congenital hypertrophy of, 326–327, 326*f*
   degenerations, 15–16, 16*f*, 181, 183*f*, 191, 191*f*, 194–199, 195*t*, 196*f*, 197*f*, 198*f*, 199*f*
   deposits, 161
   developmental anomalies, 173*f*, 175–176, 175*f*, 220*f*
   dystrophies, 194, 200–203, 201*f*, 202*f*, 203*f*
   inflammation, 176, 177*f*, 221, 221*f*, 222*f*
   leopard spots and, 385, 387*f*
   macular holes and, 158, 159*f*
   neoplasia
      adenomas and adenocarcinomas, 339–340, 339*f*
      choroidal nevus and, 314, 315*f*
      of choroid and, 227, 228*f*, 236–237, 236*f*
      hamartomas, 212–213, 213*f*, 339*f*, 340
      intraocular lymphoma and, 162–163, 163*f*
      osseous metaplasia, 16, 16*f*, 237
      posterior uveal melanoma and, 318, 321*f*, 323

retinal detachment sequelae, 181
retinal tears and, 157
staining, 30f
systemic malignancies and, 391
topography, 167–169, 168f, 169f, 170f, 172, 218, 218f
trauma to, 53–55, 54f, 55f
wound repair, 48
Retinal vasoproliferative tumor (VPT), 346t, 350–352, 351f
Retinitis. *See under* Retina
Retinitis pigmentosa (RP), 153, 203, 203f
Retinoblastoma, 353–379
    about, 353–354
    associated conditions, 376–377
    classification, 365, 366–367t, 368t
    clinical aspects, 308, 337
    diagnostic evaluation, 354–364
        ancillary imaging, 358–359, 359f, 360f, 361f
        clinical examination, 354f, 355t, 357f
        differential diagnosis, 360–364, 362t, 363f, 364f, 376
    differential diagnosis, 18, 209–210
    extraocular extension of, 273, 359, 361f
    genetics and counseling, 208–209, 209f, 374–376
    histological features, 204–208, 207f
    metastases of, 358–359, 361f, 378
    molecular diagnosis and prognosis, 308
    prognosis and prognostic factors, 377–379
    specimen handling and processing, 33
    spontaneous regression of, 374
    treatment, 368–373
        about, 308, 368
        chemotherapy, 369–371, 369f, 370f
        enucleation, 369
        local consolidation therapy, 371–373
    treatment overview, 308
Retinoblastoma *(RB1)* gene, 208–209, 308, 356f, 373–379
Retinocerebral angiomatosis. *See* Von Hippel–Lindau (VHL) syndrome
Retinocytoma, 209, 210f, 376
Retinopathy
    chorioretinopathy, 327, 328f
    diabetic, 186f, 187f, 190–191, 191f
    of prematurity, 183, 362t
    proliferative vitreoretinopathy, 157, 158f
    radiation-induced, 183, 390
    sickle cell-related, 183
    vitreoretinopathy, 53, 54f
Retinoschisis, 179, 180f
Retraction of eyelid, 247t
Retrobulbar optic nerve, 131, 358
Retrolaminar nerve, 290f
RGCs. *See* Retinal ganglion cells
RH. *See* Retinal hemangioblastoma
Rhabdomyosarcoma, 17f, 38t, 273, 283–285, 284f
Rhegmatogenous retinal detachment (RRD), 157, 158f, 179
Rheumatoid arthritis, 100, 135f
Rhinocerebral mucormycosis, 271–272, 272f
Rhizopus spp, 271–272
Rhodopsin *(RHO)* gene, 203

Rho kinase (ROCK) inhibitors, 46
Riboflavin (vitamin B_2), 108
Ring infiltrate, 97, 98f
Ring melanoma, 230, 230f, 233, 236, 319f, 320, 343–345, 343f
Riolan muscle, 240
Rituximab, 392–393
RLH (reactive lymphoid hyperplasia). *See* Primary uveal lymphoma
ROCK inhibitors. *See* Rho kinase (ROCK) inhibitors
Rosenthal fibers, 302
Rosettes, 205–206, 205f, 210, 211f
Roswell Park Memorial Institute (RPMI) medium, 20, 23t
Roth spots, 396, 397f
RP. *See* Retinitis pigmentosa
RPCD. *See* Reticular peripheral cystoid degeneration
RPD. *See* Reticular pseudodrusen
RPE. *See* Retinal pigment epithelium
RPMI medium. *See* Roswell Park Memorial Institute (RPMI) medium
RRD. *See* Rhegmatogenous retinal detachment
Rubella, 142, 176
Rubeosis iridis, 224, 224f, 357
Russell bodies, 10, 13f
Ruthenium 106, 333, 372

S-100 protein, 38t, 286
"Salmon patch," 36, 395f
"Salt-and-pepper" chromatin, 258
Salzmann nodular degeneration, 101, 101f
Sarcoidosis
    conjunctivitis and, 64–65, 65f
    eyelid manifestations of, 247t
    optic nerve and, 294t, 297, 297f
    of uveal tract, 221–222, 223f
Sarcomas, 17f, 17t, 397
SARS-CoV-2-related conjunctivitis, 61
Sattler layer, 218
"Sawtooth" pattern, 110–111, 112f, 125, 126f
Scarring
    of choroid, 179
    of cornea, 92f, 95f, 96f, 108, 111f
    laser photocoagulation and, 181, 191, 191f
    of macula, 159
    of optic nerve, 203, 293, 298
    of retina, 176, 178–179, 181, 184, 191, 191f
    wound repair and, 43–45, 44f, 46f, 47–49
SCC. *See* Squamous cell carcinoma
SCCIS. *See* Squamous cell carcinoma in situ
Schaumann bodies, 222
Schlemm canal, 119, 120f, 124
Schnabel cavernous optic atrophy, 298, 300f
Schwalbe line, 119, 120f, 121–122, 123f
Schwann cells, 285–286
Schwannoma, 38t, 238, 238f, 275t, 286, 287f
Schwannomatosis, 286
Sclera, 131–137
    about and overview, 131
    degenerations, 16, 16f, 136–137, 136f, 137f
    developmental anomalies, 132–133, 291, 292f
    inflammation, 268
    inflammation (scleritis), 133–134, 134f, 135f, 136f, 394

neoplasia, 137, 207f, 230, 231f
posterior uveal melanoma extension into, 319f, 320
retinoblastoma extension of, 359
topography, 58–59, 119, 131, 132f, 215, 218, 218f, 290, 290f
wound repair, 47–48
Scleral spur, 50–51, 51f, 52f, 119, 120f, 121, 121f, 131, 215
Scleral staphyloma, 134, 136, 136f
Scleritis, 133–134, 134f, 135f, 136f, 394
Sclerocornea, 93, 94f
Scleroderma, 247t
Scleromalacia perforans, 134
Sclerosing basal cell carcinoma. See Morpheaform basal cell carcinoma
Sclerosing nonspecific orbital inflammation (NSOI), 270
Sclerosing orbititis, 267
Sclerosis, 364
Scotoma, 172
Sebaceous carcinomas, 30f, 32t, 118
Sebaceous glands
cysts, 266, 266f
developmental anomalies, 241
inflammation, 242, 244
neoplasia, 30f, 32t, 118, 250t, 255–258, 256f, 257f
specialization of, 240
topography of, 240
Seborrheic keratosis, 248–250, 249f
Sebum, 266–267, 267f
Secondary acquired melanosis, 78, 83t, 85
Secondary aphakia, 142
Secondary glaucoma. See under Glaucoma
Secondary localized amyloidosis, 68
Secondary orbital meningiomas, 303
Secondary tumors. See Lymphomas; Metastases
Secondary vitreous, 152
Sectoral cataract, 311
Selective intra-arterial chemotherapy, 369–371
Sentinel vessels, 85, 86f, 319, 319f
Sessile papillomas, 71
SF3B1 gene, 234, 234t
SFT. See Solitary fibrous tumor
Shaken baby syndrome. See Abusive head trauma
Sickle cell retinopathy, 183
Siderosis bulbi, 129, 147
Silver deposits, 145
Simple epithelial cysts. See Epidermoid (inclusion) cysts
Simple hamartoma, 339f, 340
Sinus infections (sinusitis), 271–272, 272f, 293
Skin
of eyelids, 239–240, 240f
metastases from, 383t, 384f
metastases to, 330
SLC4A11 gene, 114
Slender spindle nevus cells, 227, 228f
Slides. See Specimen handling, processing, and testing
Slit-lamp biomicroscopy, 310f, 311, 312f, 320, 355, 385
SMA. See Smooth muscle actin
Small blue cell tumor. See Retinoblastoma
Smooth muscle actin (SMA), 238
"Snowballs," in vitreous, 154

Soemmering ring secondary cataract, 147, 147f
Soft drusen, 195t, 196f, 197
Soft-tissue tumors, 280, 282
Solar (actinic) elastosis, 67, 68f, 72, 74f, 250, 251f
Solitary fibrous tumor (SFT), 282–283, 283f
Specimen handling, processing, and testing
about and overview, 6, 19, 21
communication with pathologists, 21–23, 29, 152
for differential diagnosis, 18
glossary of terminology, 19–20
gross examination and dissection, 24–29, 25f, 26f, 27f, 28f
special diagnostic testing, 36–42, 37f, 38t
special techniques and procedures, 23t, 32–36, 33f, 35f
tissue handling and transfer, 22–24, 23t
tissue processing, 20, 29, 29f
tissue staining, 18, 29–31, 29f, 30f, 31–32t
Sphenoid bone, 265, 286
Spheres (vitreous seed type), 206. See also Vitreous seeds
Spheroidal degeneration, 102, 103f
Sphincter muscle, 216, 216f, 224f
Spindle cell carcinoma, 72
Spindle cell melanoma, 228, 231
Spindle cell rhabdomyosarcoma, 284
Spindle cells
choroidal nevus, 227, 228f
iris nevus, 225–226, 226f
melanomas, 229t, 231, 262f
neurofibroma, 285
rhabdomyosarcoma, 284, 284f
schwannoma, 286, 287f
solitary fibrous tumor, 282–283, 283f
Spitz nevus, 259
Split nevus. See Kissing nevus
Spontaneous hyphema, 222, 223f, 225
Squamous cell carcinoma (SCC)
actinic keratosis and, 250
of conjunctiva, 72–73, 73f, 74f, 85
differential diagnosis, 256–258
direct intraocular extension of, 390
of eyelid, 35, 252–253, 253f, 254f
invasive, 73, 73f, 74f
of lacrimal sac, 288
metastases from, 386f
specimen handling and processing, 22, 73
Squamous cell carcinoma in situ (SCCIS), 72–73, 73f
Squamous eddies, 73, 249, 249f
Squamous epithelial lesions, 70–73, 71f, 73f, 74f
Squamous epithelium, 240
Squamous papilloma, 70–71, 71f
S-shaped eyelid deformity, 285
"Staghorn" sinusoidal blood vessels, 282, 283f
Staining of specimens, 18, 29–31, 29f, 30f, 31–32t
Standardized ultrasonography
about, 323
of choroidal hemangioma, 342f, 343
of iris melanoma, 311, 312f
for posterior uveal melanomas, 321f, 322f, 323, 324f, 325, 333
for retinoblastoma, 355, 358, 360f
Staphylococcus aureus, 95, 242

Staphylococcus epidermidis, 143
Staphylococcus spp, 271
Staphyloma, 134, 136, 136*f*
"Star" pattern of exudates, 171, 293
Stargardt disease, 200, 201*f*
STAT6 gene, 282
Stem cell deficiency, 91
Stereotactic radiotherapy, 344
Steroids, 352
Strabismus, 50, 172, 354, 355*t*
Streptococcus pneumoniae, 95
Streptococcus spp, 271
Streptococcus viridans, 99
Striate melanokeratosis, 78
Stroma
    of choroid, 218
    of conjunctiva, 76
    of cornea
        degenerations, 101–102, 105*f*
        dystrophies, 108–113, 112*f*, 113*f*, 114*f*, 115*f*, 116*f*, 116*t*
        ectatic disorders, 106–108, 107*f*
        edema, 104, 104*f*
        infections, 95*f*, 96*f*, 97
        topography, 92, 92*f*
    cysts, 313*t*
    depositions, 106, 106*f*
    of iris, 207*f*, 216, 216*f*, 220, 222, 225–226, 226*f*, 227*f*
    of sclera, 131, 132*f*
    wound repair and, 44*f*, 45–46, 49
Stromal keratitis, 96*f*, 97
Stromal nevus. *See* Subepithelial nevus
Sturge-Weber syndrome. *See* Encephalofacial angiomatosis
Stye. *See* Hordeolum
Subepithelial nevus, 76
Subhyaloid hemorrhages, 184
Subretinal drusenoid deposits. *See* Reticular pseudodrusen
Subretinal fluid
    choroidal melanoma and, 318, 320, 322*f*, 323–325
    choroidal nevus and, 316, 318, 325
    vascular tumors and, 343–344, 352
Subretinal hemorrhage, 53, 193, 317*f*, 319, 323, 328*f*, 387
Substantia propria, 45, 57–58, 58*f*
"Sulfur granule," 273, 273*f*
Superficial keratectomy, 109, 110*f*
Superficial spreading melanoma, 262*f*, 263
Superior hypophyseal artery, 291
Suprachoroidal hemorrhage, 51, 52*f*
Surgery and surgical sites
    cataract surgery complications, 143
    epithelial inclusion cysts at, 69
    for medulloepitheliomas, 364
    for posterior uveal melanoma, 335
    pyogenic granulomas at, 66*f*, 67
    sympathetic ophthalmia, postoperative, 221
    wound repair and scar prevention, 43–45, 44*f*, 46*f*, 47–49
Sweat glands, 247, 255, 255*f*, 266
Swept-source optical coherence tomography, 323

"Swiss cheese" pattern of growth, 277, 277*f*
Sympathetic ophthalmia, 221, 221*f*, 222*f*, 394
Sympathizing eye, 221
Synaptophysin, 38*t*, 39, 258
Synchysis, 155, 160, 177*f*
Syncytial growth pattern, 303, 304*f*
Syneresis, 155, 156*f*
Syphilis, 99–100, 100*f*
Syringoma, 255, 255*f*
Systemic intravenous chemotherapy, 369–370, 369*f*
Systemic lupus erythematosus, 247*t*
Systemic lymphoma, 68
Systemic malignancies, 381–398
    leukemia, 396–398, 397*f*, 398*f*
    lymphoid tumors, 390–396, 391*f*, 393*f*, 395*f*
    metastatic carcinomas, 381–390. *See also* Metastases

T-cell lymphomas, 87, 88*f*, 162–163, 164*f*, 279, 390
T cells, 10, 38*t*
Tachyzoites, 179, 179*f*
Taenia solium, 272
Tapioca pudding pattern, 311, 312*f*
TAP trial. *See* Treatment of Age-Related Macular Degeneration With Photodynamic Therapy (TAP) trial
Tarsal plate, 240
Tarsus, 239–241, 240*f*
TBCD. *See* Thiel-Behnke corneal dystrophy
TCGA. *See* Cancer Genome Atlas (TCGA) classification
Tears, production of, 240, 355*t*
TED. *See* Thyroid eye disease
Telangiectasias
    Coats disease and, 362, 363*f*
    of eyelids, 246*f*
    retina, 173, 174*f*, 191
    retinoblastoma and, 358
Temporal artery, 29, 30*f*, 32*t*, 297
Tenon capsule, 58–59
10% neutral-buffered formalin, 20, 22, 27, 32*t*
Teratoid medulloepithelioma, 210, 211*f*
Teratomas, 8, 9*f*, 266
Tertiary vitreous, 152
Testing of specimens. *See* Specimen handling, processing, and testing
TFSOM-DIM (to find small ocular melanomas doing imaging) mnemonic, 325
TGFB1 dystrophies, 108–111, 111*f*, 112*f*, 113*f*, 114*f*, 115*f*, 116*t*
Thiel-Behnke corneal dystrophy (TBCD), 110–111, 112*f*, 116*t*
Thioflavin T (ThT) stain, 32*t*
Thromboembolism, 189
Thyroid, hamartomas of, 250*t*
Thyroid eye disease (TED), 247*t*, 267, 268*f*
Tinea faciei, 243–244
Tingible body macrophages, 278
Tissue microarrays, 41
Tissue specimens. *See* Specimen handling, processing, and testing
TNM (tumor, node, metastasis) staging system. *See* American Joint Committee on Cancer (AJCC) staging system

To find small ocular melanomas doing imaging (TFSOM-DIM) mnemonic, 325
"Tomato ketchup" fundus, 343, 343*f*
Tonsil, squamous cell carcinoma of, 386*f*
Topical medication toxicities, 99–100
Topography (general), 6–8, 7*t*, 18. *See also under specific structures*
Topotecan, 370, 372–373
Touton giant cells, 12, 15*f*, 222, 223*f*, 246
Toxocariasis, 360, 362–363
Toxoplasma gondii, 293
Toxoplasmic retinochoroiditis, 178–179, 179*f*
Toxoplasmosis, 40, 220, 362*t*
TPCD. *See* Typical peripheral cystoid degeneration
Trabecular meshwork, 119–130
  degenerations, 50, 124–129, 127*f*, 128*f*, 129*f*
  developmental anomalies, 121, 121*f*, 122*f*, 123*f*
  glaucoma and, 144
  neoplasia, 130, 130*f*, 207*f*, 231
  topography, 119–120, 120*f*
  trauma, 127–129, 127*f*, 128*f*, 129*f*
Trabeculocytes, 120, 128
Trachoma, 31*t*, 68
Tractional retinal detachment, 53
Transforming growth factor beta–induced dystrophies. *See* TGFB1 dystrophies
Transillumination, 25, 26*f*, 320, 323, 324*f*
Transpupillary thermotherapy (TTT), 336, 343, 390
Transthyretin, 160–161, 246
Trauma. *See also* Foreign bodies
  abusive head trauma, 192–194, 193*f*, 194*f*
  to anterior chamber, 122, 127–129, 127*f*, 128*f*, 129*f*
  to cornea, 97, 102
  to eyelid, 242, 247
  to lens, 143, 146
  vitreous detachment and, 157
  wound repair, 50–55, 50*f*, 51*f*, 52*f*, 53*f*, 54*f*, 55*f*
Treacher Collins syndrome. *See* Mandibulofacial dysostosis
Treatment of Age-Related Macular Degeneration With Photodynamic Therapy (TAP) trial, 344
Treponema pallidum, 99–100, 100*f*, 293
Triamcinolone acetonide, 186
Trichilemmomas, 250*t*
Trichophyton rubrum, 243–244
Trigeminal nerve, 268
Trilateral retinoblastoma, 358, 361*f*, 376
Trophic ulcer. *See* Metaherpetic ulcer
Trophozoites, 98, 98*f*
TTT. *See* Transpupillary thermotherapy
Tuberculosis, 271
Tuberous sclerosis, 364
Tumor, node, metastasis (TNM) staging system. *See* American Joint Committee on Cancer (AJCC) staging system
Tumor suppressor genes, 67
Tunica vasculosa lentis, 153
Type IV collagen genes, 142–143
Typical degenerative retinoschisis, 179, 180*f*
Typical peripheral cystoid degeneration (TPCD), 179, 180*f*

UBM. *See* Ultrasound biomicroscopy
Ulcers, of cornea, 45–46, 46*f*, 47*f*, 93, 94*f*, 95–97, 95*f*, 96*f*, 100
Ultrasonography
  of iris melanoma, 311, 312*f*
  of lymphomas, 391–392, 394, 395*f*
  of posterior uveal melanoma, 321*f*, 322*f*, 323, 324*f*, 325, 333
  for retinoblastoma, 355, 358, 360*f*
  of secondary tumors, 385–387
  vascular tumors, 342*f*, 343
Ultrasound biomicroscopy (UBM), 310*f*, 311, 312*f*, 320, 323, 385
Ultraviolet (UV) radiation, 102, 210, 258, 316
Upper respiratory tract infections, 281
Uterine fibroid, 238
UV radiation. *See* Ultraviolet (UV) radiation
UVA light, 108
Uveal lymphoid hyperplasia (infiltration). *See* Primary choroidal lymphomas
Uveal lymphoma, 393–396, 395*f*
Uveal tract (uvea), 215–238. *See also* Choroid; Ciliary body; Iris
  degenerations, 134, 136–137, 137*f*, 224, 224*f*, 225*f*
  developmental anomalies, 218–220, 219*f*, 220*f*
  inflammation (uveitis)
    degenerations and, 129
    developmental anomalies and, 153
    differential diagnosis, 362*t*
    infectious, 143–144, 145*f*, 179, 220, 363
    noninfectious, 154, 155*f*, 221–223, 221*f*, 222*f*, 223*f*
  leukemia and, 397
  lymphoma of, 393–396, 395*f*
  neoplasia, 225–238, 229*t*, 234*t*
    clinical aspects, 307–308
    differential diagnosis, 18, 394
    hemangioma, 236, 236*f*
    leiomyoma, 238
    lymphoid proliferation, 237, 237*f*
    melanocytic lesions, 85
    melanocytoma, 227–228
    melanoma, 228–234, 316–338. *See also* Posterior uveal melanoma
    metastatic tumors, 234–235, 235*f*
    molecular diagnosis and prognosis, 307–308
    neural sheath tumors, 238, 238*f*
    nevi, 225–227, 226*f*, 228*f*
    osteoma, 236–237, 237*f*
    specimen handling and processing, 33
  systemic malignancies and, 396
  topography, 131, 215–218, 216*f*, 217*f*, 218*f*
  trauma to, 51, 52*f*
  wound repair, 48, 49

Vaccine therapy, 335
Varicella-zoster virus (VZV), 40, 176, 293
Varix, of the vortex vein, 328*f*, 329
Vascular developmental anomalies, 172–173
Vascular endothelial growth factor (VEGF), 186, 189, 199, 350
Vascular endothelial growth factor (VEGF) inhibitors, 186, 199, 334, 344, 350, 352

Vascular occlusions, 183, 183f, 187–190, 188f, 190f, 301. *See also* Ischemia, of retina
Vascular tumors, 341–352. *See also* Hemangiomas
    about, 341
    of eyelid, 347
    of iris, 345–347, 348f
    of optic nerve head, 345, 347–350, 349f
    of orbit, 275t, 280–281, 281f, 282f, 347
    of retina, 345–352, 346t
        about, 341, 345
        postnatal vascular (leaking), 347–352, 348f, 349f, 351f
        prenatal vascular (nonleaking), 345–347, 347f
Vasculitis, 183, 271–272, 293
Vasoproliferative tumor (VPT), 346t, 350–352, 351f
VEGF. *See* Vascular endothelial growth factor
VEGF inhibitors. *See* Vascular endothelial growth factor (VEGF) inhibitors
Vellus hairs. *See* Pilosebaceous units
Venous occlusion, 183, 183f, 189–190, 190f
Verhoeff–van Gieson (elastin) stain, 30f, 32t
Vermilion fundus, 200
Vernal keratoconjunctivitis, 101
Verocay bodies, 286, 287f
Verruca vulgaris (wart), 242–243, 243f
Verteporfin, 344
Verteporfin in Photodynamic Therapy (VIP) trial, 343
VHL gene, 173, 175f, 350
VHL syndrome. *See* Von Hippel–Lindau (VHL) syndrome
Vincristine, 369–370
VIP trial. *See* Verteporfin in Photodynamic Therapy (VIP) trial
Viral infections. *See also specific viruses*
    of anterior chamber, 176
    of conjunctiva, 61, 71–72
    of cornea, 95–97, 96f, 100
    of eyelid, 242–243, 243f, 244f
    of optic nerve, 293
    of orbit and lacrimal drainage system, 271, 273
    of retina, 176–177, 177f
    of uveal tract, 220
    of vitreous, 176
Vision rehabilitation, 308
Vismodegib, 252
Vitamin A deficiency, 72
Vitamin B$_2$, 108
Vitrectomy, 352, 392, 397
Vitreoretinopathy, 53, 54f
Vitreous, 151–165
    about and overview, 151
    degenerations, 155–161, 156f, 157f, 158f, 159f, 161f, 162f, 180, 181f, 185, 190
    deposits, 160–161, 162f
    detachment of, 156–159, 156f, 157f, 158f, 160
    developmental anomalies, 152–153, 153f, 154f
    embryonic development, 151–152
    hemorrhage, 53, 155, 157, 159–160, 161f, 319, 357f, 362t, 374
    inflammation (vitritis), 40, 153–154, 155f, 157, 162–163, 176
    neoplasia, 162–165, 163f, 164f, 206, 211f, 213
    posterior uveal melanoma association with, 319
    specimen handling and processing, 23, 164
    systemic malignancies and, 396–397
    topography, 151–152, 152f, 157, 168f, 217
    trauma, 53, 54f
    vascular tumor extension into, 348, 349f
    wound repair, 48
Vitreous base, 53, 53f, 54f, 152f, 157, 157f
Vitreous cysts, 153
Vitreous seeding of chemotherapy, 308
Vitreous seeds
    in choroidal melanoma, 317f, 319
    classification, 206
    metastases and, 387, 388f
    retinoblastoma and, 206, 355, 356f, 357–358, 357f, 360f, 365
    treatment, 370, 372–373
Vitritis, 40, 153–154, 155f, 157, 162–163, 176
Vogt-Koyanagi-Harada (VKH) syndrome, 221, 394
Von Hippel lesions, 347
Von Hippel–Lindau (VHL) syndrome, 173, 175f, 347, 350
Von Kossa stain, 32t
Vortex veins, 51, 131, 172, 231f
Vossius ring, 52
VPT. *See* Vasoproliferative tumor
VZV. *See* Varicella-zoster virus

Wallerian degeneration, 298
Wart. *See* Verruca vulgaris
"Washout" phenomenon, 342f, 343
Wedl cells. *See* Bladder cells
Wegener granulomatosis. *See* Granulomatosis with polyangiitis
Well-differentiated SCC with keratoacanthoma-like differentiation, 253, 254f
Wet AMD. *See* Choroidal neovascularization
White flecks. *See* Glaukomflecken
White pupillary reflex. *See* Leukocoria
WHO. *See* World Health Organization
Wieger ligament. *See* Hyaloideocapsular ligament
Wilms tumor, 219
World Health Organization (WHO)
    Classification of Tumours of Haematopoietic and Lymphoid Tissues, 278
    Classification of Tumours of the Eye, 82
    CNS tumor classification, 301–303
    epithelial salivary gland tumor classification system, 274
Wound healing and repair, 43–55
    about, 43–45, 44f
    of conjunctiva, 45
    of cornea, 45–46, 46f, 47f
    of lens capsule, 48
    of optic nerve, 49
    of orbit and ocular adnexa, 49–50
    phases of, 43–44, 44f
    of retina, 48–49
    of sclera, 47–48
    trauma and sequelae, 50–55, 50f, 51f, 52f, 53f, 54f, 55f

of uveal tract, 49
of vitreous, 48
Wright-Giemsa stain, 31*t*
Wyburn-Mason syndrome (Bonnet-Dechaume-Blanc syndrome), 347

Xanthelasma, 245–246, 245*f*, 247*t*
Xanthogranuloma, 222, 223*f*, 245, 247*t*
Xanthomas, 245–246, 245*f*
Xanthophyll pigment, 171
Xeroderma pigmentosum, 72

Yeasts. *See* Fungal infections

Zeus transport medium, 23*t*
Ziehl-Neelsen stain, 31*t*
Zimmerman tumor. *See* Phakomatous choristoma
Zonal granuloma, 143, 145*f*
Zonular fibers (zonules), 52–53, 139, 140*f*, 141–142, 148, 152, 217
Zygomatic bone, 265
Zygomycosis. *See* Mucormycosis